Health Outcomes in a Foreign Land

Bernard Kwabi-Addo

Health Outcomes in a Foreign Land

A Role for Epigenomic and Environmental Interaction

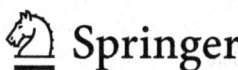 Springer

Bernard Kwabi-Addo
Department of Biochemistry and Molecular
   Biology
Howard University
Woodbridge, VA
USA

ISBN 978-3-319-55864-6   ISBN 978-3-319-55865-3 (eBook)
DOI 10.1007/978-3-319-55865-3

Library of Congress Control Number 2017935011

© Springer International Publishing AG 2017
This work is subject to copyright. All rights are reserved by the Publisher, whether the whole or part of the material is concerned, specifically the rights of translation, reprinting, reuse of illustrations, recitation, broadcasting, reproduction on microfilms or in any other physical way, and transmission or information storage and retrieval, electronic adaptation, computer software, or by similar or dissimilar methodology now known or hereafter developed.
The use of general descriptive names, registered names, trademarks, service marks, etc. in this publication does not imply, even in the absence of a specific statement, that such names are exempt from the relevant protective laws and regulations and therefore free for general use.
The publisher, the authors and the editors are safe to assume that the advice and information in this book are believed to be true and accurate at the date of publication. Neither the publisher nor the authors or the editors give a warranty, express or implied, with respect to the material contained herein or for any errors or omissions that may have been made. The publisher remains neutral with regard to jurisdictional claims in published maps and institutional affiliations.

Printed on acid-free paper

This Springer imprint is published by Springer Nature
The registered company is Springer International Publishing AG
The registered company address is: Gewerbestrasse 11, 6330 Cham, Switzerland

For we are strangers before thee, and sojourners, as were all our fathers

1 Chronicles 29:15

This book is dedicated to my mum and dad, Auntie Mary, Ben, Josh, David and Getty for your inspiration, love and support.

Foreword

The twenty-first century landmark sequencing of the 3.1 billion nucleotides in the human genome introduced a new knowledge base in biomedical research and behavioral science for biology, human identity, and population diversity. This is a knowledge base encoded in the DNA sequence of the genome that is as old as the origins of humankind, yet as new as the most recent discoveries now expressed in the epigenome. What's more, it is knowledge base grounded in the architecture, dynamics, and function of the human genome and epigenome that determines the unique phenotype of the trillions of cells that make-up the human body in health and disease. In this insightful and compelling new book on *Health Outcomes in a Foreign Land—A Role for Epigenomic and Environmental Interaction*, Dr. Bernard Kwabi-Addo, associate professor of Biochemistry at Howard University College of Medicine, skillfully presents the science on disease-specific disparities of the Africa diaspora. With a focus on common diseases categorized as health disparities, such as heart disease, cancer, stroke, chronic obstructive pulmonary disease, diabetes, kidney disease, chronic liver disease, cirrhosis and HIV/AIDS, this book addresses major public health concerns in the USA that disproportionally affect African-Americans compared to other ethnic/racial groups there. Through the lens of an African-American cancer-research scientist with a Ph.D. in Biochemistry and Molecular Biology, Dr. Kwabi-Addo knowledgably has Written an illuminating book on the evidence for genetic factors non-genetic elements and gene-environment interactions underlying disease-specific disparities of the Africa diaspora.

Combining solid scientific evidence with provocative insights, Dr. Kwabi-Addo has organized the contents of this book into three interrelated sections. Part I: Genetic Factors contains chapters on the genetic basis to health disparity and the role of epigenetics. Part II: Non-genetic Elements contains chapters on economic factors and health; social determinants; behavior and health disparities; health literacy deficits; the impact of culture, and psychological issues and how they affect disparities. Part III: Gene-Environment Interactions contains chapters on gene-environment interactions in health disparities; race, a biological or social concept, and translating health disparities. In these chapters, Dr. Kwabi-Addo provides a complete and content-rich overview of the role of epigenomic and environmental interactions in disease-specific disparities of the Africa diaspora. The information presented in these chapters shows that the behavior of a person's genes doesn't just depend on the genes' DNA sequence, but also can be influenced by the external environment's effects on genes, (i.e., epigenetic factors) that can play a critical role in disease, and in some cases these effects are inherited in the epigenome.

Dr. Kwabi-Addo is one of the few African-American science writers with an established research track record and scientific expertise in epigenetics and the African-American epigenome. In writing this foreword, it has been my distinct pleasure and privilege, as founding director of the National Human Genome Center (NHGC) at Howard University, to work collaboratively as a mentor and colleague of Dr. Kwabi-Addo at the Howard University Cancer Center, during his career development and meteoric rise as a leading cancer-research scientist in epigenetics and the epigenome. Dr. Kwabi-Addo was the first author of a ground breaking paper on the *Identification of differentially methylated genes in normal prostate tissues from African American and Caucasian men* published in the journal of Clinical Cancer Research in 2010. With a keen interest in educating people to modulate their lifestyle choices to avoid many of the cancer risk factors, the following year, Bernard wrote his first book on *Cancer Causes and Controversies: Understanding Risk Reduction and Prevention* (Praeger 2011). With increasing evidence that aberrant DNA methylation changes may contribute to prostate-cancer (PCa) ethnic disparity, in 2013, Dr. Kwabi-Addo was a senior author of a signature article on the *Identification of novel DNA-methylated genes that correlate with human prostate cancer and high-grade prostatic intraepithelial neoplasia*. This paper, published in the journal Prostate Cancer and Prostatic Diseases demonstrated how differential genome-wide DNA methylation levels influence gene expression and biological functions in African American and Caucasian PCa. In 2015, Dr. Kwabi-Addo and his research team published a landmark paper on *Genome-wide differentially methylated genes in prostate cancer tissues from African-American and Caucasian men* in Epigenetics, the official journal of the DNA Methylation Society. This landmark publication signaled Dr. Kwabi-Addo's place of authority in the science of epigenomics and unique contribution to the field in elucidating epigenomic and environmental interaction in disease-specific disparities of the Africa diaspora.

In the second decade of this third-millennium post-sequencing of the human genome project has emerged the historic Precision Medicine Initiative, sometimes known as "personalized medicine" with innovative approaches to disease prevention and treatment that take into account differences in people's genes, environments, and lifestyles; the BRAIN (Brain Research through Advancing Innovative Neurotechnologies) Initiative, a bold new research effort to revolutionize our understanding of the human mind and uncover new ways to treat, prevent, and cure brain disorders, and most recently, the twenty-first Century Cures Act passed by Congress and signed into law by the President of the United States, on December 13, 2016, a monumental new bill with the potential to seriously enhance the fights against the opioid epidemic and mental health crises and to achieve the goals of the cancer moonshot.

Into today's global marketplace of ideas and practices for patient-centered, individualized healthcare with attention to the health equity for the multicultural American population, comes this book on Health Outcomes in a Foreign Land—A Role for Epigenomic and Environmental Interaction. This new book by Dr. Bernard Kwabi-Addo is a must-read for all who aspire to learn about the enormous benefits of knowledge gained from this empowering, leading edge of biomedical research and behavioral science in the modern era of genomics-driven big data science.

December 2016

Georgia M. Dunston, Ph.D.
Professor of Microbiology
Founding & Molecular Genetics Director
National Human Genome Center
Howard University College of Medicine
Washington, D.C., USA

Preface

The word diaspora is a biblical concept that was first used for the migration of Jews from Palestine after the Babylonian captivity around the sixth century B.C. Since then, there have been many diasporas throughout the world. Perhaps the largest migration in modern human history and the most widely documented is that of the African diaspora from their native African continent to the Western Hemisphere as part of the slave trade that occurred between the sixteenth and the eighteeth centuries.

The process of migration and settling into a host country can, and in many ways does, play an adverse role in the health of the diasporic communities in comparison to the populations of either their countries of origin or their host countries. Since the days of slavery, the African diaspora in America has experienced poor health compared to Caucasians or European-Americans and all other Americans. The overriding theme is that of disparity and disadvantage. The African diaspora is disproportionately affected by conditions including: premature birth, low birth weight, high infant mortality, obesity, diabetes mellitus, HIV/AIDS, stroke, cardiovascular diseases, hypertension, Alzheimer's disease, violence, suicide, malignant neoplasms, and lead poisoning. The life expectancy for the African diaspora is shorter than that for European-Americans, and this disparity has persisted for almost 400 years.

Most people commonly think of physical health as being affected by age, gender, and biological factors, and some people also realize that health can be affected by lifestyle choices, exercise, diet, and unhealthy habits such as smoking and excessive alcohol consumption, as well as by low health literacy. Some reports suggest that social determinants are the root causes of health disparities, noting that factors such as economic hardship, psychosocial stress, and racial discrimination are causes of bad health. These social determinants derive from the environments and communities in which people are born, live, grow, work, and age. These circumstances are further shaped by the distribution of wealth, power, and resources at the global, national, and local levels, which can themselves be influenced by government policy.

However, these factors are only the tip of the iceberg of what affects health disparities. There are other factors, in particular psychological factors. There is evidence that psychological patterns such as psychosocial stress and adversity can have multi-generational consequences directly tied to low socioeconomic status, racial segregation and discrimination, incarceration rates, fatherlessness, unemployment, housing, substance abuse, under-education, poor working conditions, teen births, poor access to healthy nutrition, and the list goes on and on. There is scientific data to indicate that the maternal, in-utero conditions, as well as early life exposures, such as poor or insuffcient nutrition during critical periods of development or poor environmental exposures may set the stage for at-risk psychosocial, behavioral, and biological characteristics that correlate with increased incidences of various adult-onset diseases, including obesity and diabetes, in the African diaspora.

Genetic and biological factors contribute to virtually every human disease by way of increased susceptibility or altered resistance that affects the severity or progress of disease, with variance in different populations that can also help explain why the African diaspora disproportionately suffers from some diseases compared to other groups. Genetic studies, particularly GWAS (genome-wide association studies) that examine many common genetic variants in different individuals to seek variants associated with a trait, hold the possibility to identify common and rare variants in different populations that affect disease risk, the choices of therapeutics, and drug sensitivity/resistance profiles.

GWAS hold the promise of increasing our understanding of how genetic variants influence the differential gene expression associated with various diseases. In addition to the genetic factor, epigenetic events contribute to health disparities. The fate of a gene is not defined only by the DNA sequence per se but also by the manner by which the gene is marked and programmed by the epigenome phenomenon such as chromatin modification, DNA methylation, and noncoding RNA resuting in diversity of gene expression. At least some heritable epigenetic markers are responsive to social determinants, such as diet, psychosocial stress, or exposure to environmental toxins including drugs of abuse. Thus epigenetics has kindled excitement because nutrition, psychosocial stress, and environmental toxicant exposure can alter epigenetic markers that link environment and gene expression to physical health. In some instances, exposure effects may persist across the life course and may be transmitted to offspring via epigenetic inheritance. An emerging phenomenon posits that epigenetic processes have the potential to link social and environmental influences and patterns of health and disease found within and across societies. The current scientific data supports the notion that there cannot be health equity without an appreciation of how individual genetics or the differential genetic variation in individuals belonging to one population or different populations contributes to health. To attribute all the problems of health disparities to genetic predisposition is to ignore the underlying social and economic determinants that can influence gene expression. An appreciation of the role of epigenetic alterations is also warranted. The role of genetic variation and how different environmental exposures that affect gene expression occur by modulating epigenetic changes—the so-called 'gene-environment' interaction—is a major thread in this book that seeks to draw the reader's attention to understanding the important contribution of epigenetic alterations in addressing how social determinants can influence individual genetics and disease outcomes as well as disease disparities.

"Health Outcomes in a Foreign Land—A Role for Epigenomic and Environmental Interaction" is a book that examines the avoidable or unavoidable factors in the health disparities of the African diaspora. Regardless of causes, health disparities are unfair, because they put already disadvantaged groups at a further disadvantage in their health. Eliminating health disparities should be any nations' priority to improve the quality of health for all citizens. What if we had eliminated such disparities 100 years ago? There would be fewer black deaths, improved life expectancy, and better social determinants of health that, in their absence, otherwise may lead to drug use and homicides. Two historic periods of American history has sought to address and correct race-based health disparities. The first period (1865–1872) was linked to Freedmen's Bureau legislation, and the second (1965–1975) coincided with the Civil Rights Movement across America. Both had dramatic and positive effects on the health status and outcome of African Americans, but were discontinued too soon and failed to eliminate race-based health disparities. Although African-American health status and outcomes are slowly improving, the health status of the African diaspora as compared to that of European-Americans has generally stagnated or even deteriorated since 1980. If we are going to eliminate health disparities, there have to be dramatic changes in health-system policy, financing, and structure, and a directed effort to produce a culturally competent health system and direct health care to areas where it is needed the most, as well as to empower the workforce—all of which address health disparities at multiple points of interaction, such as the interactions of social and biological factors. There must be policies directed towards the desegregation of racial communities and/or improvment of the existing communities for African-American and other US minorities such as providing safe environments for the residents to engage in exercise and access grocery shops and fresh fruit and vegetable markets.

The book is divided into three parts: Part I contains chapters that discuss the genetic basis and the role of epigenetics in health disparities; Part II contains chapters that discuss the non-genetic determinants of health disparities, including chapters on: economic factors, social determinants, behavior, health literacy deficits, and the impact of culture and psychological issues and how they affect disparities; and, Part III contains chapters on: the role of gene-environment interactions, race—a biological or social concept; and, translating health disparities. The book is structured as such to give the reader an appreciation of the plethora of multifactorial causes of health disparities, and it discusses steps that can be taken to reduce these disparities.

Perhaps most critically, the book focuses on current scientific evidence of the potential role of epigenetic changes in linking the interactions of genetic and environmental factors and how this phenomenon can be explored to address eliminating health disparities. The goal of this book, then, is to present the simple, easy-to-understand scientific evidence underlying health disparities for public health and community workers, students, physicians, and scientists alike to gain an appreciation of the complex interaction between social determinants and genetics and its contribution to health disparities. By elucidating the genetic factors (and genetic variants) and the epigenetic events that are associated with increased risks of infectious diseases and non-communicable diseases, as well as the environmental factors such as behavioral/lifestyle choices that exacerbate these conditions, I believe we are heading in the right direction in addressing and reducing health disparities.

Woodbridge, VA, USA   Bernard Kwabi-Addo

Acknowledgments

I would like to acknowledge all the scientific authors and scholars upon whose work I have drawn. In particular, I would like to acknowledge all the research scientists who have devoted their research careers to find the underlying causes of health disparities. Though I have tried my best to present accurate and current scientific data, I apologize to the scientific experts for thus simplifying what for many represent their lifetime work; and to the others, whose work I have overlooked or about which I have not presented the most accurate or current findings.

Contents

1 Introduction: The African Diaspora and Disease-Specific Disparities 1
    1.1   The African Diaspora 1
    1.2   Disease-Specific Disparities of the African Diaspora 2
    1.3   Why the Disparity in Health? 7
    1.4   Health Disparities Are a Complex Combination of Several Causal Factors 9
    1.5   Summary 11
    References 12

Part I: Genetic Factors

2 Genetic Basis of Health Disparity 17
    2.1   Introduction: Genetic Basis of Human Diseases 17
    2.2   What Gives Rise to Genetic Variation? 20
    2.3   Tools for Studying Genetic Variants 21
    2.4   Genetic Variation in the African Population 25
    2.5   Infectious Diseases and Inherited Conditions in African Populations 27
    2.6   Non-Communicable Diseases 32
    2.7   GWAS in the African Population 32
    2.8   Genetic Variation in the African Diaspora—The African-American Population 33
    2.9   Cardiovascular Disease (CVD) Disparities 34
    2.10   Diabetes 38
    2.11   Obesity 42
    2.12   Kidney Disease 44
    2.13   Genetic Variants in Dementia (Alzheimer's) 46
    2.14   Septicemia-Sepsis 48
    2.15   Pneumonia and Influenza 49

		2.16	Cancer	50
		2.17	Summary	59
		References		62
3	The Role of Epigenetics			75
		3.1	Introduction	75
		3.2	Epigenetics and Development	80
		3.3	Neuronal Development and Disease	82
		3.4	Epigenetics Changes, Aging, and Disease Disparities	83
		3.5	Cardiovascular Disease Disparity	87
		3.6	Obesity Disparity	87
		3.7	Type 2 Diabetes Disparity	89
		3.8	Chronic Kidney Disease Disparity	90
		3.9	HIV Disease Disparity	91
		3.10	Cancer Disparities	92
		3.11	Genetic Association and Natural Human Variation	99
		3.12	Summary	100
		References		101

Part II: Non-Genetic Factors

4	Economic Factors and Health Disparities			111
		4.1	Introduction	111
		4.2	The Economic Factor	113
		4.3	Health and Human Capital	114
		4.4	Economic Investment in the Intrauterine Environment	117
		4.5	Infant Mortality	119
		4.6	Economic Investment in Childhood	120
		4.7	Investing in Child and Adolescent Health	123
		4.8	Investing in Adult Health	124
		4.9	Summary	124
		References		125
5	Social Determinants and Health Disparities			129
		5.1	Introduction: The Non-Genetic Factors that Affect Our Health	129
		5.2	Education as a Social Determinant of Health	131
		5.3	Income as a Social Determinant of Health	133
		5.4	Occupation as a Social Determinant of Health	134
		5.5	Socioeconomic Status (SES) and Family Factors	136
		5.6	SES and Neighborhood Factors	140
		5.7	SES, Interaction of Family Values, and Neighborhood Norms	142
		5.8	SES and Health Behaviors	142
		5.9	SES and Transportation	143

	5.10	SES and Access to Health Care 143
	5.11	SES and Psychosocial Factors 145
	5.12	SES and Psychological Characteristics 145
	5.13	Summary 146
	References.. 146
6	**Behavior and Health Disparities**............................ 153
	6.1	Introduction 153
	6.2	Dietary Behavior................................... 154
	6.3	Physical Activity................................... 155
	6.4	Tobacco Use....................................... 157
	6.5	Excessive Alcohol Consumption....................... 160
	6.6	Behavioral Intervention and Health Disparities............. 162
	6.7	Behavior in the Post-Genome Era...................... 165
	6.8	Summary 166
	References... 167
7	**Health Literacy Deficits**................................... 171
	7.1	Introduction 171
	7.2	Individual Self-Care 174
	7.3	Patient Navigation System 177
	7.4	Mistrust of the Healthcare System 177
	7.5	Health Literacy and Professionals...................... 178
	7.6	Health Literacy and Culture 179
	7.7	What About Cultural Competence and Acculturation? 180
	7.8	Summary 181
	References... 181
8	**The Impact of Culture on Health Disparities** 185
	8.1	Introduction 185
	8.2	Diet and Its Cultural Impact 186
	8.3	Religion and Its Cultural Impact....................... 187
	8.4	Cultural Behavior in Alternative Medicine 189
	8.5	Cultural Competence and Linguistics 191
	8.6	Culturally Sensitive Medical Care...................... 193
	8.7	Summary 193
	References... 194
9	**Psychological Factors and Health Disparities** 197
	9.1	Introduction 197
	9.2	Environmental Stressors 199
	9.3	Psychological Stress and Socioeconomic Status 200
	9.4	Biological Mechanism of Psychological Stress............. 202
	9.5	Different Categories of Stress......................... 205
	9.6	Measurement of a Stress Indicator (Allostatic Load)......... 206

9.7	Prenatal Stress		207
9.8	Parental Care and Stress		209
9.9	Cognitive Stimulation in the Home Environment		210
9.10	Community Stressors and Health		211
9.11	Psychosocial Relationships in Community and Health		212
9.12	Resilience and Psychological Impact on Health		213
9.13	Psychosocial Factors and Adverse Health Outcomes in African Americans		215
9.14	Psychosocial Factors and Psychological Implications of Health Disparities		215
9.15	Summary		222
	References		222

Part III: Gene-Environment Interactions

10 Gene-Environment Interactions in Health Disparities 233
- 10.1 Introduction 233
- 10.2 Fetal Origin of Health Disparities 236
- 10.3 Mechanisms of Epigenetic Programming and Maternal Care 247
- 10.4 Epigenetic Programming in Early Life 248
- 10.5 Infant and Child Gene-Environmental Conditions 249
- 10.6 The Role of Gene-Environment Interactions in Disease Disparities 250
- 10.7 Summary 266
- References 268

11 Race: a Biological or Social Concept 279
- 11.1 Introduction 279
- 11.2 Anthropological Rationale for the Scientific Basis of Human Classification 280
- 11.3 Skin Color as Basis for Racial Classification 283
- 11.4 The Human Genome Sequence and Race Classification 285
- 11.5 Racism and Health Disparities 286
- 11.6 Race Categorization and Health Disparities 288
- 11.7 Genetic Variation and Race Categorization 290
- 11.8 Race-Based Genetic Testing and Personalized Medicine 293
- 11.9 Summary 295
- References 296

12 Translating Health Disparities 299
- 12.1 Introduction 299
- 12.2 Life Course Programs 303
- 12.3 Community-Based Participatory Research (CBPR) 303
- 12.4 Diabetes Outcomes 305

12.5	Behavioral Intervention Approaches	305
12.6	Cancer	306
12.7	Importance of Health Literacy	307
12.8	Financial Cost of Insurance	307
12.9	Precision Medicine	309
12.10	Summary	310
	References	311

Glossary 313

Index 315

Abbreviations

%	Percentage
5'Aza-dC	5'Azacyticidine
AA	African-American
ADH	Alcohol dehydrogenase
ALDH	Aldehydyde dehydrogenase
BCa	Breast cancer
BRCA1	DNA Repair Associated Gene
CAU	Caucasian
cDNA	complementary DNA
CpG	Cytosine-phosphate-guanine
CVDs	Cardiovascular diseases
Cytochrome P450	Carcinogen detoxification family of enzymes
DNA	Deoxyribonucleic acid
DNMTs	DNA methyltransferases
EA	European-American
EST	Expressed sequence tag
GSTP1	Gluthathione S-Transferase π
GWAS	Genome-wide Association Studies
HIV	Human Immunodeficiency Virus
HOXB1	Homeobox B1
HPA	Hypothalamus Pituitary Adrenal Axis
IHC	Immunohistochemistry
IQ	Intelligence Quotient
LD	Linkage disequilibrium
miRNA	MicroRNA
MTHFR	Methylenetetrahydrofolate reductase
PCa	Prostate Cancer
PCR	Polymerase Chain Reaction
PIN	Prostatic intra-epithelial neoplasia
RNA	Ribonucleic acid

RT-PCR	Reverse transcription polymerase chain reaction
SAM	S-adenosylmethionine
SES	Socioeconomic Status
SGA	Small gestational age
siRNA	Small interfering RNA
SNPs	Single nucleotide polymorphisms
T1D	Type 1 Diabetes
T2D	Type 2 Diabetes
TSA	Trichostatin A
USA	United States of America

Chapter 1
Introduction: The African Diaspora and Disease-Specific Disparities

Abstract This introductory chapter looks at the disparities that are associated with the incidence and mortality rates for specific diseases such as cardiovascular disease, cancer, stroke, chronic obstructive pulmonary disease, unintentional injuries, pneumonia and influenza, diabetes, suicide, kidney diseases, chronic liver disease, cirrhosis, and HIV/AIDS, which are major public/health concerns in the USA. This chapter then discusses the major causes and the risk factors associated with these diseases that disproportionally affect African Americans as compared to other ethnic/racial groups in the USA.

1.1 The African Diaspora

Since the first biblical description of diaspora was used to describe the migration of the Jewish people from Israel into Babylon captivity, there have been many recorded diasporas throughout history, and several factors account for these diasporic movements. For instance, the potato famine in Ireland during the nineteenth century caused about 2 million people to migrate from Ireland to Britain, the USA, and Canada (Donnelly 2002). Colonization has caused numerous diasporic events as exemplified by the ancient Greeks who succeeded in expanding their territories through military conquest and drove people off their native lands to other parts of the world (Jackson 2010).

The last century also witnessed numerous diasporic events as a result of wars. During World War II (WWII), Nazi Germany deported and killed millions of Jews, and many millions migrated to other parts of Western Europe and the Americas. Because Germany was responsible for starting WWII, Germans who lived in other parts of Europe were deported back to Germany during the post-war period. Other forms of diaspora are the result of capture and enslavement. For instance, the Chinese diaspora, from the nineteenth century to 1940s, forced enslavements of Chinese people to work on plantation and mines in Cuba, Guyana, Trinidad and Tobago, and other parts of the world (Spence 1990). Yet other diasporic movement has been more voluntary, as people migrate to other parts of the world in search for better economic opportunities.

Perhaps the best documented diasporic movement is that of Africans as a result of enslavement from their native African continent to the Western Hemisphere. Beginning in the fifteenth century until the nineteenth century century, an estimated 15 million African slaves were forced from their native African countries to the Americas (Lifson 2002). It is estimated that about four million of the African slaves did not survive the journey across the Atlantic Ocean, the infamous "Middle Passage," as they either succumbed to disease or committed suicide. As a result, approximately 11 million survived the passage and many more died in the early years of captivity (Thomas 1998).

The African diaspora has come to be known as the population that survived enslavement and forced migration to the New World as laborers on slave plantation farms or as domestic workers or artisans. After the slave trade was eventually abolished in 1807 by parallel laws passed by the United Kingdom Parliament and the US Congress (Anon 1807), most of the British slaves of West-African origins were transported to the English-speaking Caribbean islands—Jamaica, Trinidad, Tobago, and the Bahamas. The French slaves were sent to the French colonial islands—Haiti, Martinique, and St. Martins, whereas the slaves acquired by the Dutch were sent to either St. Marten, Curacao, or Aruba, and the Spanish slaves were sent to Cuba, Puerto Rico, and the Dominican Republic (Morrison 1980). By the time slavery ended in the Americas, there were more slaves in the United States than in all other countries combined (Lifson 2002; Rachel 2004). Today, many descendants of the original African diaspora are citizens of the Caribbean islands and Brazil, but most are found in the USA.

In this book, the word African diaspora is used to describe the African population; African Americans (AA) that survived enslavement in N. America. However, in general, the African diaspora reflects the migration of Africans from their native African countries, either voluntarily or involuntarily and either recently or centuries ago, throughout the world. The diasporic movement affects every aspect of the lives of African Americans, especially their health outcomes, which is the main focus of this book.

1.2 Disease-Specific Disparities of the African Diaspora

Having been part of the African diaspora has important implications for every aspect of their lives, including religion, visual art, music, diet, and health. People of the African diaspora are disproportionally affected by major diseases in comparison to their European-Americans (EA) counterparts and other racial/ethnic groups in the USA. African Americans of all ages are more susceptible to a series of diseases and disabilities, as well as suffering premature deaths.

1.2 Disease-Specific Disparities of the African Diaspora

According to the Center for Disease Control's (CDC www.cdc.org) data and statistics on health, the top ten leading causes of death in the entire US population are heart disease, cancer, chronic lower-respiratory disease, unintentional injuries, stroke, Alzheimer's, diabetes, influenza and pneumonia, chronic kidney disease, and intentional self-harm (suicide). However, when the disease incidence and mortality rates are stratified my racial and ethnic groups in the USA, AAs are disproportionally affected by many of these diseases (Fig. 1.1).

The leading causes of death for African Americans and other minority groups in the US are cardiovascular disease (CVD) and stroke, with African Americans having disproportionally higher incidence and mortality rates than any other US racial or minority groups (Anon 2015). African Americans have a 1.3-fold higher risk of death due to heart disease in comparison with their EA counterparts in the USA (Mensah et al. 2005), especially in the so-called stroke belt of the American South. Almost 50% of AA adults develops some form of CVD, making racial disparities in these conditions a crucial public-health concern in the USA (Anon 2007). Other co-morbid conditions, such as hypercholesterolemia, hypertension, smoking, and diabetes mellitus may exacerbate the risk for CVD in AA (Adeniyi et al. 2002).

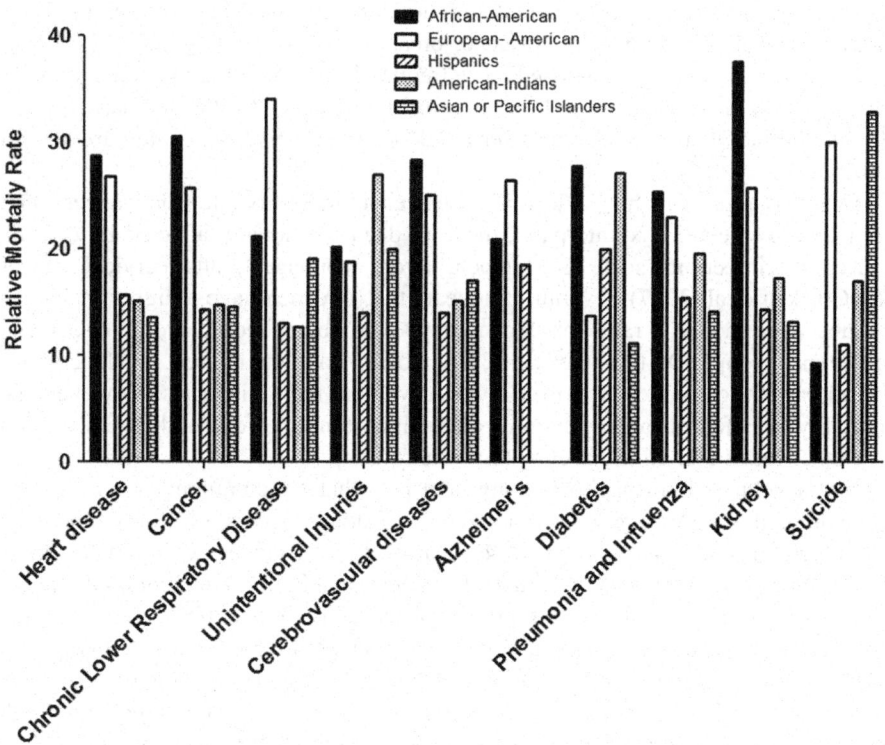

Fig. 1.1 The estimated mortality rates for the top ten leading causes of death among US racial and ethnic groups. Data used for this analysis was obtained from cdc.gov and the US Census Bureau

Another condition that increases the risk of CVD in the AA population is pneumonia infection. Although, AAs are more likely to suffer from heart diseases, they are less likely than EAs to have immunization against influenza and pneumococcal infection, which are associated with these conditions (Ross 2000). The risk of experiencing a first stroke is about two times higher for AAs than EAs with AAs more likely to die following a stroke than EAs.

Cancer is a global epidemic and the second leading cause of death in the USA. African Americans are disproportionally affected by cancer incidence and mortality rates. In particular, AA men have the highest incidence and mortality rates of cancer than any other racial or ethnic group in the USA. Prostate cancer, a leading cause of cancer death among US men disproportionally affects AA men. It is estimated that AA men suffer a 1.6-fold higher incidence rate of prostate cancer and die from the disease at twice the rate compared to their EA counterparts, who rank second with regards to incidence and mortality rates, whilst other racial and ethnic groups, such as Asian Americans and Hispanics, exhibit much lower rates of disease incidence and mortality (Powell and Bollig-Fischer 2013).

The pattern of cancer incidence and mortality rates is somewhat different among women, where EAs are reported to have a higher incidence of cancer. However, AA women are more likely to be diagnosed with aggressive forms of cancer, at later stages of disease, and die of cancer at a higher rate than any other group in the USA (Jemal et al. 2002, 2005). For instance, breast cancer, a leading cause of cancer deaths among women, is diagnosed more frequently in EA women than in any other racial and ethnic group, but AA women are more likely to die of breast cancer, despite the fact that they have a lower incidence than their EA counterparts (Anon 2005).

Even though Asians have a lower incidence and mortality rate from cancer when compared to their EA counterparts, they are disproportionally affected by cancers caused by infections such as stomach, liver, esophageal, and cervical cancer (McCracken et al. 2007). Overall, it appears that AA men have a higher incidence of cancer and mortality rates for all cancer types combined, compared to other racial and ethnic groups. On the other hand, EA women have the highest incidence rates for all cancers combined, followed by AA women, then Hispanics. However, the mortality rates for all cancers combined are highest in AA women, then EA women and other racial and ethnic groups (www.ahrq.gov).

Motor vehicular crashes, poisoning, and falls that are commonly referred to as unintentional injuries are also amongst the leading causes of morbidities and mortalities in the US population for 45-year olds and younger, with motor-vehicle crashes being the most frequent cause of unintentional injury. Unintentional injuries are ranked as the fourth leading cause of mortality in the USA. Some of the associated risk factors are car seat-belt wearing, alcohol-related crashes, distraction linked to phone usage, and aggressive driving. Herein again, ethnic minorities, including AAs, Latinos and Native American are disproportionally affected by high incidences of unintentional injuries (www.cdc.gov/unintentional-injuries).

In addition to the high incidence and mortality rates of CVD and stroke in the AA population, they also have a high prevalence of diabetes. Diabetes is ranked as the seventh leading cause of all mortality from disease in the US, and this condition affects the AA population twice as often as their EA counterparts (Ross 2000). One report estimated that the incidence of type 2 diabetes in the AA population is 1.4–2.2 higher than their EA counterparts (Harris et al. 1999). There is a direct link between obesity and conditions that constitute the so-called metabolic syndrome that contributes to an increased prevalence of diabetes and the often severe manifestation of the disease type in the AA population (Solomon and Manson 1997). Other minority groups, including Asian Americans, Hispanic/Latino Americans, American Indians, and Pacific Islander Americans are also at an increased risk of diabetes (both types 1 and 2) in comparison with their EA counterparts.

AA elders are at an increased risk of being diagnosed with diseases that commonly affect the US elderly and aging populations, such as chronic kidney disease, and are more likely to experience complications associated with these conditions. Chronic kidney disease is ranked number nine among the top-ten leading causes of morbidity, mortality, and lower quality of life in the US-elderly population. Herein again, we see that the AA population has the highest overall risk of chronic kidney disease and develops end-stage renal disease at an earlier average age (55.8 years) compared to the EA population (62.2 years). Elderly American Indians are also at increased risk of chronic kidney disease in comparison with the EA population. Other age-related diseases, such as Alzheimer's and dementias, are diagnosed at significantly higher rates among the AA elderly than in other racial and ethnic groups. African Americans over the age of 65 are two times more likely to be diagnosed with late-onset Alzheimer's when compared to their EA age-matched counterparts, whereas EA elderly are more likely to live longer with Alzheimer's and other dementias than any other US racial or ethnic group (www.alz.org).

Homicide is not ranked among the top-ten leading causes of death in the USA (currently ranked as number 13th), but the USA has the highest homicide rate in comparison with other Western industrialized societies. When stratified by age, the victimization and offender rate for homicide is highest in young adults (ages 18–24). Homicide and its associated violence, as well as drug-related complications, rank in the top-four leading causes of death. While homicide affects people of all stages of life, men are disproportionately affected by homicide than women, and it is estimated that males are at a three–four-fold higher risk to die as a result of homicide than females, among 15–34 year olds. Furthermore, AAs are at a higher risk of death as a result of homicide compared to other racial and ethnic groups in the USA (www.cdc.gov/injury/wisgars/index.html). For all age groups, AAs are disproportionately affected by homicide. Among AA youth 15–24 years old, homicide is actually the second leading cause of death (Heuveline and Slap 2002). Similarly in the aging US population, AAs are at higher risk of death from homicide than their EA counterparts (Griffith and Bell 1989), although, after adjusting for social economic status, the racial differences in homicide rates among adults decreases. Some of the risk factors for the high homicide rate include overcrowding, mass media, parental behavior, and a criminal-justice system that imposes longer and harsher sentences for AAs in comparison with EAs. The good news is that homicide rates are declining in comparison to the 1970s–1990s when the mortality rate due to homicide reached its peak.

Infant mortality is another major public-health concern—strangulation and suffocation have been attributed to be among the common causes of accidental infant death (Shapiro-Mendoza et al. 2009). The rate of accidental infant deaths among AAs or other minorities, such as American Indians or Alaskan native, is about two–three-fold higher than their EA counterparts, and factors such as sharing a bed with parents has been attributed to higher infant accidental deaths in the AA population in comparison with EA infants who do not typically share beds with their parents. Overlaying of the infant as a result of parental bed sharing with infants is believed to contribute to the accidental infant deaths, as well as the use of soft beddings (such as pillows, blankets, and bumper pads).

Infectious diseases, in particular, HIV/AIDs and tuberculosis, are the major causes of morbidity and mortality for AA men in the U.S. The incidence rates among AA men from HIV/AIDS is more than seven times that of EA men, whilst the homicide rate is six times higher, and the majority of HIV/AIDs cases are the result of male-to-male sexual contact (Ross 2000). African-American women are also disproportionally afflicted by HIV/AIDs when compared to EA women. Although AA women represented 12% of the US female population in 2001, this group accounted for an estimated 64% of HIV infections among all women in the US (Ross 2000). Another infectious pathogen of public-health concern is *Streptococcus pneumonia*. The incidence of the pneumococcal infection that causes pneumonia is estimated to be about 400,000 cases, and this is accompanied by 40,000 related deaths per year in the US. Whilst the risk factors for pneumococcal infection are not well established, race and ethnicity appear to play a role. The prevalence of pneumonia is slightly higher in AAs in comparison with EAs, and AA children are significantly more likely to be carriers of pneumococci (Meats et al. 2003) compared to other children. African-American adults, who reside with children aged less than five years or unvaccinated children, are at increased risk for developing pneumococcal disease (Metlay et al. 2010). The good news is that the incidence rate of pneumonia infection have declined over the past century, since the introduction of pneumococcal vaccine for children in 2000 (Kyaw et al. 2006).

Septicemia is another major disease that disproportionally affects the AA population. According to the CDC's healthcare-associated-infection (HAI) survey, which measures localized diseases as a result of adverse reactions in the presence of an infectious agent (https://www.cdc.gov/hai/), there is a high incidence of septicemia among hospital patients. It is estimated that one in 25 hospital patients has at least one HAI, with a higher prevalence, and more severe forms, of sepsis found among AA patients in comparison with EA patients (www.medscape.com/viewarticle/723974).

Interestingly, there are a handful of diseases and conditions for which the prevalence among AA population is lower than other ethnic groups or the EA population. The incidence and mortality rate for chronic lower-respiratory disease (COPD; emphysema, chronic bronchitis, asthma) is higher in the EA than the AA population (www.lung.org). Similarly, malignant melanoma and other skin tumors are seen in AAs but less frequently than in the EA population, presumably due to the melanin-based skin sun-screening as an evolutionary adaptation to tropical environments. Malignant melanoma and rates of dyslipidemia and hypertriglyceridemia are also lower among AAs in comparison with the EA population (Stevens et al. 2002). Furthermore, the irregular heart rhythm known as atrial fibrillation is higher in the EA population than among their AA counterparts (Upshaw 2002).

Despite the few diseases that do not disproportionately affect the AA population, in terms of the health status of the average AA in the USA, the over-riding theme is that of disparity and disadvantage (Luke et al. 2001). There is litany of health disparities among AAs when compared to EAs or other racial and ethnic groups, as highlighted by death rates from heart disease, cancer, and diabetes. As a result of the unequal disease burden in the AA population, the life expectancy for AAs is shorter than EAs, and this gap has held steady for decades, if not centuries, without any signs of narrowing (Marmot 2001). Overall, the African-American age-adjusted mortality rate for all combined causes is 1.5 times higher than for their EA counterpart (Keppel et al. 2002).

Reports from longitudinal studies and other studies have examined the impact of migration from one's native country and settlement into a new host country and how this can adversely affect health over a life-course for migrant populations, such as AAs in comparison with host EA population (Beiser et al. 2002). As we have come to realize the disparities in health that exist among the various racial and ethnic populations in the US, we find a complex combination of a multitude of environmental risk factors, social determinants, social-psychological factors, and racial discrimination among other factors that interact with the genetic makeup of the diaspora population to impact phenotypic expression associated with health and health disparities.

1.3 Why the Disparity in Health?

Health disparities are well documented in various parts of the world. The earliest observation of this phenomenon was reported in Italy over 300 years ago by Bernardino Ramazzini, who observed an unusually high frequency of breast cancer among Catholic nuns (Anon 2002). An observational report in 1775 by British surgeon Sir Perival Pott correlated scrotal cancer cases with men who in their youths were exposed to irritating soot from cleaning and sweeping chimneys. By the middle of nineteenth century, large-scale epidemiological studies began to support these earlier reports. A landmark epidemiological report by Sir Edwin Chadwick, the British civil servant who was commissioned to carry out this study on class-based differences in mortality rates between social upper and lower-class for individuals living in Liverpool, England, in the 1840s, found that the average life expectancy for the professionals was 35-years of age, whereas for the laborers, mechanics and servants the average age of death was as low as 15 years of age (Chadwick 1842). The conclusion from the so-called Chadwick report is that the disparity in life expectancy rates between the various classes could be attributed to poverty and lifestyle factors common to the poorer working classes (Macintyre 1997). Thus in Britain and other parts of Europe, the existence of class-based disparities in death rates was well known in the literature by the turn of the twentieth century (Macintyre 1997).

In European countries such as Britain, where the population is fairly homogenous (i.e., mostly European whites, Caucasians CAU), health disparity has been understood as differences in health outcomes between various socio-economic groups; where the upper-class educated and wealthy professionals are healthy and live longer compared to the lower-class and uneducated poor population (Braveman 2006). In such settings, disparities between different racial and ethnic groups, such as between the British whites and black Jamaicans immigrants has generally received less attention, although there are studies that have looked at disparities that exist in different genders (Smith and Hart 2002).

Across the Atlantic Ocean in the US, health disparities have typically been focused on racial and ethnic differences in disease incidence and mortality rates among different racial and ethnic groups of the US population. Several definitions of health disparities have evolved by policy makers and the US government, including the definition by Paula Braveman (Braveman 2006). Braveman definition is that "a health disparity/inequality is a particular type of difference in health in which disadvantaged social groups—such as the poor, racial/ethnic minorities, women, or other groups who have persistently experienced social disadvantage or discrimination—systematically experience worse health or greater health risk than more advantaged social groups".

The most widely used definition and perhaps the best description to encapsulate the concept of health disparities was articulated by Margaret Whitehead in the early 1990s as "differences in health outcomes that are not only unnecessary and avoidable but, in addition, are considered unfair and unjust" (Whitehead 1992). Several examples fit the concept of "avoidability", "injustice" and "unfairness." A child born into a minority group of lower social class is likely to have a shorter life expectancy compared to another child born into fortunate circumstance, because the parents' social class puts such a child at a disadvantage with respect to his or her health. Similarly, an adults' life expectancy is reflected by their social class. Residential segregation is unjust, for instance, compare minorities who live in poor neighborhood with limited access to healthy food and proper healthcare to individuals living in affluent neighborhoods who have access to fresh fruits and vegetables and quality healthcare. These minorities are already at a disadvantage in society because their toxic environment will likely result in adverse health outcomes. In addition, compared to the EA population, AAs receive less income at the same level of education, may pay more for home loans or are unable to negotiate a smaller mortgage loan, and have less wealth at equivalent income levels compared to their EA counterparts.

On the other hand, we cannot attribute all disparities to injustice and unfairness, as exemplified by differences in low birth weight in AA infants in comparison to EA infants. Since we do not fully know what gives rise to the differences, we cannot say the difference is unfair or unjust. However, the above definition does qualify the difference in birth weight as a "health disparity" and merits further investigation because it is an important health difference that has future health consequence for the AA population. No matter how one defines or looks at health disparity, it is unfair and unjust. However, it may not always be possible to determine whether a given difference in health or health risks is unfair or unjust in itself. Therefore, the way to overcome the disparity would require intense research to uncover the causes of the observed differences in health outcomes.

The causes of health disparities have been debated on both sides of the Atlantic Ocean, in both Europe and the US. In the late nineteenth and early twentieth centuries in Britain, the causes of social-class variations in the incidence and mortality rates of diseases were disputed between those who believed that an individual's genetically inherited natural abilities contributed to his/her social standing in society and those who believed that socio-economic factors played a major role in the health outcomes of individuals (Szreter 1984).

Similar debates were going on in the US (Krieger et al. 1993). Nineteenth-century and early twentieth-century physical anthropologists in the USA chose measurement of the human skull as the basis to gauge intellectual hierarchical rankings of social standing among different racial and ethnic groups in the USA with individuals of European descent (Caucasoids) at the top of the social class, whereas Africans (Negroids) were placed at the bottom, and Asians and Native Americans (Mongoloids) were somewhat intermediary between the top and bottom. However, such arguments have long since been refuted by other findings (Blakey 1996, 2001). Nonetheless, these social rankings formed the hideous basis of the racism that is pervasive and has contributed significantly at different levels to health disparities. Health disparities are now well documented all over the world.

1.4 Health Disparities Are a Complex Combination of Several Causal Factors

Most prominent among the causes of health disparities are social determinants and environmental risk factors, access to healthcare, utilization, and quality of health status or health outcomes. More recent findings from scientific studies that focused on the role of genetics in health disparities has provided additional insight into the complex interactions of gene–environment and social determinants in defining health outcomes. Complex gene–gene and gene–environment interactions may explain differences in disease risk or outcomes among various racial/ethnic groups and the extent to which environmental exposures can affect gene expression to modify disease risk that are differentially distributed across populations.

1.4.1 Environmental Quality

African Americans and other minorities or low-income groups who live in segregated neighborhoods, such as slums or the poorest parts of urban areas, are disproportionately affected by air pollution and other environmental stresses. Even when social class and other confounding factors are eliminated, belonging to a minority race/ethnicity group alone has been found to be associated with increased risk to toxic exposure as was recently documented for lead poisoning in Flint, Michigan (http://www.cnn.com/2016/01/26/us/flint-michigan-water-crisis-race-poverty/). In Flint, a city with 57% AA population, which is also low SES (as measured by education, income and occupation), AAs were particularly hard hit because they reside in the poorest neighborhoods, in particular, in old houses with lead water pipes. So, poor AAs were disproportionally affected by the lead poisoning. Many children in these communities who drank the unfiltered pipe water tested positive for high levels of lead contamination in their blood. Lead is known to adversely affect brain development, the nervous system, and muscle movement, and it could cause long term health consequences on childhood development and adult health. Similarly, the AA population are exposed to other environmental risk such as fish contamination, hazards in the workplace, abandoned toxic waste-dumps, and proximity to municipal landfills and incinerators in comparison to the EA population (Bullard and Wright 1993).

1.4.2 Social Effects

There is extensive evidence for the role of social determinants in the origin of premature and low birth-weight infants, and such an early life course is directly linked to future health outcomes in the AA population, for instance, childhood obesity is directly linked to increased risk of CVD. The accumulating evidence suggests an association of early life exposure, indeed intrauterine conditions such as diet and maternal stress during pregnancy, and susceptibility to diseases such as CVD, hypertension, diabetes, and stroke, which disproportionally affect the AA population (Kuzawa and Sweet 2009). Psychological stress caused by perceived racism has adverse health outcomes, including disproportionally high incidence of depression and high blood pressure in AA and other minority groups (Halpern 1993; Krieger 1990).

1.4.3 Genetics

The focus on genetic research for understanding health disparities has been met with skepticism (Cooper et al. 2003; Krieger 2005). This is because many causes of disease mortality in the US have direct links to social, environmental, and lifestyle

1.4 Health Disparities Are a Complex Combination of Several Causal Factors

behaviors, such as smoking, excessive alcohol consumption, and a sedentary lifestyle. Yet, when all these confounding social and environment factors are accounted for, there are still disparities in many diseases, suggesting that biology is also important in addressing health disparities.

Few diseases or conditions are caused mainly by genetic factors, however, and a large and growing number of common genetic risk factors associated with diseases exhibiting most important disparities are now being recognized. This is made possible largely due to the completion of the human genome sequences and technological advances in genomic studies, coupled with statistical tools for querying large-scale data on genetic variation and disease association. Genetic changes (mutations) can affect protein synthesis that plays a role in all normal biological processes in the human body, and such changes are implicated in the vast majority of human diseases. Differences in genetic variations at high frequency in one population compared to the other can contribute to health disparities causing differential susceptibility to disease for various racial and ethnic groups exposed to the same environmental risk factors.

Geneticists recognize that the genetic basis for most common diseases such as cystic fibrosis and Duchenne Muscular Dystrophy are simple mutations in genes. However, complex diseases such as diabetes and hypertension are caused by the interaction of genes and the environment and require careful examination of each contributing factor in addressing health disparities. In addition to the role of genetic variation, epigenetic alterations are increasingly reported to play an important role in health disparities. Epigenetic processes can influence which genes are expressed and which are not, and plays an important role during development, so that embryos and infants are more susceptible to epigenetic changes. Epigenetic processes can be altered by environmental factors such as diet, lifestyle choices, and other social effects and could potentially explain how environmental "nurture" controls genetic "nature" in health disparities.

1.5 Summary

In 1900, the average life expectancy in the USA was a mere 47 years. Today average life expectancy is over 77 years. Much of this improvement in life expectancy has come through changes in lifestyle and living conditions and also advances in healthcare. Despite extensive progress in improving life expectancy, disparities in health of the AA population and other ethnic minorities when compared to EA population still persist. The causes of health disparities are not fully known but involve a complex combination of social, environmental, and genetic factors.

In Britain, where health disparities refer to differences that exist as a result of social-class gradients, the approach to eliminating health disparities has been the institution of a welfare state—a system of social security to provide benefits to address the five "giant evils" of society: want (poverty); disease (medical treatment), ignorance (education), squalor (housing) and idleness (employment) (Macintyre 1997). By instituting the welfare system, Britain has abolished inequalities in access to healthcare, yet there remain persistent inequalities in health suggesting that other social inequalities persist, such as poor residential areas, demonstrating that other factors play an important role in inequalities. For instance, what good does it do to treat people's illnesses and send them back to environmental conditions that made them sick in the first place?

In the US, where health disparities refer to disparities in health outcomes that exist in different racial and ethnic groups, several interventions on the individual, community, local, and governmental policy levels are needed in order to reduce and eliminate health disparities. A major barrier to access in healthcare for AAs and other minorities is lack of insurance. On March 23, 2010, after the US Congress passed and reconciled the complex legislation, President Barack Obama signature revised the US healthcare system by enacting into law the Affordable Care Act (ACA; http://www.hhs.gov/healthcare/about-the-law/). One of the main objectives of the ACA is to mandate affordable and better health insurance to all Americans. While this approach is a step in the right direction towards the elimination of health disparities, lessons from Britain would suggest that this is not enough in addressing health disparities.

The purpose of this book is to shine light on the biological and non-biological contributing risk factors to health disparities and to address why health disparities must take into consideration to understand the multi-complex interactions of gene–environmental factors that contribute to health disparities.

References

Adeniyi, A., Folsom, A. R., Brancati, F. L., Desvorieux, M., Pankow, J. S., & Taylor, H. (2002). Incidence and risk factors for cardiovascular disease in African Americans with diabetes: The Atherosclerosis Risk in Communities (ARIC) study. *Journal of the* National Medical Association, *94*(12), 1025–1035. Available from: PM:12510702).

Anon. (1807). Congress abolishes the African Slave Trade.

Anon. (2002). *Cancer and the environment; Gene-environment interaction*. New York: National Academy Press.

Anon. (2005). *American Cancer Society (ACS) cancer fact & figures for African Americans 2005–2006*. Atlanta, GA: American Cancer Society.

Anon. (2007). *AHA, American Heart Association heart facts 2007: All Americans*. Dallas, TX: American Heart Association.

Anon. (2015). www.cdc.gov/minorityhealth/populations/REMP/black.html

Beiser, M., Hou, F., Hyman, I., & Tousignant, M. (2002). Poverty, family process, and the mental health of immigrant children in Canada. *American Journal of Public Health, 92*(2), 220–227. Available from: PM:11818295).

Blakey, M. L. (1996). Skull doctors revisited: Intrinsic social and political bias in the history of American physical anthropoplogy, with special reference to the work of Ales Hrdlicka. In L. Reynolds & L. Lieberman (Eds.), *Race and other misadventures: Essays inhonor of Ashley Montagu in his ninetieth year* (pp. 64–95). New York: General Hall.

References

Blakey, M. L. (2001). Bioarchaeology of the African diaspora in the Americas: Its origins and scope. *Annual Review of Anthropology, 30,* 387–422.

Braveman, P. (2006). Health disparities and health equity: Concepts and measurement. *Annual Review of Public Health, 27,* 167–194. Available from: PM:16533114).

Bullard, R. D. & Wright, B. H. (1993). Environmental justice for all: Community perspectives on health and research needs. *Toxicology and Industrial Health, 9*(5), 821–841. Available from: PM:8184445).

Chadwick, E. (1842). *Report of an enquiry into the sanitary conditions of the labouring population of Great Britain.* London: Poor Law Commission.

Cooper, R. S., Kaufman, J. S., & Ward, R. (2003). Race and genomics. *The New England Journal of Medicine, 348*(12), 1166–1170. Available from: PM:12646675).

Donnelly, J. (2002). *The Great Irish Potato Famine.* Stroud: Sutton Publishing.

Griffith, E. E. & Bell, C. C. (1989). Recent trends in suicide and homicide among blacks. *JAMA, 262*(16), 2265–2269. Available from: PM:2677427).

Halpern, D. (1993). Minorities and mental health. *Social Science and Medicine, 36*(5), 597–607. Available from: PM:8456329).

Harris, M. I., Eastman, R. C., Cowie, C. C., Flegal, K. M., & Eberhardt, M. S. (1999). Racial and ethnic differences in glycemic control of adults with type 2 diabetes. *Diabetes Care, 22*(3), 403–408. Available from: PM:10097918).

Heuveline, P., & Slap, G. B. (2002). Adolescent and young adult mortality by cause: Age, gender, and country, 1955 to 1994. *Journal of Adolescent Health, 30*(1), 29–34. Available from: PM:11755798).

Jackson, R. L. II (Ed.). (2010). *Encyclopedia of identity.* London: SAGE Publications.

Jemal, A., Murray, T., Ward, E., Samuels, A., Tiwari, R. C., Ghafoor, A., et al. (2005). Cancer statistics, 2005. *CA: A Cancer Journal for Clinicians, 55*(1), 10–30. Available from: PM:15661684).

Jemal, A., Thomas, A., Murray, T., & Thun, M. (2002). Cancer statistics, 2002. *CA: A Cancer Journal for Clinicians, 52*(1), 23–47. Available from: PM:11814064).

Keppel, K. G., Pearcy, J. N., Wagener, D. (2002). Trends in racial and ethnic-specific rates for the health status indicators. Healthy People Statistical Notes 23 (pp. 1–16). United States, 1990–98.

Krieger, N. (1990). Racial and gender discrimination: risk factors for high blood pressure? *Social Science and Medicine, 30,* 1273–1281.

Krieger, N. (2005). Stormy weather: Race, gene expression, and the science of health disparities. *American Journal of Public Health, 95,* 2155–2160.

Krieger, N., Rowley, D. L., Herman, A. A., Avery, B., & Phillips, M. T. (1993). Racism, sexism, and social class: Implications for studies of health, disease, and well-being. *American Journal of Preventive Medicine, 9*(6 Suppl), 82–122. Available from: PM:8123288).

Kuzawa, C. W., & Sweet, E. (2009). Epigenetics and the embodiment of race: developmental origins of US racial disparities in cardiovascular health. *American Journal of Human Biology, 21*(1), 2–15. Available from: PM:18925573).

Kyaw, M. H., Lynfield, R., Schaffner, W., Craig, A. S., Hadler, J., Reingold, A., et al. (2006). Effect of introduction of the pneumococcal conjugate vaccine on drug-resistant *Streptococcus pneumoniae*. *The New England Journal of Medicine, 354*(14), 1455–1463. Available from: PM:16598044).

Lifson, A. (2002). Voices of the slave trade. *Humanities, 23,* 28–31.

Luke, A., Cooper, R. S., Prewitt, T. E., Adeyemo, A. A., & Forrester, T. E. (2001). Nutritional consequences of the African diaspora. *Annual Review of Nutrition, 21,* 47–71. Available from: PM:11375429).

Macintyre, S. (1997). The black report and beyond: What are the issues? *Social Science & Medicine, 44*(6), 723–745. Available from: PM:9080558).

Marmot, M. (2001). Inequalities in health. *The New England Journal of Medicine, 345*(2), 134–136. Available from: PM:11450663).

McCracken, M., Olsen, M., Chen, M. S., Jr., Jemal, A., Thun, M., Cokkinides, V., et al. (2007). Cancer incidence, mortality, and associated risk factors among Asian Americans of Chinese,

Filipino, Vietnamese, Korean, and Japanese ethnicities. *CA: A Cancer Journal for Clinicians, 57*(4), 190–205. Available from: PM:17626117).

Meats, E., Brueggemann, A. B., Enright, M. C., Sleeman, K., Griffiths, D. T., Crook, D. W. (2003). Stability of serotypes during nasopharyngeal carriage of *Streptococcus pneumoniae*. *Journal of Clinical Microbiology, 41*(1), 386–392. Available from: PM:12517877).

Mensah, G. A., Mokdad, A. H., Ford, E. S., Greenlund, K. J., & Croft, J. B. (2005). State of disparities in cardiovascular health in the United States. *Circulation, 111*(10), 1233–1241. Available from: PM:15769763).

Metlay, J. P., Lautenbach, E., Li, Y., Shults, J., & Edelstein, P. H. (2010). Exposure to children as a risk factor for bacteremic pneumococcal disease: Changes in the post-conjugate vaccine era. *Archives of Internal Medicine, 170*(8), 725–731. Available from: PM:20421560).

Morrison, L. R. (1980). "Nearer to the brute creation": The scientific defense of American slavery before 1830. *Southern Studies, 19*(3), 228–242. Available from: PM:11633242).

Powell, I. J., & Bollig-Fischer, A. (2013). Minireview: The molecular and genomic basis for prostate cancer health disparities. *Molecular Endocrinology, 27*(6), 879–891. Available from: PM:23608645).

Rachel, E. S. (2004). *Cultural diversity in health and illness* (6th Ed.). Upper Saddle River, NJ: Prentice Hall.

Ross, H. (2000). Growing older: Health issues for minorities. *Closing the Gap*. A Newsletter of the Office of Minority Health. Washington, DC: U.S. Department of Health and Human Services. 1–2.

Shapiro-Mendoza, C. K., Kimball, M., Tomashek, K. M., Anderson, R. N., & Blanding, S. (2009). US infant mortality trends attributable to accidental suffocation and strangulation in bed from 1984 through 2004: Are rates increasing? *Pediatrics, 123*(2), 533–539. Available from: PM:19171619).

Smith, G. D., & Hart, C. (2002). Life-course socioeconomic and behavioral influences on cardiovascular disease mortality: The collaborative study. *American Journal of Public Health, 92*, 1295–1298.

Solomon, C. G., & Manson, J. E. (1997). Obesity and mortality: A review of the epidemiologic data. *American Journal of Clinical Nutrition, 66*(4 Suppl), 1044S–1050S. Available from: PM:9322585).

Spence, J. D. (1990). *The search for Modern China* (pp. 1–49). Lanham: Rowan and Littlefield Publishers Inc.

Stevens, J., Juhaeri, Cai, J., & Jones, D. W. (2002). The effect of decision rules on the choice of a body mass index cutoff for obesity: Examples from African American and white women. *American Journal of Clinical Nutrition, 75*(6), 986–992. Available from: PM:12036803).

Szreter, S. (1984). The genesis of the Registrar General's social classification of occupations. *British Journal of Sociology, XXXV*, 522–546.

Thomas, H. (1998). *The Slave Trade—The history of the Atlantic Slave Trade. 1440–1840*. London: Macmillian.

Upshaw, C. B., Jr. (2002). Reduced prevalence of atrial fibrillation in black patients compared with white patients attending an urban hospital: An electrocardiographic study. *Journal of National Medical Association, 94*(4), 204–208. Available from: PM:11995632).

Whitehead, M. (1992). The concepts and principles of equity in health. *International Journal of Health Services, 22*, 429–445.

Part I
Genetic Factors

Chapter 2
Genetic Basis of Health Disparity

Abstract People of the African diaspora often have a high prevalence of certain common and complex diseases, and genetic predisposition has been proposed as one of the causes. Genetic studies have identified variation or mutations in genes that are commonly associated with both common and complex diseases. The completion of the human genome sequence and technological advances, including the so-called genome-wide association studies, have identified genetic variants that are associated with increased disease risks/resistance in individuals of the African diaspora. The patterns of genetic variations in different populations could shed some light on the biological mechanisms underlying health disparities.

2.1 Introduction: Genetic Basis of Human Diseases

Our understanding of the important role of genes in determining physical traits and susceptibility to diseases can be traced back to the pioneer work carried out by Gregor Mendel (Mendel 1866) on the transmission of certain traits in the common pea plant (*Pisum sativum*). Mendel studied the inheritance of simple and obvious traits beginning with pure-breeding populations of yellow seeds that produced only plants with yellow seeds and green seeds that produced plants with only green seeds, over several generations. When he crossed a yellow seed with a green seed, all he saw was green seeds in the first generation, but then, when he crossed the green seeds to themselves or with each other, they produced yellow and green seeded plants. Mendel reasoned that these traits (now known as genes) were transmitted with precision from one generation to the next, a discovery that formed the foundations of the genetics of heredity. Mendel's work clearly demonstrated that a single trait (as in the case of pea-plant color) can be determined by a single gene, and we now know that most genes in eukaryotic organisms follow this Mendelian pattern of inheritance. Gregor Mendel's work lead to two important principles governing heredity, namely the laws of segregation and independent assortment also referred to as the Mendelian laws of heredity (Strachan and Read 1999).

How the genetic information is stored or the mechanism of transmitting this information from one generation to the next was not known until the discovery of deoxyribonucleic acid (DNA) as the genetic material by Watson and Crick in 1943. This milestone scientific breakthrough set the stage for understanding how genetic information could be successfully passed down from one generation to the next, how changes in the DNA structure could give rise to variation in gene expression, differences in physical phenotypes, and changes in metabolic pathways, as well as give rise to disease susceptibility or resistance.

DNA consists of four sugar (nucleotide) bases: Adenine (A), Cytosine (C), Guanine (G), and Thymine (T) that can be linked together in any number of combinations as a linear polymer by a phosphodiester bond. With the exception of some viruses and prokaryotic organisms, the DNA structure in most organisms exists as double-stranded molecules in which complementary strands pair together, such that the As on one strand will always pair with the Ts on the second strand, whereas the Cs will always pair with the Gs forming base pairs. Based on the completion of the human genome sequence, it is now known that the human genome contains approximately three billion base pairs of DNA arranged on 46 chromosomes (22 autosome pairs plus the X and Y chromosomes).

The Watson and Crick discovery paved the way for a detailed understanding of how DNA is transcribed into RNA, which is in turn translated into protein that perform all the biological functions for normal physiological processes in living organisms. Thus changes in DNA structure, such as mutations that affect protein encoding genes, could affect gene expression and ultimately lead to heritable changes in organisms, as well as contribute to disease susceptibility. Although DNA is made up of only four bases, there are remarkably different combinations of base nucleotides that encode for all the information needed to make all proteins inside a cell. Thus, the structure and hence the properties of all the enzymes and proteins, in essence all the components that make up a living organism including human beings, are contained in genes. It is estimated that there are between 20,000 and 25,000 protein-coding genes in the human genome necessary for all physiological functions.

The DNA molecule encodes for all the proteins expressed inside cells, making this molecule very important for normal cellular processes. The genes encoded by DNA are involved in determining normal phenotypic characteristics such as skin color, hair, body form, and sex. Alterations in the DNA molecule can lead to changes at the protein expression level, such as insufficient expression, absence of expression, or over-expression of proteins, which consequently alter their normal biological functions, and this is one way that genetic alteration can lead to the development of disease. For example, a single nucleotide change in a beta-globin gene creates a mutant form of beta-globin protein, which, under an environmental situation such as oxygen stress, creates a condition known as sickle cell anemia. This condition causes the shape of normal blood cells to "sickle," impeding blood flow and causing severe pain and, in some extreme cases, even death.

2.1 Introduction: Genetic Basis of Human Diseases

Some genetic diseases are directly caused by mutations in a single gene (monogenic), and this type of disease follows the Mendelian pattern of inheritance. This Mendelian pattern of inheritance may be the result of an affected individual having a mutation in one copy of the gene (autosomal dominant mutation), and, alternatively, mutations in both copies of the gene may be necessary for the disease to manifest itself (autosomal recessive). In some instances, there is no dominant or recessive phenotype, but both alleles are present and expressed equally (co-dominant). Other genetic disorders that follow this Mendelian pattern of inheritance are associated with the X (female) or Y (male) chromosome and known as sex-linked mutations. An example is the classical hemophilia (X-linked dominant mutation) condition whereby mutated genes associated with this condition in an affected male (because he has only one X chromosome) can cause him to bleed uncontrollably, although such conditions are relatively rare.

Studies in humans with these inheritable defects have shed light on the normal function of the protein product encoded by these genes and the pathways that are implicated in genetic disorders. Another classic example of such an inherited disease is cystic fibrosis. The cystic fibrosis transmembrane conductance regulator gene (CFTR) encodes for a protein that functions in channeling chloride ions across cell membranes in cells that produce mucus, sweat, saliva, or digestive enzymes. A common mutation, a three nucleotide deletion in cystic fibrosis Delta-F508 that removes a phenylalanine codon (Goossens 1991), results in patients being unable to produce this essential protein and causes severe problems in lung and pancreatic function, a condition known as cystic fibrosis. Another genetic disease that follows the Mendelian law of inheritance is Duchenne muscular dystrophy (DMD). The DMD encodes for a protein called dystrophin whose biological function is maintaining muscle integrity. Mutations in the DMD gene cause the most common type of hereditary muscle-wasting diseases, collectively called muscular dystrophies (Tidball and Wehling-Henricks 2004).

There are a large number of other diseases that do not follow the Mendelian pattern of inheritance. These are considered polygenic or complex diseases in the sense that they tend to cluster in families but do not follow Mendelian inheritance patterns, and in some instances there are multiple gene–gene interactions that underlie one particular disease phenotype. For instance, it was discovered that genes on the same chromosome (linkage) are passed along in tandem unless meiotic crossover occurs such that some diseases tend to be caused by two or more genetic factors that contribute to a trait, and there is also a strong influence by the environment.

Therefore, complex diseases can arise as a result of multiple gene–gene interactions and/or gene–environmental interactions in susceptibility genes that act together and contribute to both the occurrence and the severity of a disease in an individual. Examples of complex diseases include diabetes, obesity, heart disease, some types of cancer, a variety of mental disorders that have at least some heritable properties, and many more. There are also instances where mutations in any one of multiple different genes can cause the same disease. This is exemplified by retinitis pigmentosa, a disease that causes degeneration of the retina that, if not treated, can ultimately lead to blindness. More than 40 different genes with varied biological functions have been associated with retinitis pigmentosa (Ferrari et al. 2011). Several of the genes are expressed in the epithelium of the retinal pigment or encode for photoreceptors.

2.2 What Gives Rise to Genetic Variation?

All human beings, regardless of race, ethnicity, or sex, share 99.5% similarity in their DNA sequence. Thus, the 0.5% difference in the DNA sequence in individuals belonging to the same or different ethnic population is what contributes to the surprising diversity in human phenotypic differences, including hair and skin color, height, and body shape. In addition, this sequence difference is responsible for variations in disease susceptibility and resistance and accounts for differential responses to therapeutic interventions.

With the completion of the human genome project (discussed in Sect. 2.3), it is now known that there are between ten million to 15 million variants in common sequences with sufficient frequency in one or more populations to be polymorphic in humans. The majority of these sequence variants are single nucleotide polymorphisms (SNPs), whilst others are insertions or deletions of short sequence fragments and copy-number variations. Sequence variations, and in particular SNPs, have been around for a long time as a result of natural selection. Some of these sequence variations are natural variations in the human genome that are associated with the phenotypic differences observed in individuals such as hair, eye, and skin color, as well as height or body shape, but other variations contribute to disease susceptibility and drug resistance, and these could be of biomedical and/or therapeutic interest. The challenge is how to distinguish between which genetic variants are associated with natural selection and which contribute to disease risk and susceptibility.

Single nucleotide polymorphisms are the most-frequently inherited genetic variations and usually serve as biological markers rather than as underlying causes of disease, and many of these SNPs do not have any obvious biological role. Studies carried out by the international SNP consortium on the entire human genome have identified more than four million SNPs, ~ 1 per 1–2 kb (Lander et al. 2001). However, most SNPs studies have been carried out in the EA population, and very few such studies have been reported for the African or other racial and ethnic populations.

It is important to identify SNPs across different ethnic populations because the frequency of SNPs can vary substantially between different populations, as well as their usefulness as markers for gene-mapping studies (Chakravarti 2001). Significant differences in SNP frequencies could uncover a putative disease marker that may eventually be used in diagnosis. It is estimated that it takes about 40,000 generations for a new SNP to form. It is also estimated that ancient pieces of DNA sequence segments ($\sim 5 \times 10^6$ bp long) called haplotypes, such as maternal or paternal haplotypes, are inherited intact for several hundreds of generations and can serve as useful tools to study ancestry. Thus, a small DNA segment of about 10 kB may contain approximately 40 SNPs that is enough to distinguish it from a haplotype of a different person with the same-sized fragment, and this would indicate that the second person got his/her segment of haplotype from a different ancestor (different sets of alleles have enough characteristic differences). Supposedly, we all have segments of Neanderthal DNAs in our genome, which means that we can detect ancient ancestral haplotypes. The ability to use genetic markers to predict ancestry is driving ancestry mapping using either mitochondria DNA (mtDNA; the genome within mitochondria that is passed on through the maternal lineage) or the Y-chromosome DNA that is passed on from father to son.

Human DNA sequence analysis shows that various populations differ in the frequency of both mutations of biomedical interest and polymorphisms of biological interest. There is, therefore, a need to understand the causes of these genetic variations in various populations in order to understand the biological basis of health disparities. Genetic variations or mutations in DNA occur constantly, and this can arise during DNA synthesis in replication, chromosomal crossing over as in sexual reproduction, or as a result of natural selection due to environmental pressures, such as disease, diet, or parasitic infection and even climatic changes, to create certain phenotypes. These genetic variations do not result in the creation of new species or organisms; rather, they result in the adaptation of existing organisms and their progenies to new environments through natural selection. Over time, the small alterations in cellular structures and functions may prove to be advantageous. Thus human genetic variation is the end result of diverse forces in nature.

Genetic variations that arise as a result of human migration cause adaptation and influence genetic susceptibility to diseases. An advantage to identifying the unique patterns of genes across various populations and disease susceptibility will contribute to understanding complex diseases, and that will ultimately lead to the design of novel therapies targeted to the populations that are most likely to respond. Others argue against the use of genetic variation as the basis for categorizing various populations into ethnic and racial groups and the disease prevalence and health outcomes in various groups (Cooper et al. 2003), noting that the vast majority of genetic variation (90–95%) occurs within, not across, human populations (Braun 2002) and that the *Homo sapiens* species consists of a single population. Therefore, biologically distinct human races do not exist, as genetic studies clearly demonstrate that human beings share 99.5% of their DNA in common.

2.3 Tools for Studying Genetic Variants

Genetic studies over the past century have been centered on finding traits and, in particular, disease traits and the genes that are responsible for causing these traits in populations where a particular disease is rampant. Such studies have been carried out in families that transmit the disease traits from one generation to the next.

Various molecular approaches are now used to identify chromosomes that carry the trait and then to map in detail of the chromosomal region until the gene is identified. Linkage studies have been instrumental in identifying chromosomal location of disease-associated candidate genes. This is made possible by the observation that genes that reside close together on a chromosome are linked together during meiosis. By definition, genes are said to be in linkage equilibrium if two genes/traits/loci are inherited completely independently of each generation. On the other hand, two genes are said to be in linkage disequilibrium (LD) if the frequency of association of different genes are inherited together more often than would be expected by chance. In linkage studies, data from multiple families with the same disease are compared or combined to determine whether a statistically significant linkage exists between the disease gene and other known molecular markers for the condition.

Once disease candidate genes are identified, then linkage analysis is carried out in human pedigrees. Typical protocols involve a few to large number of pedigrees, typically using many families (e.g., sibling pairs) such as twin studies, where concordance rates are compared between monozygotic (MZ) and dizygotic (DZ) twins. Twins are commonly used in these studies because it is usually assumed that twins share a common environment that lessens the impact of environmental influence (although this may not be true for studies of adult twins). For example, one study found a higher concordance for cellular immune responses to mycobacteria and other antigens in MZ compared to DZ twins, suggesting that genetic factors are important regulators of this immune response (Newport et al. 2004). There are other approaches, such as case-control association studies and family-based association, as well as linkage studies where the co-segregation of a marker with the disease phenotype are tested in families (Hill 2006).

However, genetic heterogeneity such as that exhibited by retinitis pigmentosa can confound such an approach because any statistical trend in the linkage data from one family or group tends to be canceled out by another set of data obtained from a different family with an unrelated causative gene(s). Furthermore, in the epigenetic phenomena, which are discussed in Chap. 3, environmental and numerous other factors come into play. The take-home message is that genetic factors that underlie disease often work within complicated, poorly understood, and highly nonlinear relationships. This explains why the search for signature disease genes (those with allelic variants thought to be primarily responsible for disease) has largely been a failure when the underlying gene(s) is known because, while the gene(s) may confer an increased risk, it does not directly cause the disease.

Much of the early genetic studies have led to the discovery of the alterations in genes that underlie or contribute to disease etiology and/or progression, albeit such studies were focused on finding one disease gene at a time. Beginning in the 1970s with Frederick Sanger, sequencing technology that enables reading off a DNA sequence, one nucleotide at a time, has made it possible for researchers to sequence one gene, many genes, and eventually an entire organism. This technique enabled other novel techniques for DNA, RNA, and protein analysis to follow rapidly, culminating in the era of genetic-recombination technology.

The human genome project has revolutionized the approach for searching for disease genes. The complete list of three-billion bases that make up the human genome was published in 2003. It took more than a decade and at a cost of US$3 billion in federal government funds to accomplish this feat. Nowadays, it cost about US$1000 to sequence an individual's genome. Advances in cutting-edge technologies including dense genotyping arrays and genome sequencing are driving down the cost of whole genome sequencing, making it more robust and affordable. It is estimated that in the near future, every person can have their genome sequenced for much less than US$1000.

The completion of the human genome sequence has immense scientific benefits: The speed with which the genetic basis of disease is being unraveled has largely been aided by the completion of the reference human genome sequence. This has enabled cataloging of sequence variations in individuals belonging to the same or different racial or ethnic groups (including both healthy individuals and those with various diseases). This, in turn, is providing new insight into understanding molecular processes that underlie disease and disease susceptibility. The challenge still remains as to how to distinguish sequence variations of biomedical interest (i.e., mutations that contribute to disease) from natural variations and to fully elucidate the significance and impact of sequence variations in physiological processes.

One of the potential benefits from the completed human genome sequence project is the design of genome-wide association studies (GWAS), which, in conjunction with powerful statistical and other computational tools, have become **useful for assessing genetic variants and association with traits or disease** in various individuals or populations. GWAS are useful for the study of both Mendelian patterns of disease inheritance and complex genetic diseases (many genetic and environmental factors acting together). The GWAS approach is instrumental in elucidating genetic variants associated with increased disease risk/resistance in one racial or ethnic population in comparison to another group and has the potential for being used to develop better markers to detect, treat, and prevent disease. As a result of GWAS, there is increasing insight into and the discovery of more genetic variances that are associated with the high prevalence of certain common and complex diseases in the African population and how this may contribute to disease disparities in this population when compared to other racial and ethnic populations. GWAS are increasingly being utilized in pharmacogenomics, which is driving the future of precision medicine.

2.3.1 Genome-Wide Association Studies (GWAS)

DNA sequencing (candidate gene, exome, or whole genome) and linkage analysis have been successful in the identification of germline and somatic mutations. The GWAS approach is another level of DNA sequencing that is useful in the identification of susceptible genetic variants or alleles for many diseases and traits. Unlike the classical approach of investigating genetic variation one gene at a time, the GWAS approach enables comprehensive analysis of the genetic variation across the entire human genome. GWAS take advantage of linkage disequilibrium (LD), i.e., non-random association of alleles at adjacent loci, and focus on common variations (>5% frequency) not limited to coding regions and not limited to prior biological knowledge. This approach has led to the identification of rare variants and unidentified common variants and structural variations that has eluded previous investigations.

Briefly, GWAS rely on hybridization of genomic DNA extracted from human tissues or blood obtained from patients with a particular disease (case) and individuals without the disease (control) in glass chips containing hundreds to thousands of SNP markers across the entire genome using microarrays in order to identify differential genetic variants in the case versus control groups. The approach is to scan several hundreds to thousands of genetic variants for a particular disease gene by comparing thousands of individuals with the disease with those who do not have the disease in order to link variations to particular traits and diseases in a manner that was not possible before. The data obtained from such analysis is compared to a computational database that contains the reference human genome sequence. This approach makes possible examining a large number of DNA markers in populations of individuals with a particular disease, as well as in control populations of individuals without the disease, to find statistical correlations between group phenotype and polymorphic markers. Thus, if certain variants are found to be significantly more frequent in the disease population in comparison with the non-disease population, the variants/loci are said to be associated with the disease. The associated genetic variations can serve as markers or powerful pointers to disease loci on the human genome.

This approach has been used to identify multifactorial susceptibility alleles associated with diseases. For example, GWAS have identified over 200 multigenic allelic variants to be associated with diabetes- disease susceptibility, physiological, and behavioral traits. Another GWAS has identified 18 risk loci in the EA and Asian populations to be associated with germline pancreatic cancer (Amundadottir 2016). Furthermore, GWAS have the potential for the identification of disease susceptibility variants that are associated with survival, therapeutic dosage responses, gene–gene interactions, or the environmental factors that act in concert with genes.

Various organizations, government, and private sectors including the National Institutes of Health (NIH), Pfizer, and others have formed public-private partnerships to fund GWAS. Although GWAS can be a powerful tool to identify candidate disease genes, additional studies are needed in order to determine how an individual carrying a particular genetic variant might be predisposed to the disease. Nowadays, GWAS are used in association with meta-analysis to reveal associations of heritable variations with disease risks. However, sensitivity can be a concern with the undetected heritability reported in most GWAS studies (Eichler et al. 2010). As the field advances, more complex and improved statistical tools will help in the identification of heritable variances with low penetrance. One recent statistical model that took into consideration epistasis, i.e., the interaction of multiple genetic variants in influencing a trait, found that in some studies the total frequency of heritability is much higher than reported (Zuk et al. 2012).

Some of the notable success stories of the GWAS studies are reported in a landmark paper from the Wellcome Trust Case Control Consortium, which carried out GWAS on a cohort of 2000 individuals for seven major diseases: coronary artery disease, type-1 and type-2 diabetes, hypertension, rheumatoid arthritis, bipolar disorder, and Crohn's disease (The Wellcome Trust Case Control Consortium 2007). They identified 24 independent disease risk associated loci: one in coronary artery disease, seven in type- 1 diabetes and three in type-2, three in rheumatoid arthritis, one in bipolar, and nine loci in Crohn's disease. In addition, some of the loci were associated with the risk of more than one of the diseases studied.

2.4 Genetic Variation in the African Population

Research in human evolutionary genetics and the identification of fossil remains with resemblance to modern humans in East Africa support the existence of human life in Africa about 200,000 years ago, which then gradually spread across the rest of the world within the past $\sim 100,000$ years (Campbell and Tishkoff 2008). Therefore, modern humans have continuously existed on the African continent longer than any other part of the world. The African continent has a wide range of environments, including deserts, tropical rainforests, savannas, swamps, mountain highlands, and coastal plains (Campbell and Tishkoff 2008). Climatic changes mean that some of these environments have undergone dramatic changes over the course of time (Campbell and Tishkoff 2008; Scholz et al. 2007; Trauth et al. 2007). Because of this considerable diversity, the environment has given rise to an African population with a diverse range of linguistics, cultures, and diet. Furthermore, differences in exposure to pathogens have given rise in the African populations to selection pressures that have also contributed to the most genetic adaptation and phenotypic variation (Campbell and Tishkoff 2008; Reed and Tishkoff 2006) that is not found in non-African populations. Greater genetic diversity in the African population is also reflected in higher levels of nucleotide and haplotype diversity in African populations, also not found in non-African populations, in both nuclear and mitochondrial DNA (Tishkoff et al. 2003).

2.4.1 Causes of Genetic Variation in the Human Population—A Case for Disease

The introduction of pathogens into a population with no previous exposure plays a very important role in natural selection. This can result in infectious disease epidemics where a large proportion of susceptible individuals dies, with a remnant of the surviving population, who are now adapted to the pathogenic exposure and equipped with protective allelic variants.

Natural selection can have either positive or negative consequences. A positive natural selection such as increased fitness is a positive adaptive response that gives rise to individuals with an advantageous genetic variant that makes them more likely to have more offspring than individuals with another genotype or variant, i.e., fitness benefit allele. A negative natural selection, on the other hand, leads to deleterious mutations that reduce fitness. Individuals with deleterious mutations are less likely to produce offspring, and the lineage is more likely to die off eventually. Some of the best described natural selections are restricted to infectious diseases (e.g., resistance to malaria), or nutritional adaptations (e.g., lactose tolerance). For instance, genetic variation in the Duffy gene and receptor is a classic example of a positive genetic selection and is a marker for protection against malaria (Oliveira et al. 2012).

Other studies have shown selection for genetic variation in the NADSYN1 gene on human chromosome 11q13 that may play a role in prevention of pellagra, whereas differential geographic variation in the toll-like receptor at chromosome 4p14 has been linked with differential susceptibility to autoimmune diseases, such as tuberculosis and leprosy (Todd et al. 2007). It is increasingly becoming apparent that varying frequencies of heritability and somatic genetic mutations (or variants), in addition to lifestyle and environmental factors, underlie disease etiology, as well as the disparities associated with several complex diseases. It is also increasingly becoming clear that genetic variation may be advantageous for individuals in one particular environment but can become disadvantageous in a totally different environment. Further studies of these selected variants may help to elucidate the correlation between genotype and phenotype for genes that play a role in important diseases.

A classic example of the effect of natural selection on a population is described by the work of a Danish physiologist Dr. P.L. Panum. In Dr. Panum's published report entitled "Observations made during the epidemic of measles on the Faroe Islands in the year 1846" (Poland 1998), he described an epidemic of measles on the Faroe Islands where 6000 of the 7800 people of that island developed measles and more than 200 died from the disease. A previous measles epidemic had occurred in 1781, and it was discovered that none of the people previously exposed in the 1781 epidemic (many still living in 1846) developed the disease. Some of the questions that arose from Dr. Panum's studies pertain to why some people survived the measles epidemic while others died, why the mortality was so high, and why the protective effect from the past epidemic was so high. Some of these issues can be resolved by understanding the role of innate susceptibility and resistance, as well as the acquired immunity conferred by previous exposure. The human leukocyte antigen (HLA) is important in disease susceptibility, resistance, and progression (Bodmer 1996).

The HLA gene complex encodes for HLA antigens that are expressed as white blood cells, antigen-presenting cells, and other tissues. The HLA proteins play a very important role in binding and presenting pathogens to T cells for destruction.

2.4 Genetic Variation in the African Population

Therefore, the ability of an individual to respond to viral infection (or vaccination) by antibody production is partly under the control of immune-response genes within the HLA complex. Genetic variations in HLA genes and their interactions with other factors (such as host or environmental pathogens) are increasingly recognized as playing a significant role in disease susceptibility and resistance, as well as disease progression (Bodmer 1996). Genetic variation in HLA isoforms is not only crucial in immune responses but also linked to various diseases including diabetes, Hepatitis C virus (HCV) or HIV infection, cancer, and spontaneous abortion, as well as the outcomes of organ transplantation.

Immune adaptation to infectious disease as a result of previous exposure in combination with genetic susceptibility or resistance underlies the disparities associated with infectious diseases. Natural selection may give rise to protective alleles in individuals or populations exposed to adverse environmental exposures, such as infectious epidemics for the progeny of those that survive; however, this process may take decades to several hundreds of years of constant and high exposure (Ramsay 2012). Genetic variations that are associated with disease risk could be geographically restricted as a result of new mutations, genetic drift, or region-specific pressures (Campbell and Tishkoff 2008). All we know is the pattern of variation we see today, which we can use to trace what happened in the past.

2.5 Infectious Diseases and Inherited Conditions in African Populations

Historically, infectious diseases have been the most important cause of morbidity and mortality globally until recently when non-communicable diseases started to rival or even exceed that of infectious diseases in many parts of the world. For instance, infectious diseases were the number one killer in the US until the early twenty-first century, when scientific breakthroughs in immunization significantly reduced mortality rates from infectious diseases. However, mortality rates as a result of infectious disease continue to disproportionately affect individuals on the African continent as compared to any other part of the world. Africans have an extremely high mortality rate from infectious diseases, with malaria and HIV alone responsible for millions of deaths per year (http://www.cdc.gov/malaria/index.htm) (Anon 2006a).

Malaria is a major killer of children in Africa and also in other parts of the world. Malaria is also perhaps the most important evolutionary driving force for natural selection of other commonly known genetic diseases that have evolved as a by-product to protect against malaria. For instance, sickle cell, glucose-6-phosphatase deficiency, and other erythrocyte defects are all diseases that may have been selected evolutionary to protect against malaria (Weatherall and Clegg 2001). Given that malaria exerts such a powerful evolutionary force on human genetic variation, malaria protective variants are likely to be in high frequencies in affected populations. Thus, the patterns of genetic variations and association with neighboring genetic markers (such as strong LD if recently selected) could contribute to understanding any immunologic, inflammatory, or chronic diseases that are more prevalent in the African population, African diaspora, or other racial and ethnic populations.

2.5.1 Malaria

Malaria accounts for one in five childhood deaths in Africa and one million deaths per year globally, making it a serious global health issue. The World Health Organization (WHO) estimated that almost 74% of the African population live in areas endemic with malaria, with about 19% in epidemic-prone and only 7% in malaria-free areas (Anon 2006b). Malaria is a complex disease whereby the malaria parasite infects the host red blood cells (RBCs) and induces changes that can ultimately destroy the RBCs (discussed below). Clinically, malaria can be either uncomplicated or severe. In the severe cases, various organs and tissues can be affected, and this can lead to death. Genetic studies have identified polymorphisms or variants in the disease pathways that contribute to protection against malaria as mentioned in Sect. 2.4.1.

The molecular mechanisms of erythrocyte invasion by malaria parasites is central to the disease process. The signal transmission involves binding of the malaria parasite to Duffy glycoproteins, cytokine receptors that are expressed on RBCs. The importance of Duffy signaling is demonstrated by the observation that RBCs that do not express the Duffy antigens (encoded by the FY gene) are resistant to invasion by the malaria *Plasmodium vivax (P. vivax)* parasite. The absence of Duffy expression is the result of a SNP variant in the Duffy promoter that alters the binding interaction and transcription from the GATA-1 transcription factor (Tournamille et al. 1995). Thus, individuals that are Duffy (negative; homozygous mutant) are fully protected against invasion by this parasite. However, other reports indicate that individuals who are heterozygous carriers of the Duffy-negative allele have some susceptibility to *P. vivax* infection. The *P. vivax* is one of many malaria parasite species and the non-lethal form of malaria parasites. To complicate matters further, other reports indicate that *P. vivax* can infect RBCs and cause clinical manifestation of malaria in Duffy-negative individuals, suggesting that the relationship between *P. vivax* and Duffy antigen are more complex than previously described (Zimmerman 2013).

It appears that, in some populations, alpha-thalassemia, another common genetic disorder of erythrocytes, has been naturally selected for protection against malaria. Here again a complication is the observation that, through cross-immunity, alpha-thalassemia may increase susceptibility to *P. vivax* that could be beneficial to humans because it confers some natural immunity by protection against infection of the more severe *Plasmodium falciparum (P. falciparum)* (Williams et al. 1996). However, one recent report challenges this notion of cross -immunological protection between *P. vivax* and *P. falciparum* against the more severe *P. falciparum* in alpha-thalassemia patients (Rosanas-Urgell 2012). Additional studies are warranted to clarify these inconsistencies between the cross-immunological protections of one parasite and another.

Knowledge of the genetic basis for disease resistance or susceptibility to infectious disease in the oldest human population can guide research and medical intervention, and these benefits are not limited to African populations. The following section will describe some of the genetic disorders that have resulted from selection by, and protection against, malaria, a common and perhaps the single most important public health concern in Africa. Understanding the biology of genetic variations and association with susceptibility to infectious diseases is crucial in improving the overall health of people on the African continent, but it is also important in understanding the role of genetic susceptibility and the higher disease prevalence among the US AA population.

2.5.2 Sickle Cell Disease

Sickle cell disease has been extensively studied as a classic single gene disease that fits the Mendelian pattern of inheritance. Sickle cell disease is predominantly seen in individuals of African descent; however, sickle cell disease is common in other geographic areas where malaria is also common, such as Arabian Peninsula. The disease is caused by point mutation in the beta-globin gene, an important subunit of hemoglobin, the protein molecule in RBC that plays a role in binding oxygen and the transport of oxygen throughout the body. The disease is inherited in an autosomal recessive pattern, in that individuals who are homozygous for the mutant gene have the full-blown disease, whereas individuals heterozygous for the mutation do not have the disease but instead are referred to as "carriers." Individuals with sickle cell disease have an abnormal variant of hemoglobin called HbS in their red blood cells that clump together, unable to bind oxygen, and change from a smooth circular disc-like shape to sickle shape. The clinical symptoms of HbS include hemolysis and microvascular occlusion that destroy RBC and cause tissue damage and bone pain. Despite intense research in this field, there is no cure for sickle cell disease.

Another disease that is caused by mutation in hemoglobin C (HbC) is thalassemia. Interestingly, a variation in the HbC gene is associated with the protection of RBCs from infection by the malaria parasite. For example, one report suggests that a variant of HbC has a protective effect against the severe *P. falciparum* malaria in W. African population and the protection from this variant may be greater than that from the HbS variant (Agarwal 2000). The beta thalassemia (HbB) sickle-cell trait or HbA/HbS heterozygosity is associated with a ten-fold reduction in malaria risk. Variations in HbC and alpha thalassemia (HbA) genes have also been reported to confer protection against the severe form of malaria, as well as malarial anemia (Williams et al. 1996). The HbB gene has also been reported to have some protective effect against malaria; however, this protective effect has only been reported in isolated pockets of W. Africa population (Willcox et al. 1983). Clearly, differential genetic variants in the hemoglobin genes can influence malaria risk, but the currently known gene variants vary significantly among various populations and do not explain all the disease risks or protection. Further studies are required to investigate the distribution of genetic defects that are associated with the manifestations of the severe form of malaria. Other contributing factors to the differences in susceptibility or resistance to malaria disease includes genetic variants in the immune response genes which are associated with the parasitic invasion of malaria, or some environmental factors (Torcia et al. 2008).

2.5.3 Glucose-6-Phosphate Dehydrogenase Deficiency

Glucose 6-phosphate dehydrogenase (G6PD) is an enzyme that catalyzes the first step in the pentose phosphate pathway for the production of nicotinamide adenine dinucleotide phosphate (NADPH). In RBCs, NADPH is required for maintaining the integrity of RBC shape. Deficiency of G6PD protein, which is the result of X-linked recessive mutation, is commonly observed in men of African ancestry and reported in about 11% of the AA male population. However, deficiency in G6PD is protective against *P. falciparum* malaria infection, a mutation that has risen to high frequency in populations exposed to malarial infection, despite the negative consequences associated with this deficiency (Sabeti et al. 2002).

Deficiency in G6PD plays another role in the protection of RBCs. Infection of RBCs by the malaria parasites induces oxidative stress in the infected cell; this compromises the pentose pathway and ultimately the cells and parasites die from oxidative damage. Thus, G6PD mutation is a natural selection mechanism of protection against malaria, which accounts for its high frequency among individuals of African descent. The ability of G6PD deficiency to protect against malaria does, however, create a public-health conundrum in that the use of primaquine to treat malaria has an adverse hemolysis effect in patients with G6PD mutation.

2.5.4 Tuberculosis

A relatively recent infectious disease in comparison to malaria is tuberculosis (TB). It is estimated that about eight million people develop TB disease and about three million patients die from TB every year. The TB causative agent, *Mycobacterium tuberculosis,* has infected over two billion people worldwide, without any clinical symptoms. In Africa alone, there were ~3.8 million cases of TB in 2005, and this was accompanied by almost 550,000 deaths (http://www.who.int/mediacentre/factsheets/fs104/en/).

However, the molecular mechanisms causing TB infection is largely unknown. Twin studies in the African population, comparing MZ and DZ twins, have provided evidence of a significant role for host genetic factors in the innate immune-response pathways that may contribute to TB susceptibility (Jepson et al. 2001). Other reports have demonstrated that variants in several genes including SLC11A1 (NRAMP1) (Awomoyi et al. 2002), IL1B (Awomoyi et al. 2005), and vitamin D receptor (Bornman et al. 2004) with diverse cellular functions are associated with TB susceptibility. Candidate gene studies have also provided some evidence for major TB susceptibility loci in specific populations, but few candidate genes have consistently shown strong association of TB in Africans, suggesting that several loci may determine or modulate susceptibility to TB. Elucidating the biological mechanisms underlying TB infection is further complicated by co-morbid conditions including HIV and HBC infections.

A GWAS study of 96 Moroccan multiplex families including 227 siblings identified a single region on human chromosome 8q12-q13 to be significantly associated with TB. The linkage was strong if one parent was also affected with TB, suggesting an autosomal dominant TB susceptibility loci on human chromosome 8q12-13 (Baghdadi et al. 2006). Several malaria and TB GWAS, such as the MalariaGEN initiative funded by the Gates Foundation (www.malariagen.net) and the African TB Genetics Consortium and the Wellcome Trust Case Control Consortium (University of Oxford, UK; www.well.ox.ac.uk/aug-10-tb-susceptibility-locus), are ongoing to determine the etiological and associated genetic risk variants for these diseases.

2.5.5 HIV/AIDS

Approximately 10% of the world's population resides in sub-Saharan Africa, and 68% of adults and nearly 90% of children infected with HIV-1 virus live in this region. So, approximately 22.5 million Africans are estimated to be infected with the HIV-1 virus, and about 12 million AIDS orphans live on the continent, making Africa the worst affected region in the AIDS pandemic (www.whosis/database/core/core_select.cfm). Without antiretroviral treatment, the great majority of infected individuals will progress to full-blown AIDS and die following HIV infection. Although the asymptomatic period averages ten years and ranges from a few years to 20 years, there are rare instances of infected individuals who do not progress to AIDS at all. For instance, a group of female sex workers in Nairobi, Kenya who are at risk of HIV infection (Kimani et al. 2008). Such cases demonstrate the complexities in viral infections involving multiple genetic and environmental factors and their interactions, resulting in altered disease susceptibility or resistance (Lama and Planelles 2007).

One report identified variations in interferon regulatory factor 1 (IRF1), which causes deficiency in the gene expression in a cohort of the Kenyan sex workers, is associated with resistance to HIV-1 infection, whereas other variations of the IRF1 gene were found to be associated with disease progression (Ball et al. 2007). These results suggest that the key to protection from infection lies in gene variants that do not support viral transcription and replication. Other studies have identified genetic variants in genes that play roles in the viral replication pathway including cytidine deaminase enzymes APOBEC3F, APOBEC3G, CUL5, and TRIM5 alpha that are associated with protection in AA against HIV infection, accelerated loss of CD4 lymphocytes, and progression to full blown AIDs (Lama and Planelles 2007).

Several other infectious diseases are relatively common in Africa and present serious public-health issues including leishmaniasis, leprosy, schistosomiasis, and trachoma. However, unlike malaria and HIV/AIDs research, few resources have been devoted to these types of diseases. Overall, HIV/AIDs, TB, and malaria are the three major infectious diseases that continue to devastate sub-Saharan Africans. Malaria is a relatively ancient infectious disease in comparison with HIV/AIDs and TB. The host genetic diversity as a result of natural selection against malaria is well known; however, the genetic diversities associated with HIV/AIDs and TB are in their infancies, and evolutionary forces are still at play. The genetic diversity associated with this trio is not known; whether having the one disease increases protection or susceptibility to the others remains to be established. Because of the high morbidity and mortality rates from infectious diseases on the African continent, there is an urgent need for safe and effective therapeutic interventions.

2.6 Non-Communicable Diseases

Although infectious diseases are the most important public-health concerns in Africa to date, the health pattern is rapidly changing as a result of economic development and urbanization. For instance, a recent report from S. Africa indicates that over 75% of black South Africans have at least one major risk factor for heart disease (Tibazarwa et al. 2009). Other common diseases of the Western world such as obesity, diabetes, and hypertension are increasingly becoming prevalent on the African continent as the general population transitions from a rural to an urban lifestyle (Abubakari et al. 2008). The increasing incidences of complex diseases on the African continent correlate with known environmental risk factors, such as urbanization and sedentary lifestyle. Genomic studies including GWAS for elucidating genetic diversity are limited in the African population, although they represent the human population with the highest genetic diversity. It is, however, important to carry out genomic studies in the sub-Saharan African population because their genetic diversity is crucial to understanding the genetic origins to many diseases.

2.7 GWAS in the African Population

GWAS approaches have been used extensively to study the genetic variations associated with complex traits in individuals of European decent, but very few studies have been carried out in non-admixed African populations.

Conducting GWAS in the nascent African populations is important because the unique genome of the African populations has an important role to play in understanding human health and disease susceptibility. The challenges of doing such studies in the African population, as explained by Teo et al. (2010), include the diversity and structure of the African population, lack of funding, poor infrastructure and public-health systems, and perhaps the small pool of trained scientists to carry out this work. The International HapMap project (www.1000genomes.org) is a leader in GWAS in the African population.

Among the few GWAS that have been carried out have been conducted to identify genetic variants associated with susceptibility to malaria in West-African children. The results from this study highlighted the role of genetic variants in the HbS locus in the disease prevalence (Jallow et al. 2009). Other data from GWAS suggest higher levels of genetic diversity within the African population in comparison with non-African populations, confirming the results of previous mtDNA, X-chromosome, and Y-chromosome studies (Campbell and Tishkoff 2008; Conrad et al. 2006; Frazer et al. 2009). Recent studies have shown considerable variation in SNPs, INDELs, copy-number variations, translocations, and inversions (Scherer et al. 2007) within individuals of African descent, as well as other racial and ethnic populations, with African populations showing the highest levels within populations of genetic diversity relative to non-Africans (Tishkoff et al. 2009). The emerging observations from GWAS is that this approach can be used to roughly cluster diverse racial and ethnic populations by geographic region (Wall et al. 2008).

2.8 Genetic Variation in the African Diaspora—The African-American Population

As described in the introductory chapter and elsewhere, one of the largest migrations in modern human history involved the millions of Africans who were brought to the Americas as slaves over a 500–year period. However, the modern AA population has on average approximately 20% European ancestry (Shriver and Kittles 2004), making their genetic pool heterogeneous. The African diaspora in the US continues to share a common genetic heritage with nascent Africans, while, at the same time, being exposed to different environmental and lifestyle factors compared to Africans on the native African continent. Various populations of African descent, therefore, provide a great opportunity to compare and contrast the genetic variants underlying common disease susceptibility in these genetically related populations but in different environments.

Disease types and prevalence differ between the nascent African population in comparison with AA and other racial and ethnic populations in the Western (Europe and N. America) world. As discussed above in Sect. 2.5, infectious and communicable diseases are the most prevalent in the developing world, including in sub-Saharan Africa, whereas non-communicable diseases are most prevalent in the Western world. Genetic variation has been shown to be associated with susceptibility to various communicable and non-communicable diseases that have a genetic component (Cooke and Hill 2001).

People of the African diaspora often have a high prevalence of certain complex diseases (discussed in the following sections), such as hypertension, diabetes, and cancer for which the genetic bases are poorly understood, and many of the environmental factors that contribute to these complex diseases are not as common in the African populations (Forrester et al. 1998; Kaufman et al. 1999). This makes it possible to differentiate the relative contribution of genetic and environmental risk factors of these diseases. The following sections will discuss the genetic alterations associated with the leading causes of mortality for US racial and ethnic groups, with some reference to the sub-Saharan Africans.

2.9 Cardiovascular Disease (CVD) Disparities

According to the World Health Organization (WHO) factsheets, cardiovascular diseases (CVDs) including heart disease and stroke are the leading cause of death globally. Annual statistics indicate that more people die from CVDs than from any other disease. In 2012 alone, an estimated 17.5 million people died from CVDs, representing 31% of total global mortality in that year (http://www.who.int/mediacentre/factsheets/fs317/en/). In the US, not only are CVDs the leading cause of mortality, but there also is a disproportionate impact of CVDs in the AA population in comparison with EA counterparts, as well as other racial and ethnic groups. The good news is that the mortality rates for CVDs are on the decline among the general US population as a result of improved cardiovascular procedures such as coronary arteriography and coronary-artery-bypass graft surgery. However, the decline in mortality rates have not been seen in AA populations, whose mortality rates continue to be high (Hertz 2005). One of the factors that is attributable to the disparities in CVD mortality rates is unequal access to cardiovascular treatment procedures.

Other contributing factors to the high mortality rate of CVDs in AA are the high prevalence of associated risk factors or co-morbidities such as diabetes, hypertension (Cooper et al. 1997; Kaufman et al. 1996), and obesity (Colilla et al. 2000; Rotimi et al. 1995). These risk factors can lead to changes in vascular structure, causing vascular dysfunction followed by tissue injury/wall stress resulting in organ dysfunction, end-stage heart failure, and ultimately death. Several scientific reports demonstrate that there is a complex interaction between genetic risk factors (including familial predisposition) and environmental risk factors (including psychosocial stress, smoking, metabolic syndrome, and hypercholesterolemia) in CVD incidence and mortality rates. Other risk factors include congenital cardiac defects that are associated with abnormal blood pressure (BP) level and aberrant expression of vasodilators such as nitric oxide.

2.9.1 Cardiovascular Tissue Remodeling and CVDs

Some studies have investigated the mechanical properties of cardiovascular tissue and described decreased vasodilation of the vascular lumen, as well as reduced expression of nitric oxide in AAs when compared to the EA population, and this may be associated with the increased risk of CVDs in the AA population (for a review see Taherzadeh 2010). Other studies have focused on mediators in cardiovascular physiology and disease, including two opposing mediators linking obesity, diabetes, and vascular dysfunction in CVDs.

Endocrine signaling plays a very important role in cardiovascular physiology, as well as disease state. One of the mediators in this signal pathway is angiotensin II, which is important in aldosterone synthesis via the so-called "renin-angiotensin-aldosterone" system (RAAS). Aldosterone plays a very important role in sodium reabsorption, potassium secretion, and stabilization of blood pressure. Abnormally high-level production of aldosterone (hyperaldosteronism) is caused by tumors in the adrenal gland, or in response to other diseases, and can lead to increased blood pressure, hypertension, cardiac remodeling, fibrosis, and impaired endothelial function, and is also implicated in left ventricular hypertrophy (Vlachopoulos and Terentes-Printzios 2015). Other conditions that are associated with hyperaldosteronism are decreased blood potassium level, myocardial infarction, and increased inflammation (Vlachopoulos C and Terentes-Printzios D 2015).

Another mediator in the endocrine-signal pathway is known as peroxisome proliferator activated-receptor gamma (PPAR-gamma), which plays a role in fat-cell differentiation and is expressed in endothelial and vascular smooth-muscle cells. PPAR-gamma is believed to play diverse physiological role in endothelial cells including lowering blood pressure and improving endothelial function and has growth- inhibition and anti-inflammatory properties (Gibbons 2004). Dominant negative mutation in PPAR-gamma is associated with severe insulin resistance and is a risk factor for early-age onset of diabetes and hypertension, suggesting that genetic variants in the PPAR-gamma gene can mediate increased susceptibility to CVDs (Gibbons 2004). Other reports have identified variations in the RAAS and PPAR-gamma genes as associated with differential susceptibility to hypertension and myocardial infarction in the AA, in comparison with the EA, population. Genetic variance associated with lower plasma renin-activity was higher in individuals of African descent with hypertension (Underwood et al. 2010). Other genetic alterations in the endocrine-signaling pathway such the beta-adrenergic receptors are associated with significant increased risk of heart failure in the AA, in comparison with the EA, population.

Several reports have implicated different genetic variants in key regulatory genes in disparities of vasoconstriction and CVDs. One study reported that genetic variation in leukotriene A4 hydrolase gene is associated with a three-fold increased risk of myocardial infarction in AA patients, while the relative risk is only 1.16 in Europeans (Helgadottir et al. 2006). Other reports demonstrated a relationship between genetic factors such as platelets-aggregation and blood-coagulation factors, as well as specific polymorphisms in beta-adrenergic receptor genes, such as ADRB1, 2, 3 mediate physiological effects of epinephrine and neurotransmitter non-epinephrine, to be modestly associated with disparities in CVDs. Identification of genetic variance in genes associated with CVDs may contribute to understanding the genetic contribution to CVDs' disparity and help in developing novel therapies tailored for various populations.

Not many studies have investigated the genetic factors associated with CVDs' risk in the African population on their native continent, perhaps because this condition was uncommon until the 1970s. One South African study demonstrated that a family history of CVDs was significantly associated with myocardial infarction, hypertension, and type 2 diabetes in urban black South Africans (Loock et al. 2006). Another study that investigated genetic variants in serpin peptidase inhibitor (plasminogen activator inhibitor type 1, PAI1) and tissue plasminogen activator (PLAT), important players in the blood coagulation process, reported increased risk of these genetic variants for thrombosis, an important risk factor in heart attacks (Williams et al. 2007). They observed significant genetic variation in PAI1 and PLAT by sex, suggesting a complex pattern of genetic regulation via gene–environment interaction (Schoenhard et al. 2008).

2.9.2 Heart Failure (HF)

Heart failure is major public-health burden in the US population, particularly in individuals over the age of 20 years old. It is estimated that 5.1-million people in the US have been diagnosed and are living with the condition, and about 550,000 new cases are diagnosed each year (Dunlay 2014). In the US, the incidence and mortality rates of HF is highest in the AA population, followed by Hispanics and EAs, and then Chinese. Heart failure in AA patients occurs at an early age and has a worse prognosis compared to their EA counterparts, as well as having higher rates of hospitalization and advanced left-ventricular disease. Several risk factors are associated with this condition. For instance, excessive production of neurohormones such as vasopressin or norepinephrine, as well as nitric-oxide insufficiency, is a major risk factor for HF.

The good news is that there are current drugs on the market, such as mineralocorticoid blockers (antagonist beta blockers; renin angiotensin antagonists, aldosterone blockers), or, in the case of nitric oxide insufficiency, nitric oxide-enhancement can be orally administered to counteract the effect of neurohormonal excesses (Bansal 2009). Other risks factors that are associated with HF include oxidative stress and chronic inflammation, and there are significant racial differences in the levels of oxidative stress and inflammation in AA, EA, and Mexican populations. Although the mechanisms are unclear, diet, comorbidities (obesity, T2DM), lower blood levels of antioxidant nutrients, as well as higher levels of environmental stress, are all implicated in the increase risk of HF.

2.9.3 Hypertension

The prevalence of hypertension is increasing among the US population as a whole, but the AA population is disproportionally affected by this condition (Cooper et al. 1997). For example, AAs have a 1.5–2-fold increased risk of hypertension compared with European-descended Americans, with the largest difference being between AA and EA women (Eberhardt et al. 2001). This disparity is even more pronounced among women—African-American women have an age-adjusted incidence of 35.9% (based on data from 1988 to 1994) compared with 19.7% in female Americans of European descent. The reasons for the disparity in this disease is unknown, but several theories have been proposed, including a difference in genetic predisposition factors including differential genetic variants in susceptible disease genes, as well as differences in exposures to environmental risk factors (SES and diet).

Some of the associated risk factors include end-stage renal disease, heart failure, and stroke, risk factors that occur at higher frequencies in the AA population (Collins and Winkleby 2002; Hertz et al. 2005). Hypertension in AAs is potentially associated with high salt sensitivity, low levels of plasma renin, vascular dysfunction (e.g., vasoconstrictor hyperactivity and diminished vasodilatory function), as well higher frequencies of co-morbidities, such as diabetes mellitus and obesity. Other risk factors that are associated with hypertension are sedentary lifestyle, unhealthy diet, and family history of the condition.

Elucidating the genetic risk factors for hypertension has been a difficult task because of other co-morbidities that are associated with the disease. Studies of risk factors have focused on the molecular mechanisms involved in blood-pressure regulation, however identifying the candidate genes associated with this condition has met with little success. For instance, one report has identified a positive association of genetic variants in angiotensinogen (AGT which is involved in the renin-angiotensin pathway) that leads to vasoconstriction and increased blood pressure) with increased risk of hypertension. However, this result has not been replicated in other studies (Caulfield et al. 1995; Rotimi et al. 1994). The reasons for the conflicting observations of genetic studies in various populations are differences in the role of gene-gene and gene–environmental interactions in determining the hypertension phenotype (Kardia 2000; Moore and Williams 2002). A potential role for gene–gene interactions is supported by one study of the Ghanaian population that reported no evidence of single gene association with hypertension risk when analyzed independently. On the other hand, when multiple genes were analyzed together, they observed evidence of association with hypertension risk (Williams et al. 2000).

Despite the high prevalence of hypertension among AAs, hypertension was not considered a major health risk for individuals in sub-Saharan African until recently (Unwin et al. 2001). Studies of hypertension in both rural and urban settings in Nigeria and Cameroon estimate the incidence of hypertension at 15–20% (Cooper et al. 1997), and as high as 20–33% in Tanzanian population (Edwards et al. 2000).

In both studies, urban subjects and women had the highest prevalence, suggesting an increased incidence of hypertension as individuals convert from rural to urban living. Thus, in addition to the prevalence of infectious diseases, several complex diseases including obesity (discussed in Sect. 2.10) and associated hypertension are also becoming more common in Africa, presumably due to an increasingly urbanized Western lifestyle (Colilla et al. 2000; Morris et al. 2010).

A strong genetic component has been suggested for hypertension risk. Some reports indicate a genetic component in the etiology of hypertension with heritability that ranges 45–68% in people of sub-Saharan African descent (Gu et al. 1998; Rotimi et al. 1999a). Genetic variants in genes, e.g., angiotension-1 converting enzyme (ACE) and angiotensin II (AGTII) involved in the renin-angiotensin pathways, are highly heritable. However, there are differences in frequency of the variation in these traits in sub-Saharan Africans and AAs, as one report indicated heritability of 77% for AGT and 67% of ACE in Nigerians when compared to 18% heritability for AGT and ACE in AAs (Cooper 2000). The differences in the variants could be attributed to the admixture population of US AAs compared to the relatively homogenous Nigerian population, as well as different environmental lifestyle and dietary factors in the two different geographic populations. This observation supports a role for environmental variability across various populations that could influence disease risks and outcome.

Differential genetic variations that exist in various racial and ethnic populations can cause different responses to the same environmental risk as a result of differences in gene expression and phenotypic response. Thus, the genetic risk factors associated with hypertension underscore the difficulty associated with identifying genetic risk factors for complex diseases as allelic variants at several multiple genetic loci can independently, or as multivariant clusters, can interact to predispose individuals to the disease risk. This differs in various individuals belonging to the same population or different populations. Future studies in hypertension risks should focus on elucidating the underlying genetic architectures for various different populations.

2.10 Diabetes

Diabetes has become a global crisis, i.e., a worldwide epidemic, that requires both effective tools and therapeutic interventions to improve outcomes. Diabetes mellitus (DM) is a condition characterized by either the total lack of insulin (type 1) or the resistance of peripheral tissues to the effects of insulin (type 2, T2DM). Both diseases result from the absence of the signaling effect of insulin in the presence of normal or high glucagon and other metabolic signals. The disease DM is due to the imbalance in carbohydrate metabolism and its effects on other metabolic pathways. An estimated 246 million people world are affected by the T2DM condition, and this number is expected to increase to 380 million by 2025 (www.bio-medicine.org), unless some drastic measures are taken to reduce the disease risk.

2.10 Diabetes

According to the American Diabetes Association, 29.1 million Americans were affected with diabetes in 2012 (http://www.diabetes.org/diabetes-basics/statistics/). The prevalence of diabetes is highest in the Native American population, followed by AAs, and the lowest incidence is among Alaskan Americans. Compared to the EA population, the prevalence of diabetes, especially among adults, was about twice that in the AA population, whereas the African population had the lowest comparative rate of diabetes, until recently when there is increased incidences in various parts of the continent, as mentioned in Sect. 2.1. It is estimated that one in every eight AAs over the age of 20 is living with diabetes (CDC 2008).

Type 1 DM (T1DM) is a condition linked to autoimmune destruction of the pancreatic beta-cells that can cause partial or complete loss of insulin production. Insulin is an important hormone that plays a role in signaling the body to absorb blood glucose, for instance, after the ingestion of food. Thus in the absence of insulin, gluconeogenesis is unrestrained, and there is an increase in blood glucose. However, cells such as muscle and fat cells cannot take up the available blood glucose, even when present at very high levels in the blood, and this can lead to health problems. The only available treatment is the injection of exogenous insulin into the body. However, even with optimal control, the damaging effects of elevated blood glucose eventually lead to medical complications including heart attack, stroke, blindness, kidney failure, and nerve damage.

Type 2 DM (T2DM) is distinct from T2DM and is characterized by a disorder whereby the pancreatic cells do not produce enough insulin. Type 2 DM can also be caused by improper insulin signaling, such as insulin not being able to bind to cell surface receptors and enable glucose to enter cells, creating a resistance to insulin's effects on target tissues and cells. In that case, the body acts as if there is no insulin, even when the hormone is present at sufficient levels. This condition shares similarity with T1DM. Gluconeogenesis is unrestrained, and muscle and fat cells do not take up glucose resulting in similar disease outcomes as seen for T1DM. The physiologic picture of DM is complex and involves multiple organ systems, including the adipose, muscle, pancreatic islets, immunity, central nervous system, and the liver.

The identification and functional characteristics of genetic variants (discussed in Sect. 2.10.1) that either cause or predispose one to diabetes have provided insight to help explain early pancreatic beta-cells dysfunction in children and adolescents (Hattersley et al. 2009). Hannon et al. (2008) demonstrated that healthy AAs adolescents have 14% lower insulin clearances and 63% higher early-stage insulin concentrations, despite having similar insulin sensitivity as do EAs. Insulin clearance is defined as the ratio of the insulin-degradation rate and insulin concentration that can be used to measure the rate of insulin metabolism. Accordingly, AA adolescents are more likely to have a lower insulin degradation and a higher insulin concentration, leading to the abnormalities in insulin metabolism as compared with their EA peers. Genetic variance is a primary contributor to insulin sensitivity, fasting serum insulin, insulin resistance, and hyperinsulinemia in AAs (Hannon et al. 2008).

Obesity, which is discussed in Sect. 2.11, is the major risk factor for T2DM and appears to drive tissue- insulin resistance in part via a gain of ectopic fat deposits in abdominal regions, the liver, and the pancreas. However, ectopic fat in the pancreas may contribute to beta-cell dysfunction. It is estimated that individuals whose BMI is more than 35 kg/m^2 (obese individuals) have between a 50–80 fold increased risk of diabetes (T2DM) when compared with individuals whose BMI is less than 23 kg/m^2 (Chan et al. 1994). Indeed, the increasing prevalence of obesity is a key factor in increasing T2DM levels around the world, suggesting that measurement of adiposity (BMI, waist circumference or waist/hip ratios) can be a predictor of T2DM risk. Although diabetes is typically diagnosed in individuals with high BMI, the South Asian population with BMI of 22 kg/m^2 have an equivalent prevalence of T2DM as EAs with a BMI of 30 kg/m^2. One postulated reason for the high susceptibility to diabetes in the South Asian population is that they have a lower storage capacity for fat (Sniderman et al. 2007), whereas the high prevalence of diabetes in the AA population is because of the high obesity prevalence.

Although differences in body weight or waist circumference are strongly associated with insulin resistance and diabetes, the highest rate of developing T2DM among AAs cannot simply be explained by obesity. Ethnic differences in triglycerides (TGs) and glucagon-like peptide-1 (GLP-1) levels have been found to be significantly associated with insulin resistance and T2DM (Seeleang 2011). Some studies have investigated whether intermuscular adipose tissue (IMAT) or the fat tissue within skeletal muscle is associated with an increased risk of developing insulin resistance and T2DM. One study found both male and female AAs have greater IMAT than EAs (Miljkovic-Gacic et al. 2008). Therefore, genetic studies of IMAT may help explain why some people with lean or normal body weight are at a higher risk for the development of hyperglycemia and T2DM.

Several studies have shown that AAs are more insulin resistant and have higher glycated hemoglobin (AIC) than other ethnic groups, either at or before diagnosis (Adams et al. 2008). Accordingly, AA adolescents seem to have the highest rate of propensity to develop T2DM in comparison with other racial or ethnic groups. Obese AAs have higher resting and stimulated insulin concentrations in comparison with their obese EA counterparts. One study reported that the glucagon-like peptide 1 (GLP-1), a potent metabolite that plays a role in lowering blood glucose by regulating insulin secretion, was observed to be expressed at higher concentrations in the AA obese than the EA obese (Velasquez-Mieyer et al. 2003), findings that might be important in the emergence of GLP-1 based diabetic medications and their use across various populations.

2.10.1 Genetic Factors Associated with Type 1 Diabetes

Genomic analysis such as GWAS to identify genetic susceptibility loci associated with T1DM has indicated over 50 allelic loci (www.t1dbase.org). A major locus effect is shown in genetic variants in the HLA complex that could affect the binding interactions with antigens, and their presentation to T-cells has been identified in perhaps one of the largest T1DM studies in the AA population. High allelic frequencies of unique HLA-DRB1 genetic variants, which confers susceptibility for TIDM, was observed in AAs in comparison to EA (Howson et al. 2013), indicating a genetic basis for the increased risk of T1DM in the AA population.

2.10.2 Genetics Factors Associated with Type 2 Diabetes

Type 2 DM is currently the most common metabolic disorder in the world and among the many common diseases with a strong genetic component and strong familial aggregation. The risk of diabetes is estimated to be 50% for first-degree siblings and 100% risk for monozygotic twins among the families with history of diabetes (Rich 1990). Family history has been noted to double the risk of diabetes, which equivalent to the risk of obesity and which is also heritable. Furthermore, obesity and family history quadruple the risk of diabetes. Data in support of a strong familial component are marked by differences in T2DM prevalence across various different populations. Geographic regions of high T2DM incidence are found in the Pima and South Sea Island populations, where the incidence exceeds 50% of the population. On the other hand, the incidence of diabetes is reported to be lowest in European regions, reported to be about 5% in the European population. In the US, the incidence of T2DM in the AA population, with the highest incidence, is approaching 20% (Elbein 2007; Haffner 1998).

Complex diseases such as T2DM are influenced by a combination of genetic, lifestyle, and environmental risk factors. Several candidate gene studies has reported two genes, namely PPARy and the beta-cell potassium channel gene KCNJ11 (Das and Elbein 2006), to be associated with T2DM risk. GWAS, meant to identify obesity genetic variants that are associated with T2DM, identified only FTO, a gene whose protein product plays a role in energy metabolism (Do et al. 2008).

Other GWAS to identify susceptibility alleles with increased association with T2DM have identified more than 60 genetic variants in the EA, Asian, AA, and Hispanic populations. The genetic risk in the AA population persists even after adjusting for known environmental risk factors, such as body mass index (BMI), physical activity, and SES. One study by Keaton et al. (2014) showed that AAs carry a greater number of risk alleles at 46 established T2DM risk loci than EA patients. Cumulatively, these variants are strong predictors of diabetes risk in EAs, but poor predictors in AAs.

The prevalence of T2DM is relatively low in sub-Saharan Africans, reported to be lower than 5%. Although the prevalence of T2DM is on the rise across the continent, attributed mainly to changes in dietary and other environmental factors, obesity, which a major risk factor for T2DM, is still relatively uncommon, reflecting the high physical activity levels and a diet low in caloric intake. Obesity rates were reported to be 0% in Togo, between 4.8 and 8.0% in S. Africa, and 10% in Northern Sudan (Motala 2002).

The low incidence of T2DM in sub-Saharan African, an environment where dietary caloric intake is much lower than in the US, suggests that the incidence of T2DM might carry a proportionately greater genetic component. A multi-institutional, international collaboration was set up to create a genetic resource that can be used to find susceptibility genes for T2DM in the ancestral populations of African Americans in a African-American diabetes mellitus (AADM) study (Rotimi et al. 2001). The AADM study had the goal of collecting 800 sibling pairs affected by T2DM cases and 200 unaffected controls from families in both Ghana and Nigeria. One of the studies that utilized the useful AADM resource was a GWAS linkage analysis carried out to find genetic variants associated with three obesity-related phenotypes: body mass index (BMI); fat mass (FM); and percent of body fat (PBF) (Chen et al. 2005). Among the W. African population, PBF showed the strongest evidence of association with genetic variants chromosomes 2, 4, and 5. The FM showed evidence of association with genetic variants on chromosome 2, and BMI showed association with variants on chromosome 1 and 4. When all three phenotypes were combined, significant genetic variants on chromosomal regions 2p13, 4q23 and 5q14 were associated with obesity in the AADM patient population, providing genetic information of obesity in this less well-studied population.

Other GWAS to find susceptible chromosomal loci in AADM have focused on the downstream consequence of diabetes. Reduced renal function is associated with diabetes and hypertension, and renal function can be detected by measuring serum creatinine, creatinine clearance, and the glomerular filtration rate (GFR) (Chen et al. 2007). A GWAS to find susceptible loci in the genes encoding for serum creatinine, creatinine clearance, and GFR using the AADM resources identified variance in CYBA, NOX1, and NOX3 genes that have been implicated in diabetic nephropathy and renal damage. Other studies have identified genetic variants in two positional candidate genes: the pituitary adenylate cyclase activating polypeptide (PACAP) on 18p11 and the peroxisome proliferator-activated receptor gamma coactivator 1 (PPARGC1) on 4p15, for increased diabetes risk in the W. African population. The diversity in genetic variations between different ethnic and racial groups and an association with risk to T2DM complicates drawing clear conclusions about the role of genetic risk factors and T2DM disparities.

2.11 Obesity

There is strong epidemiological data to demonstrate obesity is associated with increased risk of not only in T2DM (Eckel et al. 2011) but also cardiovascular diseases (Folsom et al. 1989) and metabolic syndrome, as well as certain cancers.

As previously mentioned, the prevalence of obesity is relatively low in sub-Saharan Africans in comparison with the US AA population. For instance, the incidence of obesity is reported to be 10–13% in AA and Afro-Caribbean population, compared to 1–2% in the W. African Nigerian population (Colilla et al. 2000; Rotimi et al. 1995, 2001). This is in spite of the high heritability levels of obesity-related traits in many African-descended populations (Luke et al. 2001); thus, the difference could be a reflection of various environmental influences, such as a high-caloric Westernized diet and diminished physical activity.

However, over the past couple of decades, there is a rise in the incidence of obesity and associated diabetes in parts of the African continent. For instance, S. Africa and its neighboring countries, Namibia, Botswana, and Zimbabwe, have a high incidence of obesity similar to the levels to AAs, and this is correlated with an increase in socioeconomic status, urbanization, and adoption of a sedentary lifestyle (Walker et al. 2001). Similar observations of an increased incidence of obesity have been reported in the Tanzanian population, as there is a shift from a rural lifestyle to an urban environment (Aspray et al. 2000).

2.11.1 Genetic Factors Associated with Obesity

The genetic factors associated with obesity are not well characterized. One study has reported an association of genetic variants in a fat metabolism gene and obesity risk. Genetic-splice variants in exons 3 and 6 of the human uncoupling protein 3 (UCP3) gene have been shown to be associated with reduced fat oxidation and obesity in a group of African descendants who lived in the Gullah community of South Carolina in the US, with very low European admixture (Parra et al. 2001). Interestingly, similar splice variants were observed in an African population from Sierra Leon (W. Africa), whereas these variants where absent in the EA population. In addition, individuals who are heterozygote for exon 6 have basal fat oxidation rates reduced by 50%. The reduced fat oxidation would play a role in increased fat storage, suggesting that genetic variants in UCP3 could play a role in increased susceptibility to obesity by promoting fat storage.

In 2007, a GWAS analysis by Frayling et al. (2007) identified a common variant in the FTO (fat mass and obesity-associated protein) gene that is also associated with increased BMI, from childhood to adulthood across many generations. Because obesity is measured clinically with the surrogate measure of BMI, they reasoned that this common variant in the FTO gene could influence the development of obesity and predisposition to diabetes. In support of this hypothesis, they observed that 16% of the EA populations in their analysis are homozygous for high-risk variants of the FTO gene, and individuals with the homozygous trait weighed about three kilograms more and were 1.67 times more likely to be obese than individuals without this trait. The genetic variants in the FTO gene were also associated with increased T2DM (Frayling et al. 2007).

The FTO gene encodes for the nucleic acid demethylase, and the protein is highly expressed in the hypothalamus of the brain, where food intake is regulated, suggesting a role for FTO in energy homeostasis and body-weight regulation (Loos 2014). Ectopic fat leads to organ-specific insulin resistance via a process termed lipotoxicity (Cusi 2010). Individuals who are susceptible to T2DM appear to show a great tendency to accumulate visceral fat for a given BMI. On the other hand, there are several individuals, in particular females, who, despite attaining very high BMIs (as high as 50–60 kg/m^2), remain insulin-sensitive, normoglyceamic, and normolipaemic. Imaging studies show that these individuals have low levels of visceral and ectopic fat but high subcutaneous fat content (Stefan et al. 2008). Several reports have identified the association of genetic variants of the FTO gene and increased incidence of obesity. Studies shows significant differences in allele frequency in African ancestry compared to other populations. However there are no records of the frequency of genetic variants in the African population in their native countries.

Other studies searching for other genes that may be associated with increased risk of obesity in the AA population have led to the identification of a genetic variant in the G protein beta 3-subunit (GNB3), a gene whose protein product enhances signal transduction and play a role in adipogenesis. A high frequency of this genetic variant known as the 825T allele was found in the so-called old ethnicities, such as Australian aborigines, bushmen, pygmies, and all black populations, including AAs (Siffert et al. 1999). Individuals with this allele are prone to obesity. Patients with homozygous mutant allele demonstrated strong association to increased body-mass index, obesity, and the hypertension-related phenotype. Development of obesity in individuals with this allele was found to be also influenced by environmental-lifestyle factors.

Other genes that may directly be associated with obesity and increased risk of diabetes in the AA population have been identified, but their relationship is not well established. For instance, adiponectin, which is implicated in a number of metabolic disorders including T2DM and CVDs, is encoded by the ADIPOQ gene, and genetic variants of the ADIPOQ are associated with reduced plasma adiponectin protein levels (Sandy et al. 2013) in AA patients with diabetes. However, studies have not identified any significant association of ADIPOQ genetic variants with increased risk to T2DM in this population. This puts into question the role of adiponectin in T2DM pathogenesis. Whether low adiponectin levels are truly causal for T2DM in AAs or rather a consequence of T2DM remains to be determined.

2.12 Kidney Disease

According to the CDC 2014 factsheet, 10% of adults in the US have chronic kidney disease (CKD), making it the ninth leading cause of death in the USA. The condition is commonly diagnosed in individuals over the age of 50, and the risk factors associated with developing CKD includes diabetes, high blood pressure, CVDs, obesity and family history. (http://www.cdc.gov/diabetes/pubs/pdf/kidney_factsheet). The incidence of CKD and mortality from end- stage renal disease (ESRD) is higher in AAs than in any other racial and ethnic group, with AAs having a three-fold higher incidence than their EA counterparts even when adjusted for age and gender. There is ongoing debate as to the reasons for the markedly higher frequency of chronic kidney disease (CKD) in AAs versus EAs, because the condition is confounded by several interrelated risk factors, such as familial predisposition, socioeconomic status (SES), co-morbid conditions (diabetes, hypertension, and high blood pressure), and lifestyle risk factors such as smoking and excessive alcohol consumption. At the cellular level, CKD can be caused by numerous pathological assaults, such as chronic inflammation, oxidative stress, high lipid levels, viral infection, and hypertension, which affect the kidney glomerular and tubule-intestinal cells (Hu et al. 2012).

In search for susceptibility alleles that could be associated with ESRD, a GWAS was carried out on ESRD patients and control cases from both AA and EA populations (Kao 2008). The results of the studies revealed high freqeuncies of multiple genetic variants near the gene encoding for non-muscle myosin heavy chain type II isoform A (MYH9) on chromosome 22 in the AA cases in comparison with the EA population. The MYH9 gene may play a role in the cytoskeletal integrity of kidney glomerulus-capillary tubules, suggesting that this variant could be useful in screening for ESRD in the AA population.

Another study by Genovese et al. (2010) identified a strong association of two independent genetic variants within the apolipoproteinL1 (APOL1) gene with an increased risk of focal segmental glomerulosclerosis (FSGS) and hypertension-associated end-stage renal disease (ESRD). The APOL1 gene encodes for a serum protein that plays an important role in host defense and cellular homeostasis mechanisms, and alterations in gene expression is associated with other diseases, including African sleeping sickness, atherosclerosis, lipid disorders, obesity, schizophrenia, cancer, and chronic kidney disease (CKD), suggesting that disruption of this gene has important clinical implications.

Genetic variants in APOL1 are associated with a high risk of a spectrum of kidney diseases including FSGS and ESRD. The described variants are very common in individuals of African descent, including the W. African Nigerians and US AAs, but absent in individuals of European descent. The APOL1 variants most strongly associated with nondiabetic CKD were observed in 40% of the Yoruba population from Nigeria in W. African but not in European, Japanese, or Chinese populations. Statistical analysis showed that these variants might be the result of positive selection in Africa, which could be related to the fact that APOL1 is a trypanolytic factor in human serum (Perez-Morga et al. 2005; Vanhamme et al. 2003) that confers resistance to *T. brucei rhodesiense* (the parasite that causes trypanomiasis or sleeping sickness) which is transmitted by the tsetse flies. This protein is very important on the African continent because it confers resistance to sleeping sickness. The APOL1 gene provides another example of a genetic selection (discussed in Sects. 2.4 and 2.5) for resistance to one disease, in this case sleeping sickness, but is associated with increased susceptibility to another disease, CKD.

Only the disease-associated variants of APOL1 are capable of lysing trypanosome brucei *rhodesiense* parasite. Interestingly, there are two variants of the APOL1 gene located on haplotypes that contain signals of positive selection. This suggests that evolutionary APOL1 variants might have critical survival properties in certain parts of the African continent, where tsetse flies infections are rampant, to protect against infection from this parasite, but that, however, in a different environment and perhaps in combination with some lifestyle choices, may contribute to the high incidence and prevalence of nondiabetic CKD in AAs.

The HIV viral infection is linked to APOL1-associated kidney failure. It is estimated that $\sim 12\%$ of the HIV-negative and >50% of HIV-positive AAs, who are homozygote carriers of the APOL1 allele, may be susceptible to kidney disease (Freedman et al. 2010). However, not every person who is homozygous for the APOL1 variants will develop ESRD, suggesting some other factor, such as gene–gene interaction or gene-environment, may contribute to the disease risk.

2.13 Genetic Variants in Dementia (Alzheimer's)

Dementia and, in particular, Alzheimer disease (AD) afflict approximately 30 million of the aging population worldwide (Brookmeyer et al. 2007), making it a leading cause of morbidity and mortality among the elderly. There are differences in geographical prevalence: AD is very common in Western Europe and US and less prevalent in sub-Saharan Africa. In the US alone, it is estimated that one in nine persons over the age of 65 will be diagnosed with the disease. Late-onset Alzheimer's disease (LOAD) is the most common cause of dementia, making it a very important public-health issue. African Americans and Hispanics are more than twice as likely to develop LOAD as EAs (Tang et al. 2001). Epidemiological studies have shown that AAs are more likely to be diagnosed with dementia (in general) and Alzheimer's disease than EAs (Demirovic et al. 2003). Differences in AD prevalence may be caused by genetic variants, environmental factors, or both. African Americans and other minorities often receive delayed or inadequate health care services, especially for dementia, and this may contribute to the disparities in the disease incidence.

The molecular mechanisms underlying AD indicate that senile plaques (SP) and neurofibrillary tangles are key pathological hallmarks of AD, and genetic mutations in beta-amyloid gene (Aβ), SP, and presenilin (PSEN 1 and 2) have been shown to be associated with increased risk to Alzheimer disease (Reitz and Mayeux 2014). The differences in etiology of LOAD across populations are not well understood. Epidemiological findings have linked cardiovascular diseases (including elevated blood pressure in mid-life, between the ages of 40–60), T2DM, both low- and high-body weight, diabetes, coronary artery disease, and stroke, as well as traumatic brain injury and metabolic syndrome, with increased risk to AD (Reitz and Mayeux 2014). Because the US AA population is disproportionally affected by higher risks for CVD, diabetes, stroke, and many other conditions linked to AD risk, this could potentially explain the high prevalence of AD in the AA population in comparison with other US racial and ethnic groups.

In addition to the Aβ, SP, and PSEN1 and PSEN2 genes, other genes such as FE65, A2 M, SOLR1, and APP genes have been associated with increased risk for AD. So far, the unequivocal risk gene is polymorphisms in the apolipoprotein E

(APOE) gene that is associated with increased risk of AD. The APOE-gene product is involved in diverse cellular functions, including lipid metabolism, as a transport of lipid from one tissue or cell to the other, inflammation, oxidative stress, and aging. Several reports have shown that APOE is associated with hyperlipidemia and hypercholesterolemia, conditions that are linked to increase atherosclerosis, coronary heart disease, strokes, and increased risk of AD. In animal studies, high levels of cholesterol are associated with increased Aβ load (Refolo et al. 2000) and changes in amyloid precursor protein processing. There are three polymorphic alleles of APOE gene, namely ε2, ε3, and ε4 alleles that are associated with either increased susceptibility to, or protection from, AD in various populations (Liu et al. 2013). Various variants of the APOE gene are associated with either susceptibility or increased risk to AD. Individuals with the ε4 allele variants are at significantly higher risk of AD in comparison to individuals with the ε3 allele (neutral effect on AD risk), whereas the ε2 variant is associated with decreased risk of AD (Graff-Radford et al. 2002). Individuals, who are heterozygote for the APOE ε4 allele, are at two–three times higher risk of AD, and those homozygous for the allele are at 1–30 times higher risk. On the other hand, individuals homozygous for the APOE ε2 have a 25% reduction in the risk of AD. The APOE ε4 allele is well-established to be associated with increased risk to LOAD, as well as early onset of the disease in EA population (Graff-Radford et al. 2002). So far, the major findings have included apolipoprotein E e4 as a major risk factor for AD in most populations including AA, but the APOE e4 variant is not a risk factor for AD in some African populations such as the Yoruba people of Nigeria (Hendrie et al. 2006), suggesting that the differences in AD risk in Yorubas and AAs could be attributed to differences in either gene-gene or gene–environmental interactions.

Few epidemiological studies have been conducted in sub-Saharan African populations to look at the incidence of AD. One such study known as the Indianapolis-Ibadan Dementia Project (Hendrie et al. 2006) reported lower incidence of AD among the W. African Yoruba population in comparison with AAs. The AD incidence rates for AD in the Yoruba population was about half that of AAs for the same age group. With regards to genetic studies in the African diversity population, it is generally held that genetic analysis of complex diseases including AD may confer certain selective advantages. Another variant of APOE, called APOE e1Y, has been identified in the Yoruba population without AD, suggesting this could be the ancestral haplotype (Murrell et al. 2006), however this is the only report on this APOE variant in the Yoruba cohort.

Similar to the Yoruba study, another study from a Ghanaian cohort found that the allelic frequency of APOE e4 was lower compared to EAs and AAs, however there was a significant association with TOMM40'523 (Translocase of Outer Mitochondria Membrane) alleles. The TOMM40 gene encodes for the principle mitochondrial protein import pore and is therefore critically important for mitochondrial biogenesis and function (Chang et al. 2005), and alteration in gene expression has been linked to neurodegenerative and neuropsychiatric diseases. This observation suggests the presence of a possible cross-over event occurring in the Ghanaians, a distant observation in W. Africans that has been introduced in the

AA population but rarely observed in EA cohorts (Hendrie et al. 2001). This W. African TOMM40'523 allele in linkage analysis to the APOE e4 is observed in the AA population but not in EAs, suggesting that a possible cross-over occurred in the Ghanaian population that has been introduced to the AA population (Roses et al. 2014).

Thus it is possible, for example that gene–gene and gene–environment interactions may be different in Yoruba than AAs, who may have various degrees of admixture with other populations, such as EA and Native Americans. The differences in AD risk between AAs and the nascent African population can also be attributed to different environmental or lifestyle factors that can interact with AD risk genes to cause higher incidence of AD in the AA population than in the African population.

Many of the conditions that are associated with increased risk to AD, such as high cholesterol and heart disease, are not common in the African population in their native countries, allowing for the identification of the role of gene–environmental interaction in the sub-Saharan African and AA populations and the risk to AD (Tishkoff et al. 1996). For instance, AAs have high incidences of diabetes and hypertension and have hypercholesterolemia risk factors for AD, but these conditions are less frequent in the Yoruba population. Perhaps because the Yorubas consume a low-calorie, low-fat diet, consisting mainly of grains, roots, and tubers supplemented by small amounts of fish (Hendrie et al. 2006), and this may explain the low serum cholesterol level in this population. One report indicates that having an African ancestry is highly protective against AD neuropathology (neurite plaques) (Schlesinger et al. 2013). However, caution should be used in generalizing these findings to the entire Nigerian population or, for that matter, the entire African population as only a small cohort of patient samples has been used in this study.

2.14 Septicemia-Sepsis

Sepsis or severe inflammatory response is a condition associated with infection of the lungs and urinary tract, or some microbial, bacteria, or viral infection that can arise through surgical procedures, making this condition a major challenge in intensive-care units in US hospital and across the globe. According to a recent JAMA report (2014), up to 50% of all hospital deaths in the USA are linked to sepsis infection (Liu et al. 2014). This condition is more prone in individuals who have a weakened immune system. In particular, infants and elderly are most vulnerable. Sepsis is ranked the tenth leading cause of mortality in the US. Some of the risk factors associated with sepsis include access to health care, gender, and race. The presence of co-morbidity conditions such as chronic obstructive pulmonary disease (COPD), diabetes, HIV/AIDs, ESRD, cancer, and lifestyle choices (such as excessive alcohol consumption) is associated with an increased risk of sepsis. Many of these co-morbidity conditions are observed at higher rates in the AA population than other racial and ethnic groups, and this may explain why AAs also have a higher prevalence of sepsis than any other US racial or ethnic population. In addition, men are more likely than women to develop sepsis. Interestingly, one report indicates that, while there is an increased prevalence of arterial hypertension in AA patients with sepsis, mortality rates are lower, suggesting a possible protective effect of hypertension in the sepsis patients (Nunes 2003). Thus the high prevalence of hypertension in AAs may have evolved in a different environment as a protective mechanism in a population whose descendants are heavily exposed to infectious diseases.

Studies directed towards the identification of genetic risk factors associated with sepsis, the candidate microorganisms, and their interaction with the host's innate and adaptive immune system and downstream signals have focused on sepsis-associated diseases, such as acute lung injury that can occur in sepsis and other inflammatory disorders (Barnes 2005). Several sepsis-associated candidate-gene variants have been identified, including the IL-1 receptor antagonist (IL1RA), plasminogen activator inhibitor 1 (PAI1), Toll-like receptor1, 4 and 5 (TLR-1, 4, 5), tumor necrosis factor-(TNFA), TNFB, and lymphotaxin (LTA) (Barnes 2005). For instance, Mwantembe et al. (2001) found a high frequency of genetic variants in the interleukin 1 (IL-1) gene cluster associated with South African blacks with inflammatory bowel syndrome disease than in South African whites with the same condition. High TLR1 genetic variants that modulate the risk of bacterial infection were found to be associated with an increased risk of organ failure and a higher mortality rate in both AA and EA patients with sepsis (Wurfel et al. 2008). Plasminogen activator inhibitor (PAI) (Menges et al. 2001) and other cytokines, such as toll-like receptor 4 and tumor necrosis factor, are all associated with sepsis risk.

It is well documented that there are differences in genetic variants in candidate genes underlying inflammatory and immunologic responses to complex diseases such as hypertension, obesity, diabetes, myocardial infarction, Crohn's disease, asthma, and cancer. However, very few studies have looked at the role of ethnicity in the epidemiology of sepsis, therefore less is known about the frequency of the "high-risk" variants and how this differs across racial and ethnic populations. One report indicates polymorphism of IL1RA gene was significantly more frequent among black than white South Africans in a study of inflammatory bowel disease (Mwantembe et al. 2001). Ongoing studies are likely to identify more candidate genes.

2.15 Pneumonia and Influenza

Pneumonia and influenza infection were among the leading causes of mortality, particularly in infants at the beginning of the twentieth century. However, with improved immunization, the mortality rates have significantly been reduced, and they are now ranked as the eighth leading cause of death in the US (DeFrances 2008). US minority populations including AAs, Hispanics, and American Indians have higher prevalence and mortality from pneumonia and influenza infection than the EA population. This is largely attributed to low immunization rates, low SES, which is associated with living in an unhealthy environment, and higher risks of certain co-morbidities such as diabetes, heart disease, and HIV infection (DeFrances 2008). The rise of the invasive drug-resistant *Streptococcus pneumonia* infection (primarily bacteria and meningitis) in the elderly population is a major public-health concern.

There are few studies that have investigated genetic variations in the host's immune response and association with pneumonia and influenza infection. One report has indicated a role for endothelial nitric oxide synthase (eNOS) in the pathophysiology of pneumonia infection, noting increased production of nitric oxide is a host defense mechanism against the bacterial infection to modulate apoptosis and inflammation. Genetic variants in eNOS and other host immune response genes, such as Tumor Necrosis Factor-alpha (TNF-alpha), and Interleukin-10 (IL-10), are reported to be associated with increased incidence of pneumonia in patients with the A/H1N1 influenza infection (Romanova 2013). Other studies have identified genetic variants in FCGR2A and C1QBP to be associated with increased susceptibility to pneumonia in A/H1N1 influenza infection (Zuniga 2012).

Very few studies have been carried out on pneumonia and influenza infection in the African population, except that outbreaks result in high fatality rates. A systematic review of the literature by Cohen (2015) has suggested that influenza infection is rather common on the continent and that co-morbid conditions, such as sickle cell anemia, dengue fever, and measles increase the severity of influenza diseases. Pneumonia is the next most common disease after malaria to be diagnosed in African children, and malnutrition, as well as HIV infection, are associated with pneumonia infection. Infection of *S. pneumonia* or *Haemophilus influenza* type B (HiB) are the common causes of pneumonia in the sub-Saharan African population, and other bacterial infections (*Staphylococcus aureus* and gram-negative bacteria) are known to be contributing factors to pneumonia (Muro 2015).

2.16 Cancer

Cancer is a global epidemic accounting for 8.2 million deaths in 2012 (http://www.iarc.fr/en/publications/books/wcr/wcr-order.php) and is estimated to reach 21.4 million cases and 13.2 million deaths by 2030. The increased incidence and mortality rates from cancer are attributed to demographic shift, an enlarged aging population, and adoption of unhealthy lifestyles, such as poor diet, smoking, and excessive alcohol. In the USA alone, it is estimated that 1,685,210 people will be diagnosed with cancer in 2016, and this will be accompanied by 595,690 deaths, making cancer the second leading cause of mortality in the USA (http://www.cancer.gov/about-cancer/what-is-cancer/statistics). Some of the common cancers diagnosed in the US population includes: breast, lung and bronchus, prostate, colon and rectal, bladder, skin melanoma, lymphoma, thyroid, kidney and renal pelvis, leukemia, endometrial, and pancreatic cancer.

Recent cancer statistics for 1975–2011 by the North American Association of Central Cancer Registries (NAACCR) organization found that there is a decline in the number of new cases and mortality for several of the major cancer types: breast (women), prostate (men), lung, colon and rectal, throat, and brain cancer diagnosed in the US (Kohler 2015). The reduction parallels decreases in cancer risk factors such as smoking reduction in adults and improved and widespread screening and detection tools, as well as improved cancer-therapy treatment (Byers 2010). The downward trend in the incidence and mortality rates is reported for the US and other Western countries. On the other hand, several developing countries including many Africa countries have been observing upward trends in cancer incidence and mortality rates over the past two to three decades due to the adoption of unhealthy Western lifestyles, including smoking, sedentary living, and consumption of calorie-dense processed food.

Despite the decline in US cancer incidence and mortality rates, there remains persistence in cancer disparities as defined by differences in incidence, prevalence, and mortality rates in the US's racial and ethnic groups. According to the Center for Disease and Prevention Control (CDC) data and statistics on cancer (www.cdc.gov/cancer/dcpc/data/race.htm), AA men have the highest cancer incidence, followed by EA men, and the lowest rates in reported for Asian/Pacific Island men. Among women, EAs have the highest incidence, followed by AA women, and the lowest incidence is reported for Asian/Pacific Island women. The statistics on mortality rates places both AA men and women at the top, followed by EAs, with lowest incidence in other groups. Although the incidence and mortality rates are lowest for Asians in comparison with EAs and AAs, they have a high prevalence of cancer caused by infection, such as cervical cancer (women), stomach, liver, and esophageal cancers (McCracken 2007). The following sections will discuss the genetic alterations associated with common cancers in different US racial and ethnic groups.

2.16.1 Breast Cancer

Breast cancer is the most commonly diagnosed cancer in women in the US and the second leading cause of death after lung cancer. In 2016 alone, it is estimated that 246,660 women will be diagnosed with breast cancer, accompanied by 40,450 deaths (http://seer.cancer.gov/statfacts/html/breast.html). Breast cancer like prostate cancer (discussed in Sect. 2.16.4) tends to cluster in families, and it is estimated that 10–15% of all breast cancer cases may be due to familial predisposition (Pharoah 2002). Even though the incidence of breast cancer is highest among EA women in the US, AA women are more likely to present with late stages of the disease and die at a significantly high rates than any other racial and ethnic group in the US (Anon 2015). The reasons for the disparity in incidence and mortality rate is believed to be a complex combination of socioeconomic status, which is reflected in AA's predominantly residing in low income neighborhoods with less access to mammography screening for breast cancer, and lifestyle exposures to poor diet, tobacco smoke, and alcohol, as well as genetic susceptibility (Russell et al. 2012). Groundbreaking work in breast-cancer research has identified various tumor subtypes among diverse racial and ethnic groups. Large-scale gene expression analysis has identified five subtypes of breast cancers. For instance, young AA women are predominantly diagnosed with basal-like breast tumors that tend to be more aggressive with metastatic potential in the lungs and brain and also to be more resistant to therapy than luminal tumor subtypes (Carey et al. 2006; Sorlie et al. 2001). Furthermore, AA women have a thrice higher risk of being diagnosed with triple-negative disease (ER, progesterone receptor [PR], and human epidermal growth receptor 2 [HER2] negative) than EA women (Carey et al. 2006). Because triple negative breast cancers are characterized by the absence of the necessary signaling receptors, treatment strategies and drugs that target estrogen, progesterone, and HER2 remain a challenge, and this might contribute to the higher mortality rates in the AA women (Chlebowski et al. 2005). Other reports indicates that the disparities associated with breast-cancer mortality may reflect the later stage of diagnosis for AA women than intrinsic biological differences (Adebamowo et al. 2008).

Tremendous progress has been made in understanding the molecular mechanisms and pathways underlying breast cancer, from gene-specific alterations or entire tumor signatures that hold the promise to develop targeted treatments. Mutations in two heritable DNA-repair genes BRCA1 and BRCA2 are commonly associated with breast-cancer risk in various racial and ethnic populations, and high frequencies of BRCA2 and BRCA1 mutations are reported for AA and EA breast-cancer patients, respectively (Malone et al. 2006). Clinical studies have led to the development of screening tests and preventive strategies in breast-cancer patients with BRCA2 and BRCA1 mutations (Maxwell 2012). Women with BRCA1 or BRCA2 mutation have a higher risk for breast and ovarian cancer because there is a general recommendation for individuals belonging to families with a high frequency in this somatic mutations to seek genetic testing and counselling in order to make decisions about surveillance or even surgical approaches to reduce the risk of developing breast cancer (Schwartz et al. 2008). As in Western societies, strong genetic factors contribute to a subset of breast-cancer cases in Africa, including a high frequency of heritable BRCA1 and BRCA2 mutations in African women with breast cancer (Awadelkarim et al. 2007). Even though breast-cancer diagnosis is less prevalent in Africa than Europe, due to late diagnosis and poor survival, similar mortality rates have been reported for breast cancer patients in Africa as in Western societies.

Despite the high risk of breast cancer in individuals with BRCA1 and BRCA2 mutations, these genetic variants only accounts for a fraction of familial breast-cancer cases, thus additional genetic alterations must contribute to breast-cancer susceptibility. Numerous genetic alterations that impact gene expression have been described, including p53 (Rose and Royak-Schaler 2001),

H-ras-1 mutations (Weston and Godbold 1997), and overexpression of cyclin D1 (Joe et al. 2001). Loo and coworkers reported significant differences in gene copy-number variations in triple negative tumors from AA and EA women (Loo et al. 2011), and others have demonstrated differences in gene expression patterns between AA and EA breast-cancer patients in pathways related to tumor angiogenesis and chemotaxis (Martin et al. 2009). More than 67 breast-cancer susceptibility loci have been identified through GWAS on various chromosomal regions and with various provenances of breast cancer susceptibility in various racial and ethnic groups; most of these studies were carried out in Europe and in the US (Maxwell 2013).

Many of these genetic studies of breast-cancer risk have included very few samples of AA patients. Recent GWAS that analyzed breast tumors from the AA population have discovered a high frequency of variants in vitamin D biosynthetic intermediates associated with increased breast-cancer risk in AAs in comparison with the EA population (Yao 2012), and genetic variants in hormone-signaling pathways show greater susceptibility loci for increased breast cancer in AAs than EAs (Haddad 2015). The plethora of genetic variants being identified suggests that comprehensive large-population studies are necessary to identify important genetic alterations that could predict the increased breast-cancer risks in the AA population.

2.16.2 Colorectal Cancer

Colorectal cancer is the third most-commonly diagnosed cancer in men and women in the US. The US cancer statistics on colorectal cancers indicate that, in 2016, 95,270 new colon cancer cases and 39,220 new rectal cancers will be diagnosed, and this is accompanied by 49,190 deaths (http://www.cancer.org/cancer/colonandrectumcancer/detailedguide/colorectal-cancer-risk-factors). Some of the risk factors associated with colorectal cancers include: an unhealthy diet that is deficient in essential nutrients; tobacco smoke; excessive alcohol consumption, and a sedentary lifestyle. The disease is also commonly diagnosed in adults over the age of 50 and having a family member, such as a first-degree relative, such as parent, sibling, or child, associated with increased risk of colorectal cancer, reflecting heterogeneity in disease risk from genetic component and/or shared environmental factors.

Hereditary predisposition to certain genetic mutations can cause a family cancer syndrome that contributes to 5–10% of colorectal-cancer incidence. The most common inherited syndromes are familial adenomatous polyposis (FAP) and Lynch syndrome (hereditary non-polyposis colorectal cancer or HNPCC) or other colon inflammations, such as ulcerative colitis and Crohn's disease, which increase colorectal-cancer risks. That up to 20% of CC occurs in individuals under 50 years of age appears to indicate a strong familial-predisposition component (hereditary nonpolypotic colorectal cancer, i.e. HNPCC, and familial adenomatous polyposis, or FAP mutations). Studies in the native African population have reported a familial predisposition to colorectal cancer. One report identified HNPCC or Lynch syndrome in a small sample population of colorectal cancer patients in Nigeria (Adebamowo et al. 2000). Other reports indicate that a single founder mutation (g.1528C>T in the hMLH1 gene) was significantly associated with colorectal cancer in the Nama group of the far Northern Cape province of South Africa (Anderson et al. 2007). The hMLH1 gene encodes for mismatch repair and is frequently mutated in HNPCC. One report indicated mutations in glutathione S-transferase detoxifying genes: GSTM1 and GSTT1 in patients with an hMLH1 mutation and individuals with both null mutations having a three-fold increased risk of colorectal at an early age (Felix et al. 2006).

The African-American population has a significantly higher risk of colorectal cancer in comparison to the EA population. In addition, when the colorectal cancer occurs at a younger age in AAs, it turns out to be more aggressive. A certain proportion of disparity in the colorectal-cancer mortality rate can be explained by differences in screening rates and differences in stage-specific survival (Lansdorp-Vogelaar et al. 2012). There are also differences in anatomics site of disease presentation (Dimou et al. 2009): AAs are more likely to develop cancer in the colon, whereas EAs are more likely to develop cancer in the rectum, which is lower in the bowel and more easily detected by screening (Matanoski et al. 2006). Identification of precancerous lesions is more difficult for cancers of the colon (Matanoski et al. 2006). As a result, AAs are at increased risk of developing advanced colorectal cancer than EAs.

Evidence from genomic studies has identified widespread chromosomal instability with candidate genes including oncogenic *KRAS*, *APC*, and *DCC/MADH2/MADH4,* as well as tumor-suppressor PTEN and p53 genes (Vogelstein and Kinzler 1993). Like most genetic analysis, a lot of the reported studies in colorectal cancer were conducted using EA samples and included few or no samples of AA patients. GWAS for genetic variants and association with colorectal cancer identified two major variants, Y179C and G396D (formerly known as Y165C and G382D) in the MYH gene. The MYH gene encodes for DNA glycosylase, which plays a role in DNA repair by removing mispairing of 8-hydroxyguanine caused by oxidative damage during DNA synthesis. These variants were predominant in EA patients, where 90% of the patient population carried at least one of these variants; however, these variants were not found in the AA population in this analysis (Nielsen et al. 2009).

Obesity is a risk factor for colorectal cancer, and insulin resistance is commonly associated with obesity. One report that investigated genetic alterations in the insulin-signaling pathway and colorectal cancer identified an association of genetic polymorphism in insulin-signaling pathway and increased risk of colorectal cancer in the EA population, but not in the AA population (Keku et al. 2012).

Several scientific reports have suggested an important role for vitamin D in physiological processes, such as calcium homeostasis and insulin secretion, as well as cellular immunity; and they also suggest that deficiency in vitamin D levels are linked to conditions such as multiple sclerosis, cardiovascular disease, infectious disease, and cancer including colorectal cancer. Thus, maintaining an adequate level of vitamin D may have a protective effect against colorectal cancer. However, the AA population has lower serum levels of vitamin D than the EA population. One study by Pibiri et al. (2014) reported that genetic variants in genes involved in the biosynthetic pathway of vitamin D could modulate the serum level of vitamin D, noting significant association of genetic variants in 25-hydroxylase gene (CYP2R1) and increased risk of colorectal cancer in the AA population. The molecular mechanism whereby genetic variants in CYP2R1 could affect colorectal cancer risk is unknown; however, this observation indicates that genetic variants in the vitamin D biosynthetic pathway could influence susceptibility of the AA population to colorectal cancer. Other investigations have focused on the role of intestinal chronic inflammation and mediators, such as mannose-binding lectin 2 (*MBL2*). Genetic variation in the 3′-untranslated region of the MBL2 gene has been linked to increased susceptibility of colon cancer in AAs but not in EAs (Zanetti et al. 2012). Overall, it appears that various genetic alterations may contribute to the differential risk to colorectal cancers in the AA and EA populations.

2.16.3 Lung Cancer

Lung cancer is the leading cause of death worldwide across all income levels in both Westernized and developing countries, accounting for 1.6 million deaths per year (about 20% of all cancer mortality rates) (Ferlay 2015). According to the American Cancer Society statistics on cancers, lung cancer is the second most common cancer in both men and women, and, in 2016 alone, 224,390 new cases were diagnosed in both men and women combined, accompanied by 158,080 deaths (www.cancer.org/cancer/lungcancer-non-smallcell/detailedguide/non-small-cell-lung-cancer-key-statistics). It is estimated that more people die from lung cancer than colon, breast, and prostate cancers combined. The prevalence of lung cancer is about 20% higher in AA men than EA men, whereas the prevalence is about 10% less in AA women than EA women.

Lung cancer has a strong environmental risk factor associated with the disease risk. Tobacco smoke is significantly associated with lung cancer. Successful public-health campaigns about the dangers of tobacco smoke are largely responsible for the decline in lung-cancer-related mortality in the US (Kohler 2015). Unfortunately, this is not true for other places such as China and India where tobacco smoking is on the increase. Other environmental risk factors include exposure to residential radon and asbestos, as well as radiation in the workplace. One study indicates that racial residential segregation and targeted tobacco advertising in such communities may contribute to the 10% higher lung-cancer mortality rate compared to heterogeneous neighborhoods, and this difference persists even after adjustment for socioeconomic status (SES) (Hayanga and D'Cunha 2013).

Extensive genomic analysis has revealed numerous chromosomal alterations and genomic instabilities and a high frequency of mutations in tumor suppressor p53, VHL, and Rb genes and known oncogenes including EGFR, KRAS, ALK, MYC, and Her-2/NEU (Carbone and Minna 1992; Singh and Kathiresan 2014) with important prognostic significance. One report by Bauml et al. (2013) indicates a lower frequency of EGFR mutation in AA non-small-cell lung-cancer patients than in EA patients. Genetic variations in CYP1A1 and CYP2A6, which belongs to cytochrome P450 family of enzymes that functions in carcinogen detoxification, have been shown to be associated with lung-cancer risk. One report suggests high frequencies of these variants in AA lung-cancer patients (Wassenaar et al. 2015), whereas another report did not find a high prevalence of CYP1A1 and CYP2A6 genetic variance in AA patients (Shields et al. 1993). So, conclusive and well-replicated data are required before any association of CYP1A1 risk alleles in AA lung-cancer patients can be made.

2.16.4 Prostate Cancer

Prostate cancer is the most commonly diagnosed cancer among US men. The risk factors associated with the disease includes age, as most men diagnosed with the disease are over the age of 60 year. A family history of prostate disease, such as having a brother or father with the disease, increases the risk. Race is also an important risk factor as prostate cancer incidence and mortality rates are about twice as high in the AAs as in the EA population, suggesting a genetic component to the disease susceptibility. In support of a genetic basis to prostate cancer risk, men of African ancestry in various geographic regions of the world, including the Caribbean and S. American, share similar incidences and mortality rates comparable to AAs (Brawley 1998; Delongchamps et al. 2007). Similarly, data from sub-Saharan Africa estimates prostate cancer to be the third most-commonly diagnosed cancer in males, and incidence rates are increasing rapidly with urbanization and the adoption of a Western lifestyle (Magoha 2007; Parkin et al. 2003).

Prostate cancer tends to cluster within families, and there are increased rates of the disease in monozygotic twin pairs in comparison with dizygotic twin pairs, consistent with a strong genetic influence on disease risk (Johns 2001). Tremendous numbers of studies have been conducted over the past 30 years to identify the genetic basis of prostate cancer, and, as a result, multiple candidate genes that play diverse role in disease etiology and progress have been identified, including those involved in susceptibility to oxidative DNA damage, growth related pathways, androgen receptor signaling, chronic inflammatory response, and RNA processing (Rennert et al. 2005; Shand and Gelmann 2006; Zabaleta et al. 2008). Several of these candidate genes have been studied with regards to their allelic frequencies and prostate cancer risk in Africans, AA, and EA populations (Esteban et al. 2006; Kittles et al. 2001; Zeigler-Johnson et al. 2002).

Family-based linkage studies have been carried out to search for high penetrance genes, however these have met very little success. The few successful findings include rare variants in the prostate specific transcription factor HOXB13, found to be associated with increased risk of early-onset hereditary prostate cancer through an unknown mechanism, although variants accounts for a small proportion of all prostate cancers (Ewing 2012).

A GWAS comparing men with prostate cancer and those without the disease in a case-control study has identified genetic variants in several genes including MYC, NKX3,1, MSMB, and PSA to be associated with prostate-cancer risk (Isaacs 2012). Other efforts have focused on identifying genetic variants associated with prostate-cancer aggressiveness using the Gleason score as an indicator for PCa aggression and have identified variants in chromosomes 5q31-32, 7q32, and 19q12-13 as harboring aggressive prostate cancer loci (Isaacs 2012).

Despite the high prevalence of prostate cancer in the AA population, many of these genetic studies have not included this population, even though AAs present very aggressive and late stages of disease. It is important to carry out these studies in AA populations because the current data shows that indolent and aggressive prostate cancer has totally different genomic patterns or signatures, and, thus, it is necessary to know the genomic signatures of prostate cancer in the AA population to understand how their ancestry contributes to disease prevalence and to distinguish the indolent from the aggressive disease phenotype. One important candidate gene that could be associated with aggressive prostate cancer is BRCA2 gene, a well-known DNA-repair gene whose mutation is associated with breast cancer. Germline mutation in BRCA2 gene is not only a risk factor for prostate cancer, but more likely to be associated with high-grade and non-organ confined disease (Edwards 2010).

GWAS and other cutting-edge analysis, including comparative genomic hybridization (CGH) arrays in prostate cancer studies using biospecimens from multiple racial and ethnic group studies, have identified increased risks of prostate cancer with high frequencies of chromosomal losses on 6q13-22, 8p21, 13q13-14, and 16q11-24 and gains of 7p21 and 8q24 (Castro et al. 2009). Several SNPs on 8q24 with association to PCa risk are perhaps the most significant findings of risk alleles and prostate cancer. Furthermore, seven of these SNPs on 8q24 have been documented by several groups to be associated with significantly high risk of PCa in the AA population (Xu et al. 2009). However, these significant variants do not map to known genes, and the biological mechanisms underlying this association are not known. Gene rearrangement is now the center stage in PCa genetic research. Recent studies have identified chromosomal fusion of TMPRSS2-ERG that results in androgen- regulated over-expression of ERG protein to be associated with PCa progression (Petrovics et al. 2005). The TMPRSS2-ERG fusion is found in more than 50% of EA men and in less than 30% of AA men with prostate cancer (Magi-Galluzzi et al. 2011; Petrovics et al. 2005), indicating a lower frequency of the ERG-positive phenotype in AA men with aggressive prostate cancer.

Other studies have focused on the genetic variation of genes involved androgen signaling and metabolic pathways in regards to prostate-cancer risks in the AA population. Allelic frequencies of several genes in the androgen-signaling pathways have been reported to differ in AA and EA populations and could potentially contribute to the differential risk to prostate cancer (Platz and Giovannucci 2004). One study investigated genetic variants in CYP3A4-V and association with increased risk of prostate cancer in African (Nigerian) and AA and EA populations (Hainaut and Boyle 2008; Kittles et al. 2002). The CYP3A4 gene encodes for a protein which belongs to cytochrome P450 superfamily and plays a role in oxidative deactivation of testosterone (androgen signaling). The variant in CYP3A4-V that is an A–G promoter variant decreases CYP3A4 protein activity and thereby increases the availability of testosterone required for prostate growth. Kittles et al. (Hainaut and Boyle 2008; Kittles et al. 2002) found the highest frequency of this CYP3A4-V variant in Nigerian men, an intermediate frequency in AA, and low frequency in EA men. The high frequency of this variant was associated with prostate risk in AA in comparison with the EA counterpart. Interestingly, there was no association of this variant with prostate-cancer risk in the Nigerian population, although the variant was found at high frequency in this population. Because the AA population is genetically heterogeneous, with African ancestry and the later admixture with EA, some findings may be susceptible to spurious association, thus additional studies, such as the use of autosomal informatics markers (AIMs), are required to ensure that genetic-variant associations with disease risks are causal, and not just confounding, because of population stratification. Genetic variants in CYP3A4 has been reported in other cancers: lung, breast, kidney, and leukocytes (Lamba 2002), suggesting that genetic–environmental interactions as related to drug inactivation may play a role in cancer susceptibility.

Other studies that have investigated gene-expression profiles of tumors obtained by microarray technology from AA and EA patients point to prominent differences in primary prostate-cancer immunology (Wallace et al. 2008). Results from these studies demonstrated consistent differences in immunobiological gene-expression patterns in tumors from the two patient groups. An analysis of 69 micro-dissected tumors from 33 AA and 36 EA patients that were matched for clinic-pathological characteristics (patient's age, Gleason score, disease stage, PSA at diagnosis, and largest tumor nodule) identified numerous differences in the expression of genes related to immunobiology. These genes clustered in pathways related to immune response, host defense, cytokine signaling and chemotaxis, and inflammation. Most of the immune-related genes were expressed more frequently in tumors from AA patients than EA patients. Previously, low-grade chronic inflammation in the noncancerous prostate gland is observed to be more prevalent in AA men (Eastham et al. 1998). Thus, it is possible that the observed gene-expression differences in the tumors are partly due to a low-grade chronic inflammation that is more prevalent in AA tumors.

Because prostate cancer has a very strong genetic component to the disease, it is important to carry out genetic analysis in the various racial and ethnic US populations in order to decipher the genetic basis of the disease. Overall, prostate cancer displays a heterogeneous array of genetic alterations in individuals belonging to one population or different populations, as well as in the prostate tumor itself, making it very difficult to identify predominant pathways that are altered in the disease pathway for efficacious therapeutic intervention.

In addition to genetic factors, the development of PCa is also influenced by environmental factors such as diet. The disease prevalence as evidence by second and third generations of Chinese and Japanese migrants to the US, who have adopted the Western dietary lifestyle, have similar prostate cancer incidences to EA counterparts, whereas Chinese and Japanese living in their native countries have lower disease incidence and mortality rates (Brawley 1998). Other contributing factors includes access to screening and SES.

2.16.5 Other Cancers

Cancers that are associated with infection are more prevalent in sub-Saharan Africa than in the Western hemisphere. For instance, hepatocellular carcinoma is the second most common cancer in men from sub-Saharan Africa (Parkin 2003), but this type of cancer is ranked as only the fifth leading cause of cancer among US men. Hepatocellular cancer has a strong environmental component, such as the early infection with hepatitis B and C that interact with dietary exposure to aflatoxins from *Aspergillus* molds that is common in Africa (Hainaut and Boyle 2008). Bladder cancer occurs with high frequency particularly in N. Africa. Susceptibility to bladder cancer is modulated by variations in genes involved in pathways, such as metabolic detoxification, redox cycling, free radical injury, and metabolism of folate and methionine which are critical for DNA synthesis/repair and methylation (Ouerhani et al. 2007). Other studies have found some association of bladder cancer with GSTT1 and GSTM1 in Egypt (Saad et al. 2005) and Sudan (Ouerhani et al. 2006). Almost nothing is known about the influence of genetic factors on bladder cancer in sub-Saharan Africa.

2.17 Summary

Health disparities experienced by the African diaspora in the US is well documented. Whereas Africans in sub-Saharan Africa are plagued by infectious diseases, non-communicable diseases impose a huge burden on the US population and especially individuals of African descent, as well as other minority groups. The completion of the human genome sequence has made it possible for new genomic approaches, such as GWAS and next-generation sequencing, to unravel genomic variations and their association with increased risk to diseases such as CVDs, hypertension, obesity, diabetes, malaria, and cancer in various populations.

The people of continental Africa represent the oldest human populations and variations in their genetic sequence reflect influences of diet and climate and exposure to infectious pathogens that haves been naturally selected to adapt to their environment. Africa is also the origin of most the ancestors of AAs, who left the continent about 400 years ago. However, while the native African population is under-represented in studies in human genetics, it is important to know the genetic variation in the African population in order to understand their contribution to the health disparities of the African diaspora. On the other hand, the AA population represents a gene pool unique from native Africans because they have been subjected to a variety of environmental and racial influences, and have, on average, approximately 20% European ancestry (Shriver and Kittles 2004). We can predict that just as many European Americans are descendants of many different ethnic groups within Europe, so AAs are heterogeneous descendants from many different populations within Africa (and Europe).

Most GWAS have been carried out in EA populations, and few studies have been carried out in AA and other populations. Yet the inclusion of diverse populations in such studies is crucial for a more comprehensive appreciation of the role of human variation in complex diseases and for more accurate diagnosis and effective clinical management. GWAS is also a powerful tool to investigate the oldest human population, enabling accurate construction of ancestral haplotypes not found in non-African population. The few GWAS studies in this population have identified some of the genetic variants associated with susceptibility to infectious diseases such as HIV, malaria, and TB and have provided insight into the role of gene–gene and gene–environment interactions in disease susceptibility and resistance, as well as providing insights about how genetic variants have evolve to be protective against one type of disease resistance in one particular environment, but can contribute to an increase risk to another disease in a different environment.

GWAS holds promise to unravel genetic variations and disease risks and has the potential to help design more effective pharmaceutical treatments specifically targeted for various populations. However, there are several challenges to the full utilization of this approach:

1 The large population diversity means many populations would need to be studied, and one population cannot easily be used as proxy for another. Efforts to carry out such large-scale genomic research will be expensive, complex, challenging, and time consuming, but there are potential benefits for the large-scale genomic research of the African population.
2 Currently, GWAS has to be carried out on non-European populations using arrays designed for European populations that can only capture a proportion of the genomic variation in any non-European population leaving the other proportion of these variants not assayed (Spencer et al. 2009). There are efforts to develop African-diaspora arrays for GWAS. Furthermore, methods to capture gene–environment interactions are not well developed for complex diseases. This is more important for AAs and African ancestry because the AA population have evolved to live in a different environment than the continental African population. There are several natural genes, including HLA, Duffy, FTO, APOLI, and APOE, with variants that gives rise to the resistance to infectious diseases on the African continent, but, in a different environment such as in the US, is associated with increased risk to non-communicable diseases in the African diaspora (Fig. 2.1).

2.17 Summary

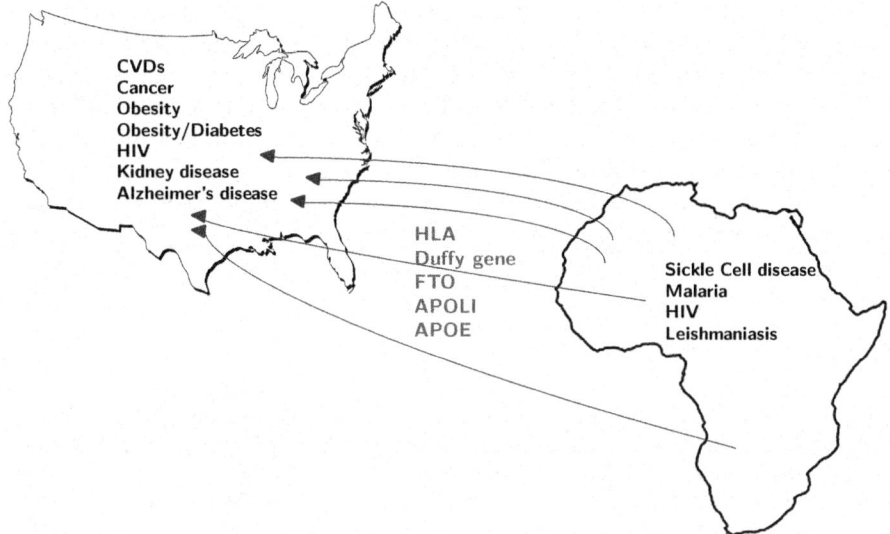

Fig. 2.1 Schematic presentation of some natural selected genes (*blue*; HLA, Duffy, FTO, APOLI and APOE) with variants that are associated with resistance to infectious diseases on the African continent. In a different environment such as the migration to USA (indicated by *red arrows*), some of these genetic variants are now associated with increased risk to non-communicable diseases among the African diaspora

Overall, some researchers attribute all of the problem of health disparities to differences in genetic predisposition (Burchard et al. 2003; Hirsch et al. 2006), assuming human genetic variation can be differentiated into conventional racial clusters (Calafell 2003; Redon et al. 2006). They suggest that disease-causing alleles are likely among the variants that can be segregated out between different groups (Burchard et al. 2003). In support, genetic studies of population substructures, in which analysis of thousands of genetic loci simultaneously, have produced clusters of genetic information that can be used to correctly to identify individuals of self-described geographic ancestry (Redon et al. 2006).

Other investigators argue that social forces drive racial health disparities, pointing to social determinants such as SES, racial segregation, psychosocial stress, and institutional and interpersonal discrimination as causes of adverse health outcomes in racial and ethnic minority groups, such as the AA population (Troxel et al. 2003; Williams and Jackson 2005). Social, economic, and contextual factors can have significant impact on health and taken into account together can diminish health disparities between AAs and whites. The ongoing debate between these competing models is described as the perfect "storm" (Krieger 2005). Scientific research cannot downplay the contributory role played by non-genetic factors (Rotimi et al. 1999b) or the onset or severity of the disease results from a complex interaction of genetic and environmental factors (Coleman 1999; Sommer et al. 1991).

These opposing forces of genetics and non-genetic causes of health disparities are basically two sides of the same coin. Genetic studies are changing the way we think about human variation, and it is important that this change has a positive impact on medicine and public health, while complete answers to many questions are beyond our grasp, some questions such as why aggregation of variants within population groups are likely to be answered in the near future, whereas other effects such as racism, with social and economic consequences of the ideology, will only be eliminated through political processes.

References

Abubakari, A. R., Lauder, W., Agyemang, C., Jones, M., Kirk, A., & Bhopal, R. S. (2008). Prevalence and time trends in obesity among adult West African populations: A meta-analysis. *Obesity Reviews, 9*(4), 297–311. Available from: PM:18179616.

Adams, A. S., Trinacty, C. M., Zhang, F., Kleinman, K., Grant, R. W., Meigs, J. B., et al. (2008). Medication adherence and racial differences in A1C control. *Diabetes Care, 31*(5), 916–921. Available from: PM:18235050.

Adebamowo, C. A., Adeyi, O., Pyatt, R., Prior, T. W., Chadwick, R. B., & de la Chapelle, A. (2000). Case report on hereditary non-polyposis colon cancer (HNPCC) in Nigeria. *African Journal of Medicine and Medical Sciences, 29*(1), 71–73. Available from: PM:11379475.

Adebamowo, C. A., Famooto, A., Ogundiran, T. O., Aniagwu, T., Nkwodimmah, C., & Akang, E. E. (2008). Immunohistochemical and molecular subtypes of breast cancer in Nigeria. *Breast Cancer Research and Treatment, 110*(1):183–188. Available from: PM:17674190.

Agarwal, A. (2000). Hemoglobin C associated with protection from severe malaria in the Dogon of Mali, a West African population with a low prevalence of hemoglobin S.

Amundadottir, L. T. (2016). Pancreatic cancer genetics.

Anderson, D. W., Goldberg, P. A., Algar, U., Felix, R., & Ramesar, R. S. (2007). Mobile colonoscopic surveillance provides quality care for hereditary nonpolyposis colorectal carcinoma families in South Africa. *Colorectal Disease, 9*(6), 509–514. Available from: PM:17477847.

Anon. (2006a). *Centers for Disease Control and Prevention (CDC): The global HIV/AIDS pandemic*. The Morbidity and Mortality Weekly Report (MMWR) 55:841–844.

Anon. (2006b). http://www.afro.who.int/malaria/publications/annual_reports/africa_malaria_report_2006.pdf

Anon. (2015). Center for Disease and Prevention Control. www.cdc.gov/cancer/dcpc/data/race.htm.

Aspray, T. J., Mugusi, F., Rashid, S., Whiting, D., Edwards, R., Alberti, K. G., et al. (2000). Rural and urban differences in diabetes prevalence in Tanzania: The role of obesity, physical inactivity and urban living. *Transactions of the Royal Society of Tropical Medicine and Hygiene, 94*(6), 637–644. Available from: PM:11198647.

Awadelkarim, K. D., Aceto, G., Veschi, S., Elhaj, A., Morgano, A., Mohamedani, A. A., et al. (2007). BRCA1 and BRCA2 status in a Central Sudanese series of breast cancer patients: interactions with genetic, ethnic and reproductive factors. *Breast Cancer Research and Treatment, 102*(2), 189–199. Available from: PM:17333343.

Awomoyi, A. A., Charurat, M., Marchant, A., Miller, E. N., Blackwell, J. M., McAdam, K. P., et al. (2005). Polymorphism in IL1B: IL1B-511 association with tuberculosis and decreased lipopolysaccharide-induced IL-1beta in IFN-gamma primed ex-vivo whole blood assay. *Journal of Endotoxin Research, 11*(5), 281–286. Available from: PM:16263000.

References

Awomoyi, A. A., Marchant, A., Howson, J. M., McAdam, K. P., Blackwell, J. M., & Newport, M. J. (2002). Interleukin-10, polymorphism in SLC11A1 (formerly NRAMP1), and susceptibility to tuberculosis. *Journal of Infectious Diseases, 186*(12), 1808–1814. Available from: PM:12447767.

Baghdadi, J. E., Orlova, M., Alter, A., Ranque, B., Chentoufi, M., Lazrak, F., et al. (2006). An autosomal dominant major gene confers predisposition to pulmonary tuberculosis in adults. *Journal of Experimental Medicine, 203*(7), 1679–1684. Available from: PM:16801399.

Ball, T. B., Ji, H., Kimani, J., McLaren, P., Marlin, C., Hill, A. V., et al. (2007). Polymorphisms in IRF-1 associated with resistance to HIV-1 infection in highly exposed uninfected Kenyan sex workers. *AIDS, 21*(9), 1091–1101. Available from: PM:17502719.

Bansal, S. (2009). Sodium retention in heart failure and cirrhosis: Potential role of natriuretic doses of mineralocorticoid antagonist?

Barnes, K. C. (2005). Genetic determinants and ethnic disparities in sepsis-associated acute lung injury. *Proceedings of the American Thoracic Society, 2*(3), 195–201. Available from: PM:16222037.

Bauml, J., Mick, R., Zhang, Y., Watt, C. D., Vachani, A., Aggarwal, C., et al. (2013). Frequency of EGFR and KRAS mutations in patients with non small cell lung cancer by racial background: Do disparities exist? *Lung Cancer, 81*(3), 347–353. Available from: PM:23806795.

Bodmer, J. (1996). World distribution of HLA alleles and implications for disease. *Ciba Foundation Symposium, 197*, 233–253. Available from: PM:8827377.

Bornman, L., Campbell, S. J., Fielding, K., Bah, B., Sillah, J., Gustafson, P., Manneh, K., et al. (2004). Vitamin D receptor polymorphisms and susceptibility to tuberculosis in West Africa: A case-control and family study. *Journal of Infectious Diseases, 190*(9), 1631–1641. Available from: PM:15478069.

Braun, L. (2002). Race, ethnicity, and health: Can genetics explain disparities? *Perspectives in Biology and Medicine, 45*(2), 159–174. Available from: PM:11919376.

Brawley, O. W. (1998). Prostate cancer and black men. *Seminars in Urology and Oncology, 16*(4), 184–186. Available from: PM:9858323.

Brookmeyer, R., Johnson, E., Ziegler-Graham, K., & Arrighi, H. M. (2007). Forecasting the global burden of Alzheimer's disease. *Alzheimers & Dementia, 3*(3), 186–191. Available from: PM:19595937.

Burchard, E. G., Ziv, E., Coyle, N., Gomez, S. L., Tang, H., Karter, A. J., et al. (2003). The importance of race and ethnic background in biomedical research and clinical practice. *The New England Journal of Medicine, 348*(12), 1170–1175. Available from: PM:12646676.

Byers, T. (2010). Two decades of declining cancer mortality: Progress with disparity.

Calafell, F. (2003). Classifying humans. *Nature Genetics, 33*(4), 435–436. Available from: PM:12665860.

Campbell, M. C., & Tishkoff, S. A. (2008). African genetic diversity: Implications for human demographic history, modern human origins, and complex disease mapping. *Annual Review of Genomics and Human Genetics, 9*, 403–433. Available from: PM:18593304.

Carbone, D. P., & Minna, J. D. (1992). The molecular genetics of lung cancer. *Journal of Advances in Internal Medicine, 37*, 153–171. Available from: PM:1348393.

Carey, L. A., Perou, C. M., Livasy, C. A., Dressler, L. G., Cowan, D., Conway, K., et al. (2006). Race, breast cancer subtypes, and survival in the Carolina Breast Cancer Study. *JAMA, 295* (21), 2492–2502. Available from: PM:16757721.

Castro, P., Creighton, C. J., Ozen, M., Berel, D., Mims, M. P., & Ittmann, M. (2009). Genomic profiling of prostate cancers from African American men. *Neoplasia, 11*(3), 305–312. Available from: PM:19242612.

Caulfield, M., Lavender, P., Newell-Price, J., Farrall, M., Kamdar, S., Daniel, H., et al. (1995). Linkage of the angiotensinogen gene locus to human essential hypertension in African Caribbeans. *Journal of Clinical Investigation, 96*(2), 687–692. Available from: PM:7635961.

Chakravarti, A. (2001). To a future of genetic medicine. *Nature, 409*(6822), 822–823. Available from: PM:11236997.

Chan, J. M., Rimm, E. B., Colditz, G. A., Stampfer, M. J., & Willett, W. C. (1994). Obesity, fat distribution, and weight gain as risk factors for clinical diabetes in men. *Diabetes Care, 17*(9), 961–969. Available from: PM:7988316.

Chang, S., ran Ma, T., Miranda, R. D., Balestra, M. E., Mahley, R. W., & Huang, Y. (2005). Lipid- and receptor-binding regions of apolipoprotein E4 fragments act in concert to cause mitochondrial dysfunction and neurotoxicity. *Proceedings of National Academic Science U S A, 102*(51), 18694–18699. Available from: PM:16344479.

Chen, G., Adeyemo, A. A., Johnson, T., Zhou, J., Amoah, A., Owusu, S., et al. (2005). A genome-wide scan for quantitative trait loci linked to obesity phenotypes among West Africans. *International Journal of Obesity (London), 29*(3), 255–259. Available from: PM:15611782.

Chen, G., Adeyemo, A., Zhou, J., Chen, Y., Huang, H., Doumatey, A., et al. (2007). Genome-wide search for susceptibility genes to type 2 diabetes in West Africans: Potential role of C-peptide. *Diabetes Research and Clinical Practice, 78*(3), e1–e6. Available from: PM:17548123.

Chlebowski, R. T., Chen, Z., Anderson, G. L., Rohan, T., Aragaki, A., Lane, D., et al. (2005). Ethnicity and breast cancer: Factors influencing differences in incidence and outcome. *Journal of the National Cancer Institute, 97*(6), 439–448. Available from: PM:15770008.

Cohen, A. L., Mc Morrow, M., Walaza, S., Cohen, C., Tempia, S., Alexander-Scott, M., et al. (2015). Potential impact of co-infections and co-morbidities prevalent in Africa on influenza severity and frequency: A systematic review. *PLoS ONE, 10*, e128580.

Coleman, A. L. (1999). Glaucoma. *Lancet, 354*(9192), 1803–1810. Available from: PM:10577657.

Colilla, S., Rotimi, C., Cooper, R., Goldberg, J., & Cox, N. (2000). Genetic inheritance of body mass index in African-American and African families. *Genetic Epidemiology, 18*(4), 360–376. Available from: PM:10797595.

Collins, R., & Winkleby, M. A. (2002). African American women and men at high and low risk for hypertension: A signal detection analysis of NHANES III, 1988–1994. *Preventive Medicine, 35*(4), 303–312. Available from: PM:12453706.

Conrad, D. F., Jakobsson, M., Coop, G., Wen, X., Wall, J. D., Rosenberg, N. A., et al. (2006). A worldwide survey of haplotype variation and linkage disequilibrium in the human genome. *Nature Genetics, 38*(11), 1251–1260. Available from: PM:17057719.

Cooke, G. S., & Hill, A. V. (2001). Genetics of susceptibility to human infectious disease. *Nature Reviews Genetics, 2*(12), 967–977. Available from: PM:11733749.

Cooper, R. S. (2000). Heritability of angiotensin-converting enzyme and angiotensinogen: A comparison of US blacks and Nigerians.

Cooper, R. S., Kaufman, J. S., & Ward, R. (2003). Race and genomics. *New England Journal of Medicine, 348*(12), 1166–1170. Available from: PM:12646675.

Cooper, R., Rotimi, C., Ataman, S., McGee, D., Osotimehin, B., Kadiri, S., et al. (1997). The prevalence of hypertension in seven populations of west African origin. *American Journal of Public Health, 87*(2), 160–168. Available from: PM:9103091.

Cusi, K. (2010). The role of adipose tissue and lipotoxicity in the pathogenesis of type 2 diabetes. *Current Diabetes Report, 10*(4), 306–315. Available from: PM:20556549.

Das, S. K., & Elbein, S. C. (2006). The genetic basis of type 2 diabetes. *Cellscience, 2*(4), 100–131. Available from: PM:16892160.

DeFrances, C. J. (2008). 2006 National Hospital Discharge Survey.

Delongchamps, N. B., Singh, A., & Haas, G. P. (2007). Epidemiology of prostate cancer in Africa: Another step in the understanding of the disease? *Current Problems in Cancer, 31*(3), 226–236. Available from: PM:17543950.

Demirovic, J., Prineas, R., Loewenstein, D., Bean, J., Duara, R., Sevush, S., et al. (2003). Prevalence of dementia in three ethnic groups: The South Florida program on aging and health. *Annals of Epidemiology, 13*(6), 472–478. Available from: PM:12875807.

Dimou, A., Syrigos, K. N., & Saif, M. W. (2009). Disparities in colorectal cancer in African-Americans vs Whites: Before and after diagnosis. *World Journal of Gastroenterology, 15*(30), 3734–3743. Available from: PM:19673013.

References

Do, R., Bailey, S. D., Desbiens, K., Belisle, A., Montpetit, A., Bouchard, C., et al. (2008). Genetic variants of FTO influence adiposity, insulin sensitivity, leptin levels, and resting metabolic rate in the Quebec Family Study. *Diabetes, 57*(4), 1147–1150. Available from: PM:18316358.

Dunlay, S. M. (2014). Understanding the epidemic of heart failure: Past, present, and future.

Eastham, J. A., May, R. A., Whatley, T., Crow, A., Venable, D. D., & Sartor, O. (1998). Clinical characteristics and biopsy specimen features in African-American and White men without prostate cancer. *Journal of National Cancer Institute, 90*(10), 756–760. Available from: PM:9605645.

Eberhardt, M. S., Ingram, D. D., Makuc, D. M., et al. (2001) Health United States, 2001 with urban and rural health chartbook. Hyattsville, MD.

Eckel, R. H., Kahn, S. E., Ferrannini, E., Goldfine, A. B., Nathan, D. M., Schwartz, M. W., et al. (2011). Obesity and type 2 diabetes: What can be unified and what needs to be individualized? *Diabetes Care, 34*(6), 1424–1430. Available from: PM:21602431.

Edwards, S. M. (2010). Prostate cancer in BRCA2 germline mutation carriers is associated with poorer prognosis.

Edwards, R., Unwin, N., Mugusi, F., Whiting, D., Rashid, S., Kissima, J., et al. (2000). Hypertension prevalence and care in an urban and rural area of Tanzania. *Journal of Hypertension, 18*(2), 145–152. Available from: PM:10694181.

Eichler, E. E., Flint, J., Gibson, G., Kong, A., Leal, S. M., Moore, J. H., et al. (2010). Missing heritability and strategies for finding the underlying causes of complex disease. *Nature Reviews Genetics, 11*(6), 446–450. Available from: PM:20479774.

Elbein, S. C. (2007). Evaluation of polymorphisms known to contribute to risk for diabetes in African and African-American populations. *Current Opinion in Clinical Nutrition and Metabolic Care, 10*(4), 415–419. Available from: PM:17563458.

Esteban, E., Rodon, N., Via, M., Gonzalez-Perez, E., Santamaria, J., Dugoujon, J. M., et al. (2006). Androgen receptor CAG and GGC polymorphisms in Mediterraneans: Repeat dynamics and population relationships. *Journal of Human Genetics, 51*(2), 129–136. Available from: PM:16365681.

Ewing, C. M. (2012). Germline mutations in HOXB13 and prostate-cancer risk.

Felix, R., Bodmer, W., Fearnhead, N. S., van der Merwe, L., Goldberg, P., & Ramesar, R. S. (2006). GSTM1 and GSTT1 polymorphisms as modifiers of age at diagnosis of hereditary nonpolyposis colorectal cancer (HNPCC) in a homogeneous cohort of individuals carrying a single predisposing mutation. *Mutatation Research, 602*(1–2), 175–181. Available from: PM:17087981.

Ferlay, J. (2015). Cancer incidence and mortality worldwide: Sources, methods and major patterns in GLOBOCAN 2012.

Ferrari, S., Di Iorio, E., Barbaro, V., Ponzin, D., Sorrentino, F. S., & Parmeggiani F. (2011). Retinitis pigmentosa: genes and disease mechanisms. *Current Genomics, 12*, 238–249.

Folsom, A. R., Kaye, S. A., Potter, J. D., & Prineas, R. J. (1989). Association of incident carcinoma of the endometrium with body weight and fat distribution in older women: Early findings of the Iowa Women's Health Study. *Cancer Research, 49*(23), 6828–6831. Available from: PM:2819722.

Forrester, T., Cooper, R. S., & Weatherall, D. (1998). Emergence of Western diseases in the tropical world: The experience with chronic cardiovascular diseases. *British Medical Bulletin, 54*(2), 463–473. Available from: PM:9830210.

Frayling, T. M., Timpson, N. J., Weedon, M. N., Zeggini, E., Freathy, R. M., Lindgren, C. M., et al. (2007). A common variant in the FTO gene is associated with body mass index and predisposes to childhood and adult obesity. *Science, 316*(5826), 889–894. Available from: PM:17434869.

Frazer, K. A., Murray, S. S., Schork, N. J., & Topol, E. J. (2009). Human genetic variation and its contribution to complex traits. *Nature Reviews Genetics, 10*(4), 241–251. Available from: PM:19293820.

Freedman, B. I., Kopp, J. B., Langefeld, C. D., Genovese, G., Friedman, D. J., Nelson, G. W., et al. (2010). The apolipoprotein L1 (APOL1) gene and nondiabetic nephropathy in African

Americans. *Journal of American Society of Nephrology, 21*(9), 1422–1426. Available from: PM:20688934.
Genovese, G., Friedman, D. J., Ross, M. D., Lecordier, L., Uzureau, P., Freedman, B. I., et al. (2010). Association of trypanolytic ApoL1 variants with kidney disease in African Americans. *Science, 329*(5993), 841–845. Available from: PM:20647424.
Gibbons, G. H. (2004). Physiology, genetics, and cardiovascular disease: Focus on African Americans.
Goossens, M. (1991). The cystic fibrosis gene: Mutation and the function of CFTR protein. *Annals of Pediatrics (Paris), 38*(9), 591–594. Available from: PM:1721508.
Graff-Radford, N. R., Green, R. C., Go, R. C., Hutton, M. L., Edeki, T., Bachman, D., et al. (2002). Association between apolipoprotein E genotype and Alzheimer disease in African American subjects. *Archives of Neurology, 59*(4), 594–600. Available from: PM:11939894.
Gu, C., Borecki, I., Gagnon, J., Bouchard, C., Leon, A. S., Skinner, J. S., et al. (1998). Familial resemblance for resting blood pressure with particular reference to racial differences: Preliminary analyses from the HERITAGE Family Study. *Human Biology, 70*(1), 77–90. Available from: PM:9489236.
Haddad, S. A. (2015). Hormone-related pathways and risk of breast cancer subtypes in African American women.
Haffner, S. M. (1998). Epidemiology of type 2 diabetes: Risk factors. *Diabetes Care, 21*(Suppl 3), C3–C6. Available from: PM:9850478.
Hainaut, P., & Boyle, P. (2008). Curbing the liver cancer epidemic in Africa. *Lancet, 371*(9610), 367–368. Available from: PM:18242399.
Hannon, T. S., Bacha, F., Lin, Y., & Arslanian, S. A. (2008). Hyperinsulinemia in African-American adolescents compared with their American white peers despite similar insulin sensitivity: A reflection of upregulated beta-cell function? *Diabetes Care, 31*(7), 1445–1447. Available from: PM:18417751.
Hattersley, A., Bruining, J., Shield, J., Njolstad, P., & Donaghue, K. C. (2009). The diagnosis and management of monogenic diabetes in children and adolescents. *Pediatrics Diabetes, 10*(Suppl 12), 33–42. Available from: PM:19754616.
Hayanga, A. J., & D'Cunha, J. (2013). Racial disparities and lung cancer care: Why the unequal playing field? *Seminars in Thoracic Cardiovascular Surgery, 25*(1), 2–3. Available from: PM:23800522.
Helgadottir, A., Manolescu, A., Helgason, A., Thorleifsson, G., Thorsteinsdottir, U., Gudbjartsson, D. F., et al. (2006). A variant of the gene encoding leukotriene A4 hydrolase confers ethnicity-specific risk of myocardial infarction. *Nature Genetics, 38*(1), 68–74. Available from: PM:16282974.
Hendrie, H. C., Murrell, J., Gao, S., Unverzagt, F. W., Ogunniyi, A., & Hall, K. S. (2006). International studies in dementia with particular emphasis on populations of African origin. *Alzheimer Disease and Associated Disorders, 20*(3 Suppl 2), S42–S46. Available from: PM:16917194.
Hendrie, H. C., Ogunniyi, A., Hall, K. S., Baiyewu, O., Unverzagt, F. W., Gureje, O., et al. (2001). Incidence of dementia and Alzheimer disease in 2 communities: Yoruba residing in Ibadan, Nigeria, and African Americans residing in Indianapolis, Indiana. *JAMA, 285*(6), 739–747. Available from: PM:11176911.
Hertz, R. P. (2005). Racial disparities in hypertension prevalence, awareness, and management.
Hertz, R. P., Unger, A. N., Cornell, J. A., & Saunders, E. (2005). Racial disparities in hypertension prevalence, awareness, and management. *Archives of Internal Medicine, 165*(18), 2098–2104. Available from: PM:16216999.
Hill, A. V. (2006). Aspects of genetic susceptibility to human infectious diseases. *Annual Reviews of Genetics, 40*, 469–486. Available from: PM:17094741.
Hirsch, C., Anderson, M. L., Newman, A., Kop, W., Jackson, S., Gottdiener, J., et al. (2006). The association of race with frailty: The cardiovascular health study. *Annals of Epidemiology, 16*(7), 545–553. Available from: PM:16388967.

Howson, J. M., Roy, M. S., Zeitels, L., Stevens, H., & Todd, J. A. (2013). HLA class II gene associations in African American type 1 diabetes reveal a protective HLA-DRB1*03 haplotype. *Diabetics Medicine, 30*(6), 710–716. Available from: PM:23398374.

Hu, C. A., Klopfer, E. I., & Ray, P. E. (2012). Human apolipoprotein L1 (ApoL1) in cancer and chronic kidney disease. *FEBS Letters, 586*(7), 947–955. Available from: PM:22569246.

Isaacs, W. B. (2012). Inherited susceptibility for aggressive prostate cancer.

Jallow, M., Teo, Y. Y., Small, K. S., Rockett, K. A., Deloukas, P., Clark, T. G., et al. (2009). Genome-wide and fine-resolution association analysis of malaria in West Africa. *Nature Genetics, 41*(6), 657–665. Available from: PM:19465909.

Jepson, A., Fowler, A., Banya, W., Singh, M., Bennett, S., Whittle, H., et al. (2001). Genetic regulation of acquired immune responses to antigens of *Mycobacterium tuberculosis*: A study of twins in West Africa. *Infection and Immunity, 69*(6), 3989–3994. Available from: PM:11349068.

Joe, A. K., Arber, N., Bose, S., Heitjan, D., Zhang, Y., Weinstein, I. B., et al. (2001). Cyclin D1 overexpression is more prevalent in non-Caucasian breast cancer. *Anticancer Research, 21*(5), 3535–3539. Available from: PM:11848520.

Johns, L. E. (2001). A systematic review and meta-analysis of familial colorectal cancer risk.

Kao, W. H. (2008). MYH9 is associated with nondiabetic end-stage renal disease in African Americans.

Kardia, S. L. (2000). Context-dependent genetic effects in hypertension. *Current Hypertension Report, 2*(1), 32–38. Available from: PM:10981124.

Kaufman, J. S., Durazo-Arvizu, R. A., Rotimi, C. N., McGee, D. L., & Cooper, R. S. (1996). Obesity and hypertension prevalence in populations of African origin. The investigators of the international collaborative study on hypertension in blacks. *Epidemiology, 7*(4), 398–405. Available from: PM:8793366.

Kaufman, J. S., Owoaje, E. E., Rotimi, C. N., & Cooper, R. S. (1999). Blood pressure change in Africa: Case study from Nigeria. *Human Biology, 71*(4), 641–657. Available from: PM:10453105.

Keaton, J. M., Cooke Bailey, J. N., Palmer, N. D., Freedman, B. I., Langefeld, C. D., Ng, M. C., et al. (2014). A comparison of type 2 diabetes risk allele load between African Americans and European Americans. *Human Genetics, 133*(12), 1487–1495. Available from: PM:25273842.

Keku, T. O., Vidal, A., Oliver, S., Hoyo, C., Hall, I. J., Omofoye, O., et al. (2012). Genetic variants in IGF-I, IGF-II, IGFBP-3, and adiponectin genes and colon cancer risk in African Americans and Whites. *Cancer Causes & Control, 23*(7), 1127–1138. Available from: PM:22565227.

Kimani, J., Kaul, R., Nagelkerke, N. J., Luo, M., MacDonald, K. S., Ngugi, E., et al. (2008). Reduced rates of HIV acquisition during unprotected sex by Kenyan female sex workers predating population declines in HIV prevalence. *AIDS, 22*(1), 131–137. Available from: PM:18090401.

Kittles, R. A., Chen, W., Panguluri, R. K., Ahaghotu, C., Jackson, A., Adebamowo, C. A., et al. (2002). CYP3A4-V and prostate cancer in African Americans: Causal or confounding association because of population stratification? *Human Genetics, 110*(6), 553–560. Available from: PM:12107441.

Kittles, R. A., Young, D., Weinrich, S., Hudson, J., Argyropoulos, G., Ukoli, F., et al. (2001). Extent of linkage disequilibrium between the androgen receptor gene CAG and GGC repeats in human populations: Implications for prostate cancer risk. *Human Genetics, 109*(3), 253–261. Available from: PM:11702204.

Kohler, B. A. (2015). Annual report to the nation on the status of cancer, 1975–2011, featuring incidence of breast cancer subtypes by race/ethnicity, poverty, and state.

Krieger, N. (2005). Stormy weather: Race, gene expression, and the science of health disparities. *American Journal of Public Health, 95*, 2155–2160.

Lama, J., & Planelles, V. (2007). Host factors influencing susceptibility to HIV infection and AIDS progression. *Retrovirology, 4*, 52. Available from: PM:17651505.

Lamba, J. K. (2002). Genetic contribution to variable human CYP3A-mediated metabolism.

Lander, E. S., Linton, L. M., Birren, B., Nusbaum, C., Zody, M. C., Baldwin, J., et al. (2001). Initial sequencing and analysis of the human genome. *Nature, 409*(6822), 860–921. Available from: PM:11237011.

Lansdorp-Vogelaar, I., Kuntz, K. M., Knudsen, A. B., van, B. M., Zauber, A. G., & Jemal, A. (2012). Contribution of screening and survival differences to racial disparities in colorectal cancer rates. *Cancer Epidemioloy, Biomarkers & Prevention, 21*(5), 728–736. Available from: PM:22514249.

Liu, V., Escobar, G. J., Greene, J. D., Soule, J., Whippy, A., Angus, D. C., et al. (2014). Hospital deaths in patients with sepsis from 2 independent cohorts. *JAMA, 312*(1), 90–92. Available from: PM:24838355.

Liu, C. C., Kanekiyo, T., Xu, H., & Bu, G. (2013). Apolipoprotein E and Alzheimer disease: Risk, mechanisms and therapy. *Nature Reviews Neurology, 9*(2), 106–118. Available from: PM:23296339.

Loo, L. W., Wang, Y., Flynn, E. M., Lund, M. J., Bowles, E. J., Buist, D. S., et al. (2011). Genome-wide copy number alterations in subtypes of invasive breast cancers in young white and African American women. *Breast Cancer Research & Treatment, 127*(1), 297–308. Available from: PM:21264507.

Loock, M., Steyn, K., Becker, P., & Fourie, J. (2006). Coronary heart disease and risk factors in Black South Africans: A case-control study. *Ethnicity & Disease, 16*(4), 872–879. Available from: PM:17061740.

Loos, R. J. (2014). The bigger picture of FTO: The first GWAS-identified obesity gene.

Luke, A., Guo, X., Adeyemo, A. A., Wilks, R., Forrester, T., Lowe, W., Jr., et al. (2001). Heritability of obesity-related traits among Nigerians, Jamaicans and US black people. *International Journal of Obesity and Related Metabolic Disorders, 25*(7), 1034–1041. Available from: PM:11443503.

Magi-Galluzzi, C., Tsusuki, T., Elson, P., Simmerman, K., LaFargue, C., Esgueva, R., et al. (2011). TMPRSS2-ERG gene fusion prevalence and class are significantly different in prostate cancer of Caucasian, African-American and Japanese patients. *Prostate, 71*(5), 489–497. Available from: PM:20878952.

Magoha, G. A. (2007). Overview of prostate cancer in indigenous black Africans and blacks of African ancestry in diaspora 1935–2007. *East African Medical Journal, 84*(9 Suppl), S3–S11. Available from: PM:18154197.

Malone, K. E., Daling, J. R., Doody, D. R., Hsu, L., Bernstein, L., Coates, R. J., et al. (2006). Prevalence and predictors of BRCA1 and BRCA2 mutations in a population-based study of breast cancer in white and black American women ages 35 to 64 years. *Cancer Research, 66*(16), 8297–8308. Available from: PM:16912212.

Martin, D. N., Boersma, B. J., Yi, M., Reimers, M., Howe, T. M., Yfantis, H. G., et al. (2009). Differences in the tumor microenvironment between African-American and European-American breast cancer patients. *PLoS One, 4*(2), e4531. Available from: PM:19225562.

Matanoski, G., Tao, X., Almon, L., Adade, A. A., & Davies-Cole, J. O. (2006). Demographics and tumor characteristics of colorectal cancers in the United States, 1998-2001. *Cancer, 107*(5 Suppl), 1112–1120. Available from: PM:16838314.

Maxwell, K. N. (2012). Cancer treatment according to BRCA1 and BRCA2 mutations.

Maxwell, K. N. (2013). Common breast cancer risk variants in the post-COGS era: A comprehensive review.

McCracken, M. (2007). Cancer incidence, mortality, and associated risk factors among Asian Americans of Chinese, Filipino, Vietnamese, Korean, and Japanese ethnicities.

Mendel, G. (1866). Versuche über Pflanzen-Hybriden. Verhandlungen des naturforschenden Vereines, Abhandlungen. *Brunn, 4*, 3–47.

Menges, T., Hermans, P. W., Little, S. G., Langefeld, T., Boning, O., Engel, J., et al. (2001). Plasminogen-activator-inhibitor-1 4G/5G promoter polymorphism and prognosis of severely injured patients. *Lancet, 357*(9262), 1096–1097. Available from: PM:11297964.

References

Miljkovic-Gacic, I., Gordon, C. L., Goodpaster, B. H., Bunker, C. H., Patrick, A. L., Kuller, L. H., et al. (2008). Adipose tissue infiltration in skeletal muscle: Age patterns and association with diabetes among men of African ancestry. *American Journal of Clinical Nutrition, 87*(6), 1590–1595. Available from: PM:18541544.

Moore, J. H., & Williams, S. M. (2002). New strategies for identifying gene-gene interactions in hypertension. *Annals of Medicine, 34*(2), 88–95. Available from: PM:12108579.

Morris, M. R., Ricketts, C., Gentle, D., Abdulrahman, M., Clarke, N., Brown, M., et al. (2010). Identification of candidate tumour suppressor genes frequently methylated in renal cell carcinoma. *Oncogene, 29*(14), 2104–2117. Available from: PM:20154727.

Motala, A. A. (2002). Diabetes trends in Africa. *Diabetes Metabolism Research and Reviews, 18* (Suppl 3), S14–S20. Available from: PM:12324980.

Muro, F. (2015). Acute respiratory infection and bacteraemia as causes of non-malarial febrile illness in African children: A narrative review.

Murrell, J. R., Price, B. M., Baiyewu, O., Gureje, O., Deeg, M., Hendrie, H., et al. (2006). The fourth apolipoprotein E haplotype found in the Yoruba of Ibadan. *American Journal of Medical Genetics B Neuropsychiatric.Genetics, 141B*(4), 426–427. Available from: PM:16583434.

Mwantembe, O., Gaillard, M. C., Barkhuizen, M., Pillay, V., Berry, S. D., Dewar, J. B., et al. (2001). Ethnic differences in allelic associations of the interleukin-1 gene cluster in South African patients with inflammatory bowel disease (IBD) and in control individuals. *Immunogenetics, 52*(3–4), 249–254. Available from: PM:11220627.

Newport, M. J., Allen, A., Awomoyi, A. A., Dunstan, S. J., McKinney, E., Marchant, A., et al. (2004). The toll-like receptor 4 Asp299Gly variant: No influence on LPS responsiveness or susceptibility to pulmonary tuberculosis in The Gambia. *Tuberculosis (Edinburgh), 84*(6), 347–352. Available from: PM:15525557.

Nielsen, M., Joerink-van de Beld, M.C., Jones, N., Vogt, S., Tops, C. M., Vasen, H. F., et al. (2009). Analysis of MUTYH genotypes and colorectal phenotypes in patients with MUTYH-associated polyposis. *Gastroenterology, 136*(2), 471–476. Available from: PM:19032956.

Nunes, J. P. (2003). Arterial hypertension and sepsis. *Revista Portuguesa de Cardiologia, 22*(11), 1375–1379. Available from: PM:14768492.

Oliveira, T. Y., Harris, E. E., Meyer, D., Jue, C. K., & Silva, W. A., Jr. (2012). Molecular evolution of a malaria resistance gene (DARC) in primates. *Immunogenetics, 64*(7), 497–505. Available from: PM:22395823.

Ouerhani, S., Oliveira, E., Marrakchi, R., Ben Slama, M. R., Sfaxi, M., Ayed, M., et al. (2007). Methylenetetrahydrofolate reductase and methionine synthase polymorphisms and risk of bladder cancer in a Tunisian population. *Cancer Genetics and Cytogenetics, 176*(1), 48–53. Available from: PM:17574963.

Ouerhani, S., Tebourski, F., Slama, M. R., Marrakchi, R., Rabeh, M., Hassine, L. B., et al. (2006). The role of glutathione transferases M1 and T1 in individual susceptibility to bladder cancer in a Tunisian population. *Annals of Human Biology, 33*(5–6), 529–535. Available from: PM:17381051.

Parkin, D. M., Ferlay, J., Hamdi-Chérif, M., Sitas, F., Thomas, J., Wabinga, H., et al. (2003). *Cancer in Africa: Epidemiology and prevention*. Lyon: IARC Press.

Parra, E. J., Kittles, R. A., Argyropoulos, G., Pfaff, C. L., Hiester, K., Bonilla, C., et al. (2001). Ancestral proportions and admixture dynamics in geographically defined African Americans living in South Carolina. *American Journal of Physical Anthropology, 114*(1), 18–29. Available from: PM:11150049.

Perez-Morga, D., Vanhollebeke, B., Paturiaux-Hanocq, F., Nolan, D. P., Lins, L., Homble, F., et al. (2005). Apolipoprotein L-I promotes trypanosome lysis by forming pores in lysosomal membranes. *Science, 309*(5733), 469–472. Available from: PM:16020735.

Petrovics, G., Liu, A., Shaheduzzaman, S., Furusato, B., Sun, C., Chen, Y., et al. (2005). Frequent overexpression of ETS-related gene-1 (ERG1) in prostate cancer transcriptome. *Oncogene, 24* (23), 3847–3852. Available from: PM:15750627.

Pharoah, P. D. (2002). Polygenic susceptibility to breast cancer and implications for prevention.
Pibiri, F., Kittles, R. A., Sandler, R. S., Keku, T. O., Kupfer, S. S., Xicola, R. M., et al. (2014). Genetic variation in vitamin D-related genes and risk of colorectal cancer in African Americans. *Cancer Causes & Control, 25*(5), 561–570. Available from: PM:24562971.
Platz, E. A., & Giovannucci, E. (2004). The epidemiology of sex steroid hormones and their signaling and metabolic pathways in the etiology of prostate cancer. *Journal of Steroid Biochemistry and Molecular Biology, 92*(4), 237–253. Available from: PM:15663987.
Poland, G. A. (1998). Variability in immune response to pathogens: Using measles vaccine to probe immunogenetic determinants of response. *American Journal of Human Genetics, 62*(2), 215–220. Available from: PM:9463343.
Ramsay, M. (2012). Africa: Continent of genome contrasts with implications for biomedical research and health. *FEBS Letters, 586*(18), 2813–2819. Available from: PM:22858376.
Redon, R., Ishikawa, S., Fitch, K. R., Feuk, L., Perry, G. H., Andrews, T. D., et al. (2006). Global variation in copy number in the human genome. *Nature, 444*(7118), 444–454. Available from: PM:17122850.
Reed, F. A., & Tishkoff, S. A. (2006). African human diversity, origins and migrations. *Current Opinion in Genetics & Developmwnt, 16*(6), 597–605. Available from: PM:17056248.
Refolo, L. M., Malester, B., Lafrancois, J., Bryant-Thomas, T., Wang, R., Tint, G. S., et al. (2000). Hypercholesterolemia accelerates the Alzheimer's amyloid pathology in a transgenic mouse model. *Neurobiology of Disease, 7*(4), 321–331. Available from: PM:10964604.
Reitz, C., & Mayeux, R. (2014). Genetics of Alzheimer's disease in Caribbean Hispanic and African American populations. *Biological Psychiatry, 75*(7), 534–541. Available from: PM:23890735.
Rennert, H., Zeigler-Johnson, C. M., Addya, K., Finley, M. J., Walker, A. H., Spangler, E., et al. (2005). Association of susceptibility alleles in ELAC2/HPC2, RNASEL/HPC1, and MSR1 with prostate cancer severity in European American and African American men. *Cancer Epidemiology, Biomarkers & Prevention, 14*(4), 949–957. Available from: PM:15824169.
Rich, S. S. (1990). Mapping genes in diabetes. Genetic epidemiological perspective. *Diabetes, 39*(11), 1315–1319. Available from: PM:2227105.
Romanova, E. N. (2013). TNF-alpha, IL-10, and eNOS gene polymorphisms in patients with influenza A/H1N1 complicated by pneumonia.
Rosanas-Urgell, A. (2012). Lack of associations of alpha(+)-thalassemia with the risk of *Plasmodium falciparum* and *Plasmodium vivax* infection and disease in a cohort of children aged 3–21 months from Papua New Guinea.
Rose, D. P., & Royak-Schaler, R. (2001). Tumor biology and prognosis in black breast cancer patients: A review. *Cancer Detection and Prevention, 25*(1), 16–31. Available from: PM:11270418.
Roses, A. D., Lutz, M. W., Saunders, A. M., Goldgaber, D., Saul, R., Sundseth, S. S., et al. (2014). African-American TOMM40'523-APOE haplotypes are admixture of West African and Caucasian alleles. *Alzheimers.Dementia, 10*(6), 592–601. Available from: PM:25260913.
Rotimi, C. N., Cooper, R. S., Ataman, S. L., Osotimehin, B., Kadiri, S., Muna, W., et al. (1995). Distribution of anthropometric variables and the prevalence of obesity in populations of west African origin: The International Collaborative Study on Hypertension in Blacks (ICSHIB). *Obesity Research, 3*(Suppl 2), 95s–105s. Available from: PM:8581794.
Rotimi, C. N., Cooper, R. S., Cao, G., Ogunbiyi, O., Ladipo, M., Owoaje, E., et al. (1999a). Maximum-likelihood generalized heritability estimate for blood pressure in Nigerian families. *Hypertension, 33*(3), 874–878. Available from: PM:10082502.
Rotimi, C. N., Cooper, R. S., Okosun, I. S., Olatunbosun, S. T., Bella, A. F., Wilks, R., et al. (1999b). Prevalence of diabetes and impaired glucose tolerance in Nigerians, Jamaicans and US blacks. *Ethnicity & Disease, 9*(2), 190–200. Available from: PM:10421081.
Rotimi, C. N., Dunston, G. M., Berg, K., Akinsete, O., Amoah, A., Owusu, S., et al. (2001). In search of susceptibility genes for type 2 diabetes in West Africa: The design and results of the first phase of the AADM study. *Annals of Epidemiology, 11*(1), 51–58. Available from: PM:11164120.

References

Rotimi, C., Morrison, L., Cooper, R., Oyejide, C., Effiong, E., Ladipo, M., et al. (1994). Angiotensinogen gene in human hypertension. Lack of an association of the 235T allele among African Americans. *Hypertension, 24*(5), 591–594. Available from: PM:7960018.

Russell, E. F., Kramer, M. R., Cooper, H. L., Gabram-Mendola, S., Senior-Crosby, D., & Jacob Arriola, K. R. (2012). Metropolitan area racial residential segregation, neighborhood racial composition, and breast cancer mortality. *Cancer Causes & Control, 23*(9), 1519–1527. Available from: PM:22825071.

Saad, A. A., O'Connor, P. J., Mostafa, M. H., Metwalli, N. E., Cooper, D. P., Povey, A. C., et al. (2005). Glutathione S-transferase M1, T1 and P1 polymorphisms and bladder cancer risk in Egyptians. *International Journal of Biological Markers, 20*(1), 69–72. Available from: PM:15832776.

Sabeti, P. C., Reich, D. E., Higgins, J. M., Levine, H. Z., Richter, D. J., Schaffner, S. F., et al. (2002). Detecting recent positive selection in the human genome from haplotype structure. *Nature, 419*(6909), 832–837. Available from: PM:12397357.

Sandy, A. S., Palmer, N. D., Hanley, A. J., Ziegler, J. T., Mark, B. W., Freedman, B. I., et al. (2013). Genetic analysis of adiponectin variation and its association with type 2 diabetes in African Americans. *Obesity (Silver Spring), 21*(12), E721–E729. Available from: PM:23512866.

Scherer, S. W., Lee, C., Birney, E., Altshuler, D. M., Eichler, E. E., Carter, N. P., et al. (2007). Challenges and standards in integrating surveys of structural variation. *Nature Genetics, 39*(7 Suppl), S7–S15. Available from: PM:17597783.

Schlesinger, D., Grinberg, L. T., Alba, J. G., Naslavsky, M. S., Licinio, L., Farfel, J. M., et al. (2013). African ancestry protects against Alzheimer's disease-related neuropathology. *Molecular Psychiatry, 18*(1), 79–85. Available from: PM:22064377.

Schoenhard, J. A., Asselbergs, F. W., Poku, K. A., Stocki, S. A., Gordon, S., Vaughan, D. E., et al. (2008). Male-female differences in the genetic regulation of t-PA and PAI-1 levels in a Ghanaian population. *Humam Genetics, 124*(5), 479–488. Available from: PM:18953568.

Scholz, C. A., Johnson, T. C., Cohen, A. S., King, J. W., Peck, J. A., Overpeck, J. T., et al. (2007). East African megadroughts between 135 and 75 thousand years ago and bearing on early-modern human origins. *Proceedings of National Academy Science U S A, 104*(42), 16416–16421. Available from: PM:17785420.

Schwartz, G. F., Hughes, K. S., Lynch, H. T., Fabian, C. J., Fentiman, I. S., Robson, M. E., et al. (2008). Proceedings of the international consensus conference on breast cancer risk, genetics, & risk management, April, 2007. *Cancer, 113*(10), 2627–2637. Available from: PM:18853415.

Seeleang, K. (2011). Genetic disparities in the development of type 2 diabetes among African Americans. *Journal of American Academy of Nurse Practitioners, 23*(9), 473–478. Available from: PM:21899642.

Shand, R. L., & Gelmann, E. P. (2006). Molecular biology of prostate-cancer pathogenesis. *Current Opinion in Urology, 16*(3), 123–131. Available from: PM:16679847.

Shields, P. G., Caporaso, N. E., Falk, R. T., Sugimura, H., Trivers, G. E., Trump, B. F., et al. (1993). Lung cancer, race, and a CYP1A1 Genetic polymorphism. *Cancer Epidemiology, Biomarkers & Prevention, 2*(5), 481–485. Available from: PM:8220094.

Shriver, M. D., & Kittles, R. A. (2004). Genetic ancestry and the search for personalized genetic histories. *Nature Reviews Genetics, 5*(8), 611–618. Available from: PM:15266343.

Siffert, W., Naber, C., Walla, M., & Ritz, E. (1999). G protein beta3 subunit 825T allele and its potential association with obesity in hypertensive individuals. *Journal of Hypertension, 17*(8), 1095–1098. Available from: PM:10466464.

Singh, C. R., & Kathiresan, K. (2014). Molecular understanding of lung cancers—A review. *Asian Pacific Journal of Tropical Biomedicine, 4*(Suppl 1), S35–S41. Available from: PM:25183110.

Sniderman, A. D., Bhopal, R., Prabhakaran, D., Sarrafzadegan, N., & Tchernof, A. (2007). Why might South Asians be so susceptible to central obesity and its atherogenic consequences? The adipose tissue overflow hypothesis. *International Journal of Epidemiology, 36*(1), 220–225. Available from: PM:17510078.

Sommer, A., Tielsch, J. M., Katz, J., Quigley, H. A., Gottsch, J. D., Javitt, J. C., et al. (1991). Racial differences in the cause-specific prevalence of blindness in east Baltimore. *New England Journal of Medicine, 325*(20), 1412–1417. Available from: PM:1922252.

Sorlie, T., Perou, C. M., Tibshirani, R., Aas, T., Geisler, S., Johnsen, H., et al. (2001). Gene expression patterns of breast carcinomas distinguish tumor subclasses with clinical implications. *Proceedings of National Academic Science U S A, 98*(19), 10869–10874. Available from: PM:11553815.

Spencer, C. C., Su, Z., Donnelly, P., & Marchini, J. (2009). Designing genome-wide association studies: Sample size, power, imputation, and the choice of genotyping chip. *PLoS Genetics, 5*(5), e1000477. Available from: PM:19492015.

Stefan, N., Kantartzis, K., Machann, J., Schick, F., Thamer, C., Rittig, K., et al. (2008). Identification and characterization of metabolically benign obesity in humans. *Archives of Internal Medicine, 168*(15), 1609–1616. Available from: PM:18695074.

Strachan, T., & Read, A. P. (1999). Mendelian pedigree patterns. *Human Molecular Genetics, 2* (Garland Science).

Taherzadeh, Z. (2010). Function and structure of resistance vessels in black and white people.

Tang, M. X., Cross, P., Andrews, H., Jacobs, D. M., Small, S., Bell, K., et al. (2001). Incidence of AD in African-Americans, Caribbean Hispanics, and Caucasians in northern Manhattan. *Neurology, 56*(1), 49–56. Available from: PM:11148235.

Teo, Y. Y., Small, K. S., & Kwiatkowski, D. P. (2010). Methodological challenges of genome-wide association analysis in Africa. *Nature Reviews Genetics, 11*(2), 149–160. Available from: PM:20084087.

The Wellcome Trust Case Control Consortium. (2007). Genome-wide association study of 14000 cases of seven common diseases and 3000 shared controls. *Nature, 447*, 661–678.

Tibazarwa, K., Ntyintyane, L., Sliwa, K., Gerntholtz, T., Carrington, M., Wilkinson, D., et al. (2009). A time bomb of cardiovascular risk factors in South Africa: Results from the Heart of Soweto Study "Heart Awareness Days". *International Journal of Cardiology, 132*(2), 233–239. Available from: PM:18237791.

Tidball, J. G., & Wehling-Henricks, M. (2004). Evolving therapeutic strategies for Duchenne muscular dystrophy: Targeting downstream events. *Pediatric Research, 56*(6), 831–841. Available from: PM:15531741.

Tishkoff, S. A., Dietzsch, E., Speed, W., Pakstis, A. J., Kidd, J. R., Cheung, K., et al. (1996). Global patterns of linkage disequilibrium at the CD4 locus and modern human origins. *Science, 271*(5254), 1380–1387. Available from: PM:8596909.

Tishkoff, S. A., Gonder, K., Hirbo, J., Mortensen, H., Powell, K., Knight, A. et al. (2003). *The genetic history of linguistically diverse Tanzanian populations: A multilocus analysis*. Tempe: American Association of Physical Anthropology.

Tishkoff, S. A., Reed, F. A., Friedlaender, F. R., Ehret, C., Ranciaro, A., Froment, A., et al. (2009). The genetic structure and history of Africans and African Americans. *Science, 324*(5930), 1035–1044. Available from: PM:19407144.

Todd, J. A., Walker, N. M., Cooper, J. D., Smyth, D. J., Downes, K., Plagnol, V., et al. (2007). Robust associations of four new chromosome regions from genome-wide analyses of type 1 diabetes. *Nature Genetics, 39*(7), 857–864. Available from: PM:17554260.

Torcia, M. G., Santarlasci, V., Cosmi, L., Clemente, A., Maggi, L., Mangano, V. D., et al. (2008). Functional deficit of T regulatory cells in Fulani, an ethnic group with low susceptibility to *Plasmodium falciparum* malaria. *Proceedings of National Academic Science U S A, 105*(2), 646–651. Available from: PM:18174328.

Tournamille, C., Colin, Y., Cartron, J. P., & Le Van, K. C. (1995). Disruption of a GATA motif in the Duffy gene promoter abolishes erythroid gene expression in Duffy-negative individuals. *Nature Genetics, 10*(2), 224–228. Available from: PM:7663520.

Trauth, M. H., Maslin, M. A., Deino, A. L., Strecker, M. R., Bergner, A. G., & Duhnforth, M. (2007). High- and low-latitude forcing of Plio-Pleistocene East African climate and human evolution. *Journal of Human Evolution, 53*(5), 475–486. Available from: PM:17959230.

References

Troxel, W. M., Matthews, K. A., Bromberger, J. T., & Sutton-Tyrrell, K. (2003). Chronic stress burden, discrimination, and subclinical carotid artery disease in African American and Caucasian women. *Health Psychology, 22*(3), 300–309. Available from: PM:12790258.

Underwood, P. C., Sun, B., Williams, J. S., Pojoga, L. H., Chamarthi, B., Lasky-Su, J., et al. (2010). The relationship between peroxisome proliferator-activated receptor-gamma and renin: a human genetics study. *Journal of Clinical Endocrinology & Metabolism, 95*, E75–E95.

Unwin, N., Setel, P., Rashid, S., Mugusi, F., Mbanya, J. C., Kitange, H., et al. (2001). Noncommunicable diseases in sub-Saharan Africa: Where do they feature in the health research agenda? *Bulletin of World Health Organisation, 79*(10), 947–953. Available from: PM:11693977.

Vanhamme, L., Paturiaux-Hanocq, F., Poelvoorde, P., Nolan, D. P., Lins, L., Van Den Abbeele, J., et al. (2003). Apolipoprotein L-I is the trypanosome lytic factor of human serum. *Nature, 422* (6927), 83–87. Available from: PM:12621437.

Velasquez-Mieyer, P. A., Cowan, P. A., Umpierrez, G. E., Lustig, R. H., Cashion, A. K., & Burghen, G. A. (2003). Racial differences in glucagon-like peptide-1 (GLP-1) concentrations and insulin dynamics during oral glucose tolerance test in obese subjects. *International Journal of Obesity and Related Metabolic Disorders, 27*(11), 1359–1364. Available from: PM:14574347.

Vlachopoulos, C., & Terentes-Printzios, D. (2015). Thyroid, aldosterone, and cardiovascular disease.

Vogelstein, B., & Kinzler, K. W. (1993). The multistep nature of cancer. *Trends in Genetics, 9*(4), 138–141. Available from: PM:8516849.

Walker, A. R., Adam, F., & Walker, B. F. (2001). World pandemic of obesity: The situation in Southern African populations. *Public Health, 115*(6), 368–372. Available from: PM:11781845.

Wall, J. D., Cox, M. P., Mendez, F. L., Woerner, A., Severson, T., & Hammer, M. F. (2008). A novel DNA sequence database for analyzing human demographic history. *Genome Research, 18*(8), 1354–1361. Available from: PM:18493019.

Wallace, T. A., Prueitt, R. L., Yi, M., Howe, T. M., Gillespie, J. W., Yfantis, H. G., et al. (2008). Tumor immunobiological differences in prostate cancer between African-American and European-American men. *Cancer Research, 68*(3), 927–936. Available from: PM:18245496.

Wassenaar, C. A., Ye, Y., Cai, Q., Aldrich, M. C., Knight, J., Spitz, M. R., et al. (2015). CYP2A6 reduced activity gene variants confer reduction in lung cancer risk in African American smokers—Findings from two independent populations. *Carcinogenesis, 36*(1), 99–103. Available from: PM:25416559.

Weatherall, D. J., & Clegg, J. B. (2001. Inherited haemoglobin disorders: An increasing global health problem. *Bulletin of the World Health Organisation, 79*(8), 704–712. Available from: PM:11545326.

Weston, A., & Godbold, J. H. (1997). Polymorphisms of H-ras-1 and p 53 in breast cancer and lung cancer: A meta-analysis. *Environmental Health Perspectives, 105*(Suppl 4), 919–926. Available from: PM:9255581.

Willcox, M., Bjorkman, A., & Brohult, J. (1983). Falciparum malaria and beta-thalassaemia trait in northern Liberia. *Annals of Tropical Medicine and Parasitology, 77*(4), 335–347. Available from: PM:6357119.

Williams, S. M., Addy, J. H., Phillips, J. A., III, Dai, M., Kpodonu, J., Afful, J., et al. (2000). Combinations of variations in multiple genes are associated with hypertension. *Hypertension, 36*(1), 2–6. Available from: PM:10904004.

Williams, D. R., & Jackson, P. B. (2005). Social sources of racial disparities in health. *Health Affairs (Millwood), 24*(2), 325–334. Available from: PM:15757915.

Williams, T. N., Maitland, K., Bennett, S., Ganczakowski, M., Peto, T. E., Newbold, C. I., et al. (1996). High incidence of malaria in alpha-thalassaemic children. *Nature, 383*(6600), 522–525. Available from: PM:8849722.

Williams, S. M., Stocki, S., Jiang, L., Brew, K., Gordon, S., Vaughan, D. E., et al. (2007). A population-based study in Ghana to investigate inter-individual variation in plasma t-PA and PAI-1. *Ethnicity & Diseases, 17*(3), 492–497. Available from: PM:17985503.

Wurfel, M. M., Gordon, A. C., Holden, T. D., Radella, F., Strout, J., Kajikawa, O., et al. (2008). Toll-like receptor 1 polymorphisms affect innate immune responses and outcomes in sepsis. *American Journal of Respiratory and Critical Care Medicine, 178*(7), 710–720. Available from: PM:18635889.

Xu, J., Kibel, A. S., Hu, J. J., Turner, A. R., Pruett, K., Zheng, S. L., et al. (2009). Prostate cancer risk associated loci in African Americans. *Cancer Epidemiology, Biomarkers & Prevention, 18*(7), 2145–2149. Available from: PM:19549807.

Yao, S. (2012). Variants in the vitamin D pathway, serum levels of vitamin D, and estrogen receptor negative breast cancer among African-American women: A case-control study.

Zabaleta, J., Lin, H. Y., Sierra, R. A., Hall, M. C., Clark, P. E., Sartor, O. A., et al. (2008). Interactions of cytokine gene polymorphisms in prostate cancer risk. *Carcinogenesis, 29*(3), 573–578. Available from: PM:18174250.

Zanetti, K. A., Haznadar, M., Welsh, J. A., Robles, A. I., Ryan, B. M., McClary, A. C., et al. (2012). 3′-UTR and functional secretor haplotypes in mannose-binding lectin 2 are associated with increased colon cancer risk in African Americans. *Cancer Research, 72*(6), 1467–1477. Available from: PM:22282660.

Zeigler-Johnson, C. M., Walker, A. H., Mancke, B., Spangler, E., Jalloh, M., McBride, S., et al. (2002). Ethnic differences in the frequency of prostate cancer susceptibility alleles at SRD5A2 and CYP3A4. *Human Heredity, 54*(1), 13–21. Available from: PM:12446983.

Zimmerman, P. A. (2013). Red blood cell polymorphism and susceptibility to *Plasmodium vivax*.

Zuk, O., Hechter, E., Sunyaev, S. R., & Lander, E. S. (2012). The mystery of missing heritability: Genetic interactions create phantom heritability. *Proceedings of National Academic Science U S A, 109*(4), 1193–1198. Available from: PM:22223662.

Zuniga, J. (2012). Genetic variants associated with severe pneumonia in A/H1N1 influenza infection.

Chapter 3
The Role of Epigenetics

Abstract Genetic variations among individuals and populations are providing insights into how information in the DNA sequence is executed at the cellular level. However, phenotypic differences between individuals cannot be entirely explained by genetic differences. Epigenetic events such as DNA-methylation changes have increasingly been found to be associated with health disparities. Social and environmental determinants, such as diet, stress, infection, and exposure to toxins can cause epigenetic changes. The epigenome of the developing fetus is especially sensitive to maternal nutrition, exposure to environmental toxins and psychological stress, and this can result in differences in health outcomes later in life. The emerging epigenetic model of health disparities points to social determinants and environmental exposures as key to addressing racial differences in disease burdens.

3.1 Introduction

The Greek prefix *epi,* which means 'above,' in the word epigenetics was first used by Waddington (1942) to describe how the environment can influence the genome through a gene-environment interaction during development and embryogenesis. Nowadays, epigenetics has come to mean the molecular mechanisms that are mitotically stable and regulate gene expression or cellular phenotype without altering the DNA sequence itself (Skinner et al. 2010). Epigenetic processes play important roles in marking genes for either activation or inactivation and are essential in establishing cellular identity, as well as maintaining cell and tissue-type diversity. Thus epigenetic processes play an important role during all stages of development for establishing cell, tissue, and organism phenotypes. The consequence of epigenetic changes is modification at the phenotypic level without changes in the genotype.

There are at least three types of epigenetic mechanisms that influence human development and health outcomes: histone modification, noncoding RNA (RNA associated gene silencing), and DNA methylation, and there are possible interactions between all three types of epigenetic mechanisms to regulate gene expression in the human cell.

3.1.1 Histone Modification

Very little of the genomic DNA exists as naked double-helical structure inside the nucleus of cells. Instead, DNA sequences are wrapped around protein structures called histones, the basic building block of chromatin that is involved in packaging the approximately two-meter-long DNA helix into the cell nucleus. There are five basic forms of histone proteins: H1, H2A, H2B, H3, and H4 (Finch et al. 1977), and X-ray crystallography at the level of atomic resolution has demonstrated that two copies each of H2A, H2B, H3, and H4 form an octamer around which 146 bp of double-stranded DNA molecule wraps itself to form a nucleosome, the smallest unit of chromatin. The H1 protein plays a role in linking nucleosomes together to form structures, like beads on a string, called nucleosomes. The histone proteins undergo complex and reversible post-translational modifications at their N-terminal tail including methylation phosphorylation, acetylation, and ubiquitination tags (Shilatifard 2006). These modifications are dynamic and reversible reactions that can change the chromatin structure to determine how tightly or loosely they can package DNA to regulate gene expression. Some modifications are added by "writers" such as the addition of acetyl groups to lysine amino acids, other modifications are "erasers" that remove acetyl groups, whilst other post-translational modifications are "readers" that bind and engage the chromatin in different conformations. Specific patterns of histone modification form a "histone code" to delineate gene expression in spatial and temporal in a given cell type (Jenuwein and Allis 2001).

The importance of histone modification in regulating chromatin dynamics is exemplified by diverse array of modifying enzymes linked to transcriptional regulation. For instance, several transcriptional regulators have histone acetyltransferases (HATs) and deacetylases (HDACs). The HATs catalyzes acetylation of histone tail and thereby increases access for transcription. The acetylation of histone proteins is a predominant signal for the active chromatin (euchromatin) configuration (Lee et al. 1993; Perry and Chalkley 1982). The HDACs, on the other hand, catalyze deacetylation, removing acetyl groups from the histone tails, exposing the positively charged histone tail that interacts tightly with negatively charged DNA backbone and limit access to transcription [Heterochromatin or inactive state (Kuo and Allis 1998)] as depicted in Fig. 3.1. However, this is an over-simplistic explanation of the molecular mechanisms controlling histone modification as many

3.1 Introduction

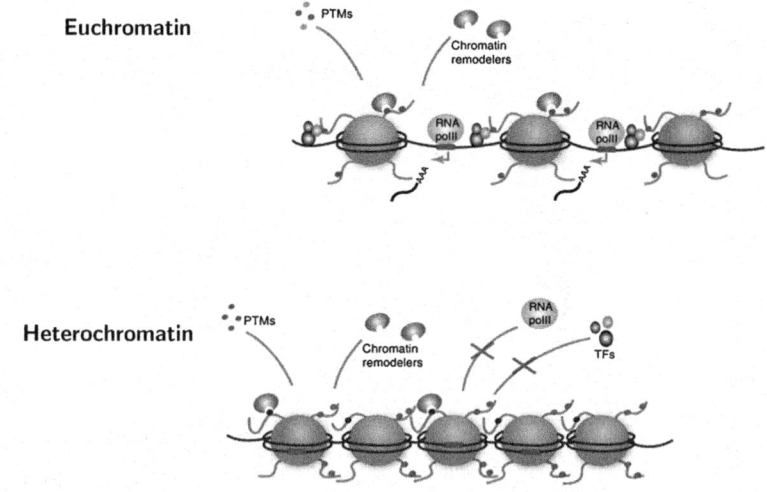

Fig. 3.1 Histone modification that creates euchromatin and heterochromatin states. Euchromatin is the active chromatin state that is maintained by post-translational modification (*PTMs*) of histones proteins by enzymes including Histone Acetylases (*HATs*) and enables access for transcription factors and the RNA-polymerase complex to direct transcription. Heterochromatin state is maintained by PTMs of the histone proteins by enzymes including Histone Deacetylases (*HDACs*), which prevent the access of transcription factors and RNA polymerase complex to ensure transcription. For simplicity in this diagram, chromatin remodelers are depicted as histone-modifying enzymes but would include ATP-dependent remodelers, histone-modifying enzymes, and other specialized macromolecular complexes that are important for maintaining a heterochromatin or euchromatin state. Copyright with permission: *Trends in Parasitology* 2012 28, 202–213. doi: (10.1016/j.pt.2012.02.009)

repressors and repressor-complexes play a role in recruiting HDACs that are responsible for the deacetylation of the histone proteins to inactivate chromatin and associated genes (Wolffe 1996).

3.1.2 microRNAs (miRNAs)

Another important epigenetic mechanism is the role of small non-coding RNA, termed "miRNA" (Bergmann and Lane 2003). The miRNAs are increasingly recognized as important players in gene regulation. The miRNAs are endogenous microRNAs, only 21–22 nucleotides in length, and function by binding to target mRNAs through sequence-specific base pairing and blocking translation (Alvarez-Garcia and Miska 2005), see Fig. 3.2. MiRNAs can inhibit the translation of multiple mRNAs because of imperfect pairing. Another non-coding microRNA referred to as siRNA is exogenous to the host cell (typically of viral origin). Unlike miRNAs, siRNAs binds perfectly to mRNA and therefore can only inhibit the

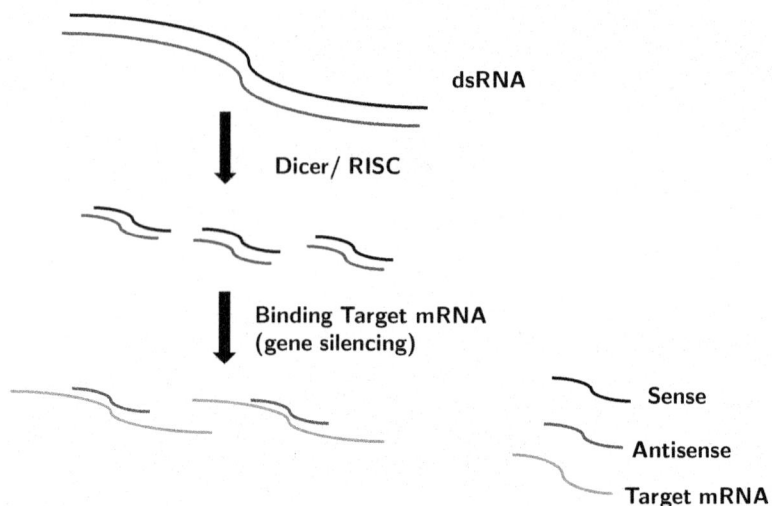

Fig. 3.2 Schematic diagram of microRNA function. Double stranded (*dsRNA*) RNA is processed into sense and antisense RNA, a processed catalyzed by dicer. The microRNAs then associate with RISC (RNA-induced silencing complex) and unwind. The antisense microRNA then associates with complementary single-stranded mRNA and degrade it to stop gene expression and subsequent translation

translation of its target mRNA. In addition, there are other less sequence-specific non-coding short and long RNAs with similar biological functions in blocking translation. Several reports have shown evidence of function for microRNAs and non-coding RNAs in embryogenesis, cell differentiation and organogenesis, cellular growth, programmed cell death, and human diseases (Alvarez-Garcia and Miska 2005) as discussed in Sects. 3.2–3.10.

3.1.3 DNA Methylation

DNA methylation is a heritable epigenetic process with diverse roles in cellular physiology including gene expression during development, genome stability, and imprinting, as well as the repression of endogenous retroviral and transposable elements. DNA methylation is perhaps the best known of the three epigenetic processes and the most studied with regards to its role in gene regulation. DNA methylation is a process whereby a methyl group donated by S-adenosyl-methionine is covalently added to a cytosine nucleotide to form 5-methylcytosine (5mC), a process catalyzed by DNA methyltransferases (DMNTs) (Razin 1998). In mammals and higher eukaryotes, the addition of methylation only occurs on a cytosine that precedes a guanine in a cytosine-phosphate-guanine (CpG) context. However, not all CpG are methylated, methylation occurs on distinct CpG sites, and there are cell- and tissue-type specific DNA methylation marks. This process generates cell-type specific patterns of methylation which contribute to the cellular phenotypic identity. There are at least three well-characterized DNMTs. DNMT1 whose substrate is hemimethylated DNA is referred to as the maintenance methyltransferase responsible for copying the methylation pattern to daughter cells during replication (Probst et al. 2009). In contrast to DNMT1, the other 2 DNMTs, namely, DNMT3A and DNMT3B, catalyze methylation on unmethylated CpG sites (Okano et al. 1999).

However, recent evidence indicates that there are redundancies in the biological activities of these DNMTs. The DNMT1 can catalyze de novo methylation and DNMT3A, and DNMT3B can also catalyze methylation on hemimethylated DNA during replication (Riggs and Xiong 2004). The DNMTs proteins are part of a growing list of over 100 genes including HATs, HDACs, histone methyltransferases (HMTs), histone demethylases (HDMTs), and chromatin remodeling enzymes that mediate the epigenetic events causing dynamic transcriptional control of gene expression (Miremadi et al. 2007). All of these enzymes play diverse roles in regulating gene expression (Miremadi et al. 2007). Similar to histone modification, the DNA methylation is a reversible biological process which has generated attention in developing therapeutic agents that can mimic the demethylase activity for disease treatment, e.g., 5-azacytidine which has been approved by the FDA for treatment of certain types of cancers including leukemia.

DNA methylation in association with histone modification and the cross-talk between these two processes play a key role in controlling biological processes and differentiation through influencing gene expression. Experimental findings demonstrate that the human genome is compartmentalized into the active euchromatin structure, which is loosely packed and associates with hypomethylated DNA, whereas the inactive heterochromatin structure is tightly packed and associates with hypermethylated DNA. This pattern of methylation is maintained by a dynamic balance of methylation and demethylation enzymes and specific histone modifications directed by gene-specific trans-acting factors that recruit chromatin-modifying enzymes to the local sites for regulating gene expression throughout life (Cervoni and Szyf 2001).

The process whereby DNA methylation leads to gene silencing can occur either by the direct binding inhibition of transcription factors that are sensitive to the methylation of their cognate CpG sequence (Comb and Goodman 1990). Or, an alternative process through which DNA methylation can lead to gene silencing is in response to DNMTs, in which case methylated DNA binding proteins such as MeCP2 and other proteins including HDACs are recruited to compact the chromatin structure making the DNA inaccessible for gene expression (Nan et al. 1997).

It is estimated that 0.75–1% of all the nucleotides in the normal human genome constitute 5mC, and approximately, 3–4% of all cytosines are methylated in the normal human genome (Esteller 2005). The CpG dinucleotides are not randomly distributed throughout the human genome; the majority of the human genome is depleted of CpG dinucleotide, and only a small region usually associated with 5′ untranslated region (UTR) and gene promoters for ∼60% of genes have dense CpG

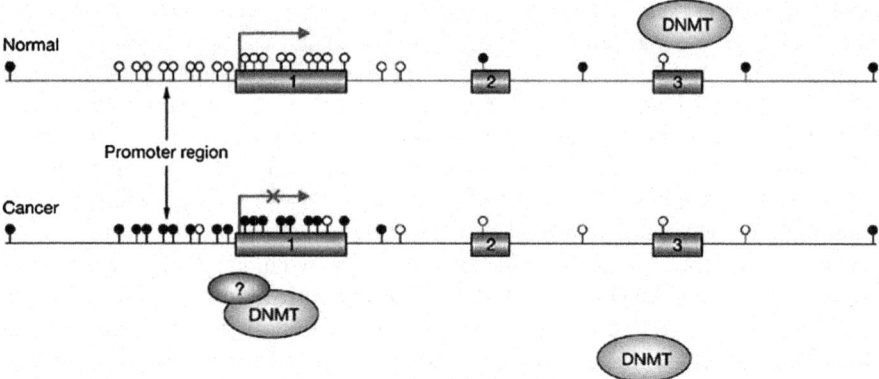

Fig. 3.3 Schematic diagram of DNA methylation process. A CpG site is depicted as a *circle*. The *solid circle* indicates DNA methylation catalyzed by DNMTs. *Open circles* depict unmethylated CpG sites. Majority of genome is depleted of CpGs. Only a small region associated with 5′ untranslated (5′ UTR) region has dense CpG sites known as CpG islands. In normal cells, the majority of the region is methylated, whereas in cancer cells the genome is no longer methylated but the 5′ UTR region associated with over 60% of genes are now methylated and leads to gene silencing. Copyright with permission: Nature Clinical Oncology (2005) 2; S4–S11

dinucleotides, these are referred to as CpG-rich regions or CpG islands, and DNA methylation of these CpG islands is associated with control of gene expression (Bird 2002). For instance, in almost all mammalian cells, there is a high level of methylation in repetitive sequences such as transposon. Transposons are specialized intragenic parasites, and methylation of their promoter region is associated with inactivation of transposable elements (Bird 2002). Eckhardt et al. (2006) have shown that one-third of the gene-specific promoter regions analyzed on three different chromosomes demonstrated an inverse correlation of DNA methylation and gene expression. The DNA promoter hypermethylation was associated with down-regulation of gene expression, whereas promoter hypomethylated correlated with increased gene expression. Thus, the current scientific evidence demonstrates an important role for DNA methylation in normal human development, and defects in the DNA methylation process is increasingly found to be associated with the development of a number of diseases, particularly cancers (Fig. 3.3).

3.2 Epigenetics and Development

During embryogenesis, the embryonic stem (ES) maintains unlimited replicative potential while retaining the ability to differentiate into functionally distinct cell types (Bibikova et al. 2008). Since the DNA sequence information is the same, the pluripotency capacity indicates that these processes are controlled by epigenetic mechanisms in conjunction with transcriptional regulatory machinery for proper development.

3.2 Epigenetics and Development

A role for microRNAs in embryonic development has been reported that is based on the observation that several transcription factors, namely: OCT4, SOX2 and NANOG that play essential roles in early development, are targets for multiple miRNAs to regulate their transcriptional activity (Boyer et al. 2005). Additional evidence of a role for miRNAs in development comes from the observation that ES cells that are deficient in dicer, the enzyme required to process double stranded RNA into miRNA transcript were unable to differentiate ES cells. On the other hand, re-expression on dicer into these mutant ES cells was able to rescue this phenotype, demonstrating that miRNA plays a role in ES differentiation (Kanellopoulou et al. 2005). The role for miRNA in development is not well understood, but there is increasing interest in its role in development and disease states.

The enzymes that catalyze histones modification have also been shown to play important roles in embryonic development. Transgenic mice that have been engineered to have a mutant HDAC1 gene causes a variety of embryonic lethality with several growth defects and retardation. Similarly, transgenic HDAC2 mutant mice are only able to survive for 24 h and die from severe cardiac malformation (Haberland et al. 2009). In addition, the polycomb group (PcG) of proteins, which play biological roles in gene repression by catalyzing histone modification, have also been reported to be required for ES cell self-renewal and pluripotency (Boyer et al. 2005). The PcG proteins were originally discovered to be key regulators of homeotic (Hox) genes during development for the normal body segmentation of *Drosophila melanogaster*.

In addition to miRNAs and histone modifications, an essential role for DNA methylation during embryonic development is well established, and programmed changes in patterns of the cytosine methylation during embryogenesis suggest that methylation may play an important role in cell-fate specification. Direct evidence that DNA methylation is involved in embryonic development is demonstrated by transgenic mice studies where deficiency in DNMTs activity resulted in embryonic lethality at approximately day E9 (Razin and Shemer 1995). Different embryonic developmental stages are associated with different genome-wide pattern of DNA methylation that may serve as general signals for gene activation/inactivation. For instance, early embryonic stages of development are characterized by dramatic changes of genome-wide DNA demethylation, and, then during later stages in development, there is methylation in most tissue-specific genes.

Additional evidence for the importance of DNA methylation during embryogenesis is provided by other studies on mice, which demonstrates that parental genomes undergo dramatic reprogramming of DNA methylation patterns after fertilization (Mayer et al. 2000). For instance, male sperm undergoes significant demethylation within 6–8 h after fertilization, whereas the female genome undergoes demethylation after several embryonic cell divisions (Mayer et al. 2000). It is hypothesized that the genome-wide demethylation may erase epigenetic information that was present in the highly differentiated genes, providing a new developmental program that may be required to establish a pluripotent state before specific cell-lineages can be determined. However, this global demethylation and re-establishment of the methylation status does not include imprinted genes, whose methylation status is maintained throughout this process (Branco et al. 2008).

3.3 Neuronal Development and Disease

There are reports to demonstrate epigenetic regulation of neuronal-specific genes, noting that such genes are characterized by DNA-sequence motifs known as silencer elements (RE1/NRSE). The RE1/NRSE sequence motif restricts neuronal-specific gene transcription in non-neuronal cells by transcriptional control of RE1-silencing transcription factor (REST) (Huang et al. 1999). To accomplish blocking in the expression of these neuron-specific genes, REST recruits the transcriptional co-repressor Sin3A and HDAC to the regulatory domains of genes containing RE1/NRSE elements to form heterochromatin and silence the expression of these genes. Other recent findings support an important role for REST in neurogenesis. This is demonstrated by the expression of REST that correlates with normal aging of human cortical and hippocampal neurons, whereas the loss of REST is linked to mild cognitive impairment and Alzheimer's disease (Lu et al. 2014). In addition, REST is reported to play a role in activating genes that protect neurons from oxidative stress and B-amyloid protein toxicity, as well as repressing genes that promote cell death (Lu et al. 2014) by modulating histone modifications and associated co-repressors.

The importance of epigenetic mechanisms in neuronal development is exemplified by aberrant epigenetic alterations and neurological diseases. A role for aberrant epigenetic changes in neurological diseases has been known for more two decades, when it was first discovered that an X-linked dominant mutation in methyl-CpG-binding protein 2 (MeCP2) was responsible for causing the progressive neurological condition known as Rett syndrome (Amir et al. 1999). Other reports have described an association of DNA mutations in MeCPs or loss of expression with conditions such as autism (Ben Zeev 2007; Nagarajan et al. 2006). Mutations in a family of protein called SNF2, which has a biological function in chromatin remodeling, have been shown to be associated with a severe X-linked form of mental retardation known as ATRX (ATR-X syndrome associated with alpha thalassemia) (Picketts et al. 1996). The role of epigenetic changes in neuronal development and disease states is providing new insights into the nervous system in health and disease states. Because epigenetic changes are reversible with pharmacological interventions, the role of epigenetics in neuronal diseases holds great promise for the development of epigenetic-based, novel diagnostic and therapeutic approaches for targeting neurological diseases.

Other reports have implicated epigenetic changes in learning and a variety of neuropsychiatric disorders including depression. The process of learning includes memory encoding, storage, and retrieval of information; this process requires signals and the molecular cascade activation of NMDA receptors, protein kinases, and phosphatases, as well as specific transcription factors. In addition, epigenetic DNA methylation and histone modifications, which together regulate chromatin structure, are also important players in this cascade reaction.

Research data on the role of epigenetics in neuronal development has largely come from animal studies. To demonstrate a role for epigenetics in neuronal plasticity, rat models were induced to exhibit a conditional fear-freezing phenotype (Levenson et al. 2006; Miller and Sweatt 2007). To accomplish this, rats were treated with the pharmacological DNMT inhibitor 5-aza-deoxycytidine and the histone deacetylase inhibitor Trichostatin A, drugs that are able to reverse epigenetic DNA methylation and histone modification respectively and to reactivate gene expression. In the rats treated with the drugs, the treatment was able to rescue rats from the fear-freezing condition in comparison to control animals that were not treated with the drugs, suggesting that these drugs can enhance memory and synaptic plasticity. Other reports indicate that epigenetics play a role in another mental disorder, schizophrenia. In vitro studies demonstrated that treatment of mammalian cells with 5-azacytidine and/or Trichostatin A induces the expression of reelin whose deficiency is associated with schizophrenia (Chen et al. 2002; Costa et al. 2002).

Although there have been advances in elucidating the role of epigenetics in neuronal development and diseases, the role of epigenetic changes associated with adult neurodegenerative diseases such as Alzheimer's, which is ranked in the top-10 leading causes of health disparities in USA, falls behind genomic studies where tremendous advances have been made in identifying may loci linked to Alzheimer's-disease disparity. Thus research focus needs to be directed towards unraveling epigenetic changes in Alzheimer's disease for effective therapeutic intervention.

3.4 Epigenetics Changes, Aging, and Disease Disparities

Aging is a phenomenon which involves a host of cellular processes including senescence and telomere shortening. It is well known that the epigenome is quite stable and heritable, but it can also be dynamic, with changes overtime suggesting that epigenetic changes may constitute an important component of the aging process. There are few reports that have looked at the epigenetic changes throughout childhood and adolescence, whereas most of the studies have focused on either developmental stages and/or disease states. A study by Adkins et al. (2011) that investigated genome-wide methylation changes in cord blood from newborn African-American (AA) and European-American (EA) babies identified significant differences in DNA methylation patterns for several gene loci suggesting that perhaps exposure associated with maternal diets or other in utero environmental exposures (discussed in Sect. 10.2) may have caused the observed differences in the newborns.

The association between epigenetic changes with aging has been observed in fish, rat, mice, and humans. In humans, global and gradual decrease of genomic DNA demethylation (hypomethylation), as well as the hypermethylation of gene specific-promoter regions in combination with histone modification and non-coding RNAs (e.g., miRNAs), have been shown to contribute to aging (Rodriguez-Rodero et al. 2010). This author and others have reported an increase in DNA methylation changes as a function of age in prostate and colon tissues (Issa 2000; Kwabi-Addo 2007). In addition, significant differences in DNA methylation of gene-specific loci in various ethnic and racial groups have been reported. In a survey of gene-specific DNA methylation changes in normal prostate tissues from AA and EA men, we observed higher methylation for two genes: TIMP3 and NKX2-5 in the AA samples, in comparison to EA samples (Kwabi-Addo et al. 2010). The TIMP3 gene encodes for the tissue inhibitor of metalloproteinase inhibitor 3, NKX2-5 belongs to the homeobox family of transcription factors, and these have potential tumor-suppressing function in mammalian cells.

The mechanisms whereby epigenetic patterns changes as a function of age is not clear, but several reports have suggested that, as individual ages, there are changes in gene expression which correlate with changes in the expression of DMNTs, HATs, and HDACs. For instance, the expression of sirtuin family of histone deactylases have emerged as sensors of cellular energy, and this is associated with aging, age-related diseases, and diverse cellular and molecular processes including genomic stability, senescence, DNA repair, stem-cell exhaustion, and metabolic homeostasis (Carmona and Michan 2016). Studies carried out in transgenic mice models indicate that over-expression of sirtuins may be associated with normal learning and memory and may also promote longevity (Carmona and Michan 2016).

Age-related diseases such as the Hutchinson-Gilford progeria (HGP) and Werner syndrome (WS) provide excellent models to investigate the role of epigenetic alterations in these two premature-aging conditions. Scientific advances in cutting-edge and high-throughput technologies such as genome-wide DNA methylation array are making it possible to query all the methylation sites in the human genome. This technology, in addition to the next-generation sequencing tools described in Chap. 2, has made possible the characterization of DNA methylation substrates throughout the human genome and throughout lifetime, beginning at conception.

Using genome-wide DNA methylation analysis on lymphoblastoid cell lines derived from patients with age-related diseases has demonstrated profound changes in DNA methylation patterns, suggesting a role for epigenetic alteration in premature aging (Heyn et al. 2013a). Furthermore, genome-wide analysis of human peripheral blood leukocytes from healthy individuals aged 4–94 years has demonstrated small age-dependent decreases in DNA methylation, whereas similar methylation analysis in human-placenta DNA at various gestational ages exhibited a gestation-dependent increase in DNA methylation (Fuke et al. 2004). This study observed differential methylation levels at the global genomic level in individuals in the study population. Because DNA methylation is influenced by environmental factors, such as diet or exposure to infectious agents and excessive hormones, the differences in methylation levels could reflect differences in the exposure to various environmental factors (discussed in Chap. 12). In addition, differences in methylation levels observed in individuals in the study cohort could be explained by inherent genetic factors involved in metabolic processes of external exposures, as well as genetic variation in epigenetic factors, including DNMTs.

Other reports of DNA methylation analysis at the gene-specific loci or genome-wide level, in addition to histone acetylation analysis in monozygotic twins, has revealed that although twins have indistinguishable epigenetic patterns during the early years of life, older monozygotic twins' demonstrated remarkably different DNA methylation distributed throughout their genome and histone acetylation patterns (Fraga et al. 2005a). Since monozygotic twins share a common genotype, the differences in epigenetic patterns later in life suggests an environmental rather than genetic basis for the lifelong epigenetic changes, and these differences could partly demonstrate susceptibility to adult or age-related diseases.

Current findings from DNA methylation studies suggest that it may be possible to predict health outcomes based on an individual's epigenetic signature: for instance, individuals who are epigenetically old or young relative to individuals, who display concordant epigenetic and chronological ages, could be predictive of health outcomes. One report investigating DNA methylation changes and longevity found a slower age-related global DNA methylation pattern for centenarians compared to non-long-lived individuals (Gentilini et al. 2013). Interestingly, genes that were differentially methylated in the two groups included genes that function in development, nucleotide biosynthesis, metabolism, and control of signal transmission. It is well known that exposure to environmental risk factors such as diet, smoking hormones, and conditions such as obesity—factors that actually decreases life expectancy of an individual—are associated with increases in aberrant DNA methylation events and aging in both men and women, suggesting that if we can better preserve the methylation of these processes, it may be possible to slowdown aging.

The process of DNA methylation changes is under the control of several factors extrinsic to the cell and, given that epigenetic mechanisms are reversible, the epigenetic mechanism may reflect the stochastic aspect of aging. Beginning with ES cells, there are reports that the polycomb target genes that are essential in targeting ES cells to regulate cellular differentiation and development undergo DNA methylation as a function of age (Hahn et al. 2008). Adult stem cells are indispensable for normal tissue homeostasis; repair and decline in stem-cell functions are related to aging; there is evidence of epigenetic alterations in aging of adult stem cells; and this too may play a role in regulating life span (Liu and Rando 2011).

The biological consequence of DNA hypermethylation in stem cells is the gene silencing of critical genes essential for self-renewal. This can result in the depletion of the stem-cell pool in an age-dependent manner. On the other hand, DNA hypomethylation in stem cells leads to the aberrant activation of genes whose expressions are normally restricted in stem cells (Shen et al. 2007). Therefore aberrant epigenetic changes in stem cells can increase the propensity of the cellular genomic instability that is associated with several common age-related diseases. One important family of enzymes, known as the Sirtuin protein family of deacetylase (mentioned above), is responsible for the deacetylation of many proteins, including histones, and has been associated with protection from several age-related diseases. The biological activities of sirtuins are increased when the ratio between nicotinamide adenine dinucleotide and nicotinamide adenine dinucleotide dehydrogenase is high. This enzyme-substrate complex plays a role in dietary metabolism thus linking chromatin regulation to dietary restriction and exercise (Stein 2012 1336/id), suggesting environmental interventions that can target diet can slow or delay aging.

Other reports have identified key transcription factors that can regulate age-related transcriptional changes including the GATA transcription factor family. The expression levels of these transcription factors are reduced in association with aging, and this involves epigenetic processes. The *Caenorhabditis elegans* (the worm *C. elegans*) has been used as a model to study the transcriptional network that is dysregulated in association with aging. Experimentations using old *C. elegans* that have been engineered to overexpress these transcription factors reversed their aging process to a young state (Brunet 2014; Mann 2016). This model has been instrumental in studying age-dependent dysfunction of vital organs such as the heart and kidney. In the kidney, some of this age-associated transcription factors are also involved in inflammation, and, because methylation is reversible, this offers the exciting possibility to alter the trajectory of age-dependent trajectory of organ failure.

A model proposed by Jean-Pierre Issa predicts that human stem cells begin life with a relatively uniform epigenetic code. As humans develop into adulthood, the aging process and associated exposure to various environmental factors, such as diet, toxins, and infection, alters the epigenetic information in a subset of stem cells. Over time and in addition to other exposures, epigenetic mosaicism develops in patches of cells with consequential changes in gene expression. The cumulative changes in these selected patches of cells favor increased cell proliferation, reduced apoptosis, and/or altered differentiation, promoting the acquisition of further molecular changes (epigenetic and genetic) that ultimately result in various diseases, including cancer (Issa 2014).

DNA methylation is not the only epigenetic phenomenon that progresses in an age-dependent manner. At least one report has demonstrated changes in the expression of microRNAs (mir-21 and let 7) in association with age, suggesting that mir-21 and let 7 may provide a potential link between cancer and aging by modulating NF-kB signals in senescence and the inflammation that are also characteristic of the aging (Catana et al. 2015). Although there is no report of differential microRNAs expression and aging in various ethnic/racial groups, as discussed in Sect. 2.4, other reports have shown differential expression of microRNAs (including mir-21 and let-7) in AA and EA prostate cancer patients to support a role for microRNA in aging and cancer among these two groups.

Because epigenetics DNA methylation changes affect gene expression in an age-dependent and tissue specific manner (Issa 2000; Kwabi-Addo et al. 2007), this age-associated epigenetic alterations can alter cellular physiology and potentially predispose to disease. Thus, differences in DNA methylation patterns observed in individuals belonging to one population group or different populations could underlie differences in susceptibility to some epigenetically influenced age-related diseases, such as cancer, which differ in incidence and mortality rates in various racial and ethnic groups (Issa 2000).

3.5 Cardiovascular Disease Disparity

The mammalian heart consists of four chambers forming the left ventricle (LV), left atrium (LA), right ventricle (RV), and right atrium. Differential gene-expression signatures exquisitely control the complex and intricate process of the development of these heart chambers during embryonic development through to adulthood. For instance, there are activations of several genes, including the proto-oncogenes and early growth-response genes, such as atrial natriuretic peptide (ANP), as well as the beta-myosin chain during heart development, and then the silencing of these genes' expression at maturity (Lakatta and Sollott 2002). On the other hand, abnormal heart conditions, such as myocardial hypertrophy dysfunction and heart failure, is linked to the activation of multiple signaling pathways that transduce mechanical and hormonal stimuli associated with these conditions (Tan et al. 2002). However, the molecular mechanisms regulating the distinct gene expression that are critically linked to the formation of the unique heart chambers are not well known.

Recent studies by two groups (Mathiyalagan et al. 2010; Tan et al. 2002) have demonstrated that there are distinct epigenetic patterns associated with the development of LV and RV muscular chambers in mice. In their examination of epigenetic mediated gene expression, they observed increased expression of ANP and beta-type natriuretic peptide (BNP) to be associated with distinct histone modifications, including increased histone acetylation and demethylation in the LV in comparison with the RV. Since the combination of histone acetylation and demethylation is linked to increased gene expression, this suggests that distinct epigenetic markers could regulate the differential gene expression in the different chambers. Other studies have indicated a role for DNA methylation and miRNA in influencing heart diseases as observed by different epigenome patterns in patient with different disease states in comparison with control patients who do not have such conditions (Lorenzen et al. 2012; Tan et al. 2002).

While there is little evidence of the role of epigenetic alterations and CVD disparities, AA population are disproportionately affected by CVDs. The risk factors are not well known, but some reports suggest that the intrauterine environment (such as pre-natal nutrition) and other early-life exposures are important indicators of adult cardiovascular health (see Chap. 10). Thus, lifetime exposures, in particular in utero and childhood exposures, could have long-term impact on the epigenetic mechanisms involved in the disparities associated with CVDs.

3.6 Obesity Disparity

Obesity is associated with increase in adipose-tissue deposits, which can contribute to inflammation, oxidative stress, insulin resistance, and hypertension, explaining why obesity is a risk factor for diabetes, atherosclerosis, CVD, and some types of cancer. Although obesity is a commonly diagnosed condition, certain ethnic populations appear to be more susceptible than others to the condition. As a typical complex disease, obesity is associated with both external (environmental) and internal (genetic) factors (Anon 2000). Genetic defects associated with imprinting are linked to development disorders and clinical symptoms including abnormal body weight. A classic example of genetic cause of morbid obesity in children is Prader-Willi syndrome, which is caused by abnormal epigenetic imprinting of genes associated with energy balance (Shapira et al. 2005; Tan et al. 2002). However, since genetic variation does not adequately explain the variability in fat mass observed in various individuals, epigenetics has been proposed as an alternative molecular mechanism mediating this process. Despite the importance of epigenetic mechanisms, there are few reports of the role of epigenetic alterations and obesity.

One epigenome-wide-association-study (EWAS) analysis of obese and normal-weight preadolescent girls identified several differentially methylated in genes that are associated with obesity. Significant methylation changes were observed for KARS, TERF2IP, PEX1, MSI1, STON1, and BCAS3 genes in individuals who had genetic variants in fat mass and the obesity-associated (FTO) gene (Almen et al. 2012), suggesting an association between DNA methylation and genetic variants for regulating gene expression in certain conditions (discussed in more details in Sect. 3.11). The FTO gene is reported to have the strongest association with obesity. Although, its biological function is not well known, it has been shown to remove the methyl group from nucleic acids in vitro, indicating that FTO association with obesity could be mediated through epigenetic mechanisms (Almen et al. 2012). Other recent EWAS of 14,000 genes in peripheral blood leukocytes (related to obesity-induced immune dysfunction) observed differential methylation patterns for lean adolescents in comparison with obese adolescents (Feinberg et al. 2010; Wang et al. 2010).

Not many epigenetic studies have been carried out in AA populations, despite the high prevalence of obesity in this population in comparison with other racial and ethnic groups in the USA. To find out about the role of epigenetic alterations and increased obesity in AA population, Demerath et al. (2015) carried out an EWAS using genomic DNA samples extracted from blood leukocytes obtained from 2097 AA adults as part of the Atherosclerosis Risk in Community (ARIC) study, a prospective cohort study of CVD risk in four US communities (The ARIC Investigators 1989). Using various statistical models, such as mixed-effect regression models that analyze methylation frequency in association with body mass index (BMI) and waist circumference (WC), they observed significant methylation of genes that are predominantly associated with energy and other diverse signal pathways. For instance, several genes involved in lipid metabolism showed significant methylation, including: CPT1A which is involved in mitochondria uptake of long-chain fatty acids and triglyceride metabolism; ABCG1 which is involved in macrophage cholesterol and phospholipids transport; and HIF3A which regulates cells' adaptive responses to hypoxia, as well as lipid homeostasis. Other methylated genes identified in this study play key roles in immune response/cytokine signaling and diverse signaling pathways. A previous study identified and replicated methylation alterations with BMI that had been reported in an obesity study in EA blood and adipose tissue, in which methylation of the HIF3A was identified (Dick et al. 2014). Large-scale studies involving various ethnic and racial groups are needed in order to gain more insight into the role of epigenetic alterations associated with obesity, as well as to develop novel therapies to reduce or reverse this condition.

3.7 Type 2 Diabetes Disparity

Diabetes has a strong genetic-predisposition risk factor, and genetic variations associated with this condition can in part explain the differences in frequency of diabetes risk in individuals belonging to one population or different populations, as discussed in Chap. 2. In addition to genetic factors, there is also a strong environmental component to diabetes risk, such as a sedentary lifestyle and obesity (insulin-resistant obesity), suggesting that epigenetic events could provide a mechanism for translating the environmental exposures into the disease pathogenesis.

Comprehensive DNA methylation analysis of 254 genes on genome DNA samples, isolated from freshly isolated pancreatic beta-islet that were obtained from type 2 diabetes (T2D) or non-diabetic human cadaveric donors, demonstrated that significant alterations in DNA methylation are associated with T2D diabetes (Volkmar et al. 2012). Volkmar et al. observed significant methylation in genes associated with DNA damage, oxidative stress, hormonal signals, and that the metabolic pathways were enriched in the T2D samples. Specifically, aberrant hypermethylation of genes with functional roles in insulin signaling such as CDK5 and GRB10 and potassium-channel genes (KCNE2, KNNJ1, and KCNK16) were also associated with T2D. Some genes that were hypomethylation in T2D included genes related to DNA damage and oxidative stress (GSTPI and ALDH3B1). Because diabetes is significantly associated with hyperglycemia, it is likely that the aberrant methylation phenomenon observed here is secondary to hyperglycemic conditions in their study cohort. However, Volkmar et al. (2012) demonstrated that exposure of non-diabetic human cells to high glucose stress did not modify methylation patterns, suggesting that aberrant DNA methylation was probably not the causative mechanism of T2D in their study population.

Other studies suggest a role for histone modifying enzymes, specifically a role for sirtuin1, a multifunctional histone deacetylase with diverse and critical roles in stress responses, cellular metabolism, and energy metabolism as discussed in Sect. 3.4. Zheng et al. (2012) demonstrated that hyperglycemia decreased the expression of Sirtuin1, whereas the over-expression of Sirtuin1 was able to decrease hyperglycemia stress markers and reactive oxygen species, suggesting that aberrant histone modifications may be associated with diabetes.

A role for epigenetic miRNAs has been shown in diabetes. Studies have demonstrated that miRNAs are involved in normal pancreatic development and is important in insulin signals, insulin resistance, and energy metabolisms in various target organs including, adipose, liver, skeletal, endothelial and angiogenesis, as well as cardiac tissues. Specifically, the loss of miR-375 that is most abundant in islet cells leads to increase insulin secretion, whereas the over-expression of miR-375 impairs insulin secretion. Furthermore, miR-375 knockout mice are hyperglycemic and glucose intolerant demonstrating that miRNAs play a role in the pathogenesis of diabetes (Shantikumar et al. 2012).

Epigenetic studies lag behind genetic studies (such as GWAS) in elucidating a role for epigenetics in the disparity associated with diabetes and other diseases. While GWAS studies have identified genetic variants associated with increased susceptibility to diabetes in the AA population, very few epigenetic studies have demonstrated differential epigenetic changes and an association with an increased prevalence of diabetes in the AA population. Rather, epigenetic studies of complex disease disparities, such as cancer, have included diabetes as a co-morbid condition in their studies (see Sect. 3.10). For instance, a genome-wide methylation analysis of a case-control study from the Israel Diabetes Research Group identified methylation of a CpG site in the first intronic region of the FTO gene (Toperoff et al. 2012). Hypomethylation of this intronic CpG site occurred at low frequency but varied significantly in cases compared to control samples. Methylation at this CpG site could potentially influence gene expression by interfering with transcription factors that are methylation sensitive. Thus differential methylation in the FTO gene and other genes in individuals and different populations could influence individual susceptibility diabetes.

3.8 Chronic Kidney Disease Disparity

Another disease with higher prevalence among the US AA population is chronic kidney disease (CKD). The risk of CKD is associated with several factors including diabetes, hypertension, obesity, high cholesterol level, smoking, and CVD-conditions that are all linked to inflammation.

The human kidney is a heterogeneous organ consisting of various cell types. Epigenetic factors, in particular histone modification and chromatin remodeling, have been implicated in the development of the kidney organ. One study observed that DNA-binding proteins, such as Pax2/8, and cis-acting factors that are essential for differentiating intermediate mesoderm and renal epithelial lineage are also essential for establishing kidney-specific fates via mechanisms that modulate histone methylation and chromatin remodeling (Dressler 2008). Chronic renal disease is associated with age and, in the glomerulus, aging podocytes exhibit age-related epigenetic phenomenon with correlated changes in gene expression and structural morphology that is associated with renal diseases (Dressler 2008).

Typically CKD disorder is assessed by estimating blood markers, such as creatinine, in combination with demographic factors such as (age, sex, and ethnicity) as an indicator for the glomerular filtration rate (GFR; estimating GFR-eGFR), which is a reflection of kidney function. One DNA methylation study carried out by Bomotti et al. (2013) analyzed 14,000 genes using blood DNA samples from 972 AA-patient blood samples from the Genetic Epidemiology Network of Arteriopathy (GENOA) study. The GENOA study is a community-based genomic study of hypertension and arteriosclerosis complications. Bomotti et al. observed that the majority of differential methylated genes that were associated with eGFR in their AA patient population were genes encoding for proteins with biological functions in human aging, inflammation, and cholesterol pathways. One top candidate gene was KLF2, a Kruppel-like transcription factor which plays a role in regulating vasculature processing and the kidney glomerular capillary bed. This study provides an epigenetic basis to link inflammation and CKD in the AA population.

Another study investigated epigenetic changes in kidney tissue injury, also known as acute kidney injury (AKI). Acute kidney injury contributes to the decline in renal function and is a risk factor for chronic kidney disease and death. The AKI is primarily caused by chronic inflammation as host pro-inflammatory cytokines/kenokines, such as TNF-alpha, are upregulated in AKI. Several reports have suggested a role for chromatin remodeling and aberrant histone modification in the activation of pro-inflammatory cytokines, as well as aberrant DNA methylation of interferon gamma-response element in AKI (Bomsztyk and Denisenko 2013). Other reports suggest aberrant epigenetic changes in renal cell carcinoma. For instance, one report demonstrated that secreted frizzled-related protein 5, a negative regulator of Wnt signaling pathway, is down-related by DNA methylation and histone modification (Kawakami et al. 2011), and this could potentially contribute to renal-cell carcinogenesis. Thus, epigenetic mechanisms play diverse roles in kidney development, as well as in the disease state, and could potentially underlie the differential susceptibility seen in different ethnic and racial groups.

3.9 HIV Disease Disparity

A role for aberrant epigenetic changes during microbial infection has been suggested by several scientific findings. For instance *Helicobacter pylori* infection, a major causative agent in gastric cancer, has been shown to increase DNMTs expression and hypermethylation of E-Cadherin (an adhesion molecular of cell invasion and migration), thereby increasing gastric carcinogenesis. Similarly, gastric adenocarcinoma that contains Epstein-Barr virus (EBV) was observed to have loss of expression of p16 protein, as detected by immunohistochemical staining and the mechanism of gene inactivation by DNA methylation (Vo et al. 2002). In addition, Vo et al. (2002) identified differences in EBV infection by sex and ethnic group. Males were observed to have a significantly higher rate of EBV infection, and the prevalence of EBV infection was higher among Hispanics than in the AA or EA populations, suggesting that the disparity of viral-mediated gastric cancer may be caused by epigenetic alterations.

The HIV virus is a cytopathic retrovirus which causes acquired immunodeficiency syndrome (AIDs). The life cycle of the HIV virus and its ability to establish a prolonged latent period of infection in the host system are important for the pathogenesis of full-blown AIDs disease. For instance, during infection, the single-stranded HIV viral RNA is converted to double stranded, a process catalyzed by the host reverse transcriptase, which then integrates the viral DNA into the host genome (provirus) to establish latency. For latency to be established, transcription from the HIV promoter is switched off, and a potential role for epigenetic changes in repressing transcription from the HIV promoter in order to establish latency has been proposed. Some reports indicate a role for histone posttranslational deacetylation and methylation in establishing latency of HIV-1 infection by repressing gene expression from the HIV-1 (Imai 2011). The factors responsible for switching from latency to lysis are unknown. Mikovits et al. observed that HIV infection of $CD4^+$ T-cells in in vitro down-regulated interferon gamma (IFNy) expression (Mikovits et al. 1998). In parallel, there was an increase of DMNTs expression, and the methylation level of the IFN-y promoter was also elevated. Other recent observations suggest a role of microRNAs in modulating HIV-1 gene expression in favor of establishing latency, whereas HIV-1 infection increases DNMTs expression, inducing hypermethylation and silencing of several proteins, including interferon-gamma, thereby blocking host immune response (Ay 2013). Epigenetic therapy based on HIV proviral infection is currently being explored as an attractive alternative for HIV/AIDs treatment. One report has indicated differential methylation of GPR15 gene in AA and EA HIV patients who smoke (Dogan et al. 2015 1337/id). The GPR15 encodes for the chemokine receptor and the co-receptor for HIV that may facilitate efficient transport of certain strains of HIV-1, HIV-2, and SIV, suggesting that differential methylation of the GRP15 gene may contribute to differences in the prevalence of HIV infection under certain environmental exposures, such as tobacco smoke.

3.10 Cancer Disparities

Most cancers arise by multifactorial interactions of genetic, epigenetic, and environmental factors (the role of gene-environment interaction in disease is discussed in Chap. 10). Epigenetic changes affect genomic stability and gene expression, which can result in cellular growth advantage, thereby promoting carcinogenesis from initiation through progression. The role of epigenetic processes—DNA methylation, histone modification, and miRNAs during organogenesis, aging, and diseases such as CVDs, diabetes, CKD, and HIV—have been discussed in previous sections. However, most of the ground-breaking findings of the important role for epigenetic changes have come from studies in cancer research. Epigenetic alterations that are relevant to cancer risk are believed to occur early in the disease pathway, which might be the first hint in the pathway of genomic instability and associated genomic alterations, such as mutations, deletions and chromosomal amplifications, and/or translocation.

Evidence supporting that aberrant epigenetic DNA methylation occurs early in the disease pathway comes from the observation that a number of genes, the so-called epigenetic gate keepers, exhibit DNA hypermethylation in pre-invasive stages of colon and other cancers, but rarely in the pre-invasive cancers. This indicates that the normal methylation of such genes may be necessary to prevent stem/precursor cells from becoming immortalized and acquiring infinite cell-renewal capacity, whilst, at the same time, allowing genes to be activated when needed (Jones and Baylin 2007). Another example of the importance of DNA methylation changes in early stages of cancer is demonstrated for the DNA methylation of π-class glutathione S-transferase (GSTP1), whose protein product encodes for carcinogen detoxification enzyme. This gene is inactivated by hypermethylation in more than 90% of prostate cancers, with hypermethylation appearing early and more consistently than other genetic defects in the disease pathway (Nelson et al. 2003), suggesting that DNA hypermethylation may be particularly important in prostate carcinogenesis (Gonzalgo et al. 1997; Zingg and Jones 1997).

Most epigenetic studies of cancer have focused on transcriptional silencing by DNA methylation because it has been demonstrated that aberrant CpG-rich promoter regions (CpG islands) can permanently silence genes that play important physiological and pathological roles in mammalian cell cultures (Feinberg and Tycko 2004; Jones and Baylin 2002). The role of DNA methylation has been extensively studied in colon, breast, pancreatic, ovarian, and prostate cancer, as well as other cancer types. Toyota et al. (1999) used methylated CpG-island amplification (MCA) to identify a distinct methylation signature involving a group of CpG-island promoters that were differentially methylated in colorectal cancers, which they called "CpG-island methylator phenotype" or CIMP, suggesting that large stretches of DNA can become abnormally methylated in cancer.

Recent findings indicate that several genes that are repressed during ES differentiation have these CIMP loci and are candidates for reversible methylation by stem-cell-associated polycomb groups of proteins (see Sect. 3.4). Aberrant methylation at these CIMPs could lock ES cells in perpetual self-renewal and initiate carcinogenesis supporting a role for the stem-cell origin of cancer (Widschwendter et al. 2007). Other supporting reports by Hansen et al. (2011) indicate that cancer-specific differential DNA methylation regions (cDMRs) in colon, breast, lung, thyroid, and Wilms tumors are distinguishable from normal cells. Most of the genes in these methylated regions are involved in mitosis and matrix remodeling, indicating that the carcinogenesis pathway involves aberrant epigenetic alterations that increase genomic instability of well-defined genomic domains. In addition to the importance of DNA methylation in cancer, the focus in the field recently has shifted to investigate the potential roles of histone modification and miRNA, as well as nucleosome remodeling in carcinogenesis. A link between all these epigenetic processes, in particular histone modification and DNA methylation, is also established.

Recent technological advances in epigenetic tools to query the entire human genome are providing more insights into the epigenetic changes in cancer. Genome-wide changes of histone modification, in particular the deacetylation of histone H4 lysine 16 and the trimethylation of the lysine 20, are now established as a hallmark of human cancer (Fraga et al. 2005b). Other reports suggest more global histone-modification patterns in association with PCa recurrence (Seligson et al. 2005). The polycomb gene BMI, a member of polycomb repressor complex that was already mentioned, is overexpressed in multiple cancers and suggests that it may perhaps contribute to gene silencing of regulatory proteins in cancer cells by catalyzing histone methylation (Valk-Lingbeek et al. 2004).

The accumulating epigenetic data indicates that several hundreds of genes may be inactivated in a single cancer cell, suggesting a nuance of epigenetic abnormalities that affect a network of multiple genes which affect multiple signaling pathways that in turn alter key signaling intermediates via epigenetic mechanisms. However, the several hundreds of genes that are silenced by aberrant epigenetic mechanisms in any tumor cannot all happen by random. This suggests a role for abnormalities in programmed epigenetic control, including abnormal chromatin regulation that is essential for the maintenance of cells in a stem-cell state. A potential contribution of the stem-cell state is integral to current thinking, as suggested by dysregulation of the PcG system, which is associated with carcinogenesis (Valk-Lingbeek et al. 2004).

3.10.1 *Disparities in Cancer Risk and Development*

While there is abundant literature in support of epigenetic alterations in cancer initiation and progression, as well as disease aggression, limited studies have explored the role of differential epigenetic alterations in various ethnic and racial groups as a fundamental cause of differences in cancer susceptibility, as well as disease progression, among various ethnic groups. However, there are some findings of differences in methylation frequencies in various racial and ethnic groups, as subsequently discussed for organ specific cancers. Although it is not entirely clear why epigenetic patterns are corrupt in human cancers and why there are potential differences between individuals belonging to the same racial groups and/or different populations, there are possible explanations and findings from many investigations to suggest various factors may contribute to these aberrant epigenetic changes and cancer disparities.

For instance, genetic variance in the DNA methylation machinery, including DNMTs in various populations, may contribute to differences in susceptibility to DNA methylation (Hoffmann et al. 2007; Patra et al. 2002), and this is discussed in more detail in Chap. 10. In addition, differential exposure to environmental toxins, infection, or dietary carcinogens and hormonal exposures are associated with chronic and recurrent inflammation of the prostate (De Marzo et al. 2007). These endogenous and exogenous carcinogens can induce both somatic and heritable changes in DNA methylation, causing cancer. Furthermore, dietary factors, specifically components of a particular carbon metabolism including folate, vitamin B12, choline, betaine, methionine, cysteine, and elevated plasma concentrations of choline and vitamin B2 have been associated with increased prostate risk in a large prospective study (Johansson et al. 2009). Other reports indicate that depletion of folate can create imbalance of both S-adenosylmethionine and nucleotide pools, causing epigenetic and genetic changes that are capable of initiating tumorigenesis (Kim 2007).

3.10.2 Prostate Cancer Disparity

One study reported by Enokida et al. (2005) identified significantly higher methylation for GSTPI gene in AA prostate cancer in comparison with EA and Asian prostate cancers. Another study that surveyed gene-specific promoter methylation for eight genes: GSTP1, RASSF1A, CD44, RARβ2, E-cadherin, EDNRB, Annexin-2, and Caveolin-1 in AA and EA prostate biospecimens (Woodson et al. 2004), found significant association of DNA methylation for the CD44 gene but not for the GSTP1 gene in AA versus EA prostate cancers. Some of the inconsistency associated with the methylation level in various racial and ethnic groups could be attributed to differences in the methodologies used for the methylation analysis and also the different sample cohorts used in these studies. There is also the challenge of tissue heterogeneity, as well as inter-individual differences in methylation profiles, that could account for the observed differences in GSTPI methylation status by the two groups.

The author and collaborators have carried out gene-specific, as well as genome-wide DNA methylation, analysis in organ donors or radical-prostatectomy prostate-tissue samples from AA and EA patients using current sequencing technologies on modified DNA samples that is able to distinguish methylated from unmethylated cytosine in real time and quantitatively. Using this approach, we have identified differential methylation in matched normal versus prostate-tumor samples from both AA and EA populations. As would be expected for abnormal methylation in cancer samples, we have observed significantly higher methylation levels for several genes including GSTP1, RARβ2, SPARC, TIMP3, and NKX2-5 in tumor samples in comparison with matched benign samples, and the methylation level inversely correlated with the gene-expression level (Kwabi-Addo et al. 2010). Thus, in the normal samples where we observed a low methylation frequency, this correlated with higher levels of gene expression. On the other hand, in the tumor samples where there was a high methylation frequency, this correlated with a low gene-expression level, clearly demonstrating that methylation leads to loss of gene expression in the tumor samples. Furthermore, we observed that, in addition to the higher methylation frequencies in tumor samples, when the methylation patterns were stratified by AA and EA samples, there was significantly higher methylation for AR, RARβ2, SPARC, TIMP3, and NKX2-5 in prostate-tumor tissues when comparing AAs and EA, and significant differences in methylation levels of TIMP3 and NKX2-5 in the normal tissue samples from AAs in comparison with EA samples. Not all genes demonstrated this higher methylation frequency in the AA samples in comparison to the EA, as we did not see this phenomenon for GSTP1 gene.

To ascertain whether aberrant DNA methylation phenomenon observed in prostate cancer is restricted to just a few genes or is a global phenomenon, we have carried out a comprehensive genome-wide DNA methylation analysis on matched normal and prostate tumors from AA and EA patients who had undergone radical prostatectomy (Devaney et al. 2015). Genome-wide arrays have been developed that look at all CpG sites in the human genome, including CpG-islands/shores/shelves/open-sea, non-coding RNA, and sites that surround the transcription start sites for coding genes, but also for the corresponding gene bodies and the 3′-UTR. This enables the analysis of DNA methylation across the entire genome. Hierarchical clustering analysis showed that for both AA and EA samples there was genome-wide higher methylation in the tumor samples in comparison with the matched benign samples. Overall, we observed higher prevalence of differentially methylated loci scattered across the genome in AA samples when compared to EA samples. Pathway analysis to identify the top signaling pathways differentially altered by DNA methylation in the two groups was demonstrated for genes with biological roles in immune/inflammatory pathways, cellular development, DNA recombination and replication, DNA repair, and cell-to-cell signaling. This observation underscores the myriad ways through which aberrant DNA methylation can underlie disease etiology, as well as progression. Overall, the few reported studies by this author and others suggest that differentially higher methylation patterns observed in AA in comparison to EA may cause differential changes in the gene-expression patterns of key regulatory genes that can create a more aggressive disease milieu in the AA population.

A role for differential histone modification has also been reported in prostate-cancer disparity. One study by Dias et al. (2013) reported a significantly higher protein-expression level for the metastasis-associated protein 1 (MTA1) in prostate tumors from AA men in comparison to EA men. The MTA1 protein functions as a transcription factor and an epigenetic modifier that form complex with deacetylation co-repressors in regulating histone deacetylation. The overexpression of MTA1 in AA tumors may play a role in silencing gene expression, which could contribute to the prostate-cancer disparity.

A potential role for miRNAs in prostate cancer disparity has been reported by Srivastava et al. (2013). Using miRNA PCR array analysis with matched normal and prostate tumors in Formalin Fixed Paraffin Embedded samples, Srivastava et al. demonstrated differential expression of many miRNA in AA tumors in comparison with EA tumors. They observed significantly decreased expression of miR-205, mir-214, mir-221, and miR-99b in the cancer samples when compared with the matched normal samples in the two populations. Specifically, mir-99 was significantly down-regulated in AA tumors when compared to EA tumors. One of the targets of mir-99b is the mTOR pathway, an important pathway in prostate-cancer progression, suggesting that mir-99b might contribute to increased prostate-cancer aggression in AA patients.

3.10.3 Breast Cancer Disparity

Aberrant methylation may also play a role in breast cancer (BCa). There is also evidence in the literature for differential methylation and BCa disparity. One report observed significantly higher methylation frequency of four genes: *Hin*1, *Twist*, Cyclin D2 (*CCND2*), and *RASSF*1A in AA breast tumors in comparison with EA breast-cancer tumors for women under the age of 50 and with the ER-/PR-subtype (Mehrotra et al. 2004). This data was the first to suggest that differential DNA methylation could contribute to the BCa disparities observed in the AA and EA populations. The author and collaborators were interested to extend this study by asking whether differential methylation could also correlate with clinicopathological features in AA and EA breast-cancer patients by quantitatively analyzing the methylation of six gene-specific promoter regions in breast tumors from both AA and EA patients for which we had clinicopathological data (Wang et al. 2012). We observed significantly higher frequencies of DNA methylation for the under 50-year-old AA patients who are estrogen-receptor (ER) negative in comparison to EA patients. In addition, we noticed that the combined methylation frequency of three genes—*CDH*13, *SFRP*1, and *RASSF*1A—were associated with poor disease outcomes, suggesting a potential role for DNA-methylation markers and breast-cancer outcomes. The CDH13, SFRP1, and RASSF1A genes have putative tumor-suppressor functions, suggesting that inactivation by the DNA-methylation mechanism may contribute to distinct molecular signaling alterations in the early onset of breast cancer in AAs that lacks ER expression.

One group has carried out genome-wide DNA methylation in breast cancers to gain insight into the pathways altered by differential methylation changes in individual AA and EA women who are under the age of 50 and with estrogen-receptor-negative breast cancer (Ambrosone et al. 2014). While they observed a myriad of altered pathways, there was no significant enrichment for any particular pathway in this genome-wide DNA methylation analysis. A selected panel of five genes, namely, HIN1, TWIST1, CCND2, RASSF1A, and RARβ2 that has previously been reported, demonstrated significantly higher prevalence in AA cancer in comparison to EA cancers. Because AA women are more likely to be diagnosed with aggressive and ER-negative breast tumors, DNA methylation changes could provide an underlying cause for the disease's aggressiveness and help elucidate the biological basis of the disease. In addition, genes most differentially methylated in ER-negative breast tumors from various ethnic groups could provide a novel therapeutic approach for cancer prevention and therapies. To my knowledge, there is no report of differential histone-modification patterns in breast cancers in the AA population versus other racial and ethnic groups.

There is no current report of differential miRNA expression in AA and EA breast-cancer patients. However, one report by Yao et al. (2013) observed genetic variants of miRNA precursors (pre-miRNAS) and miRNA processing genes which target genes known to play biological roles in breast carcinogenesis. Yao et al. found that AGO4 genes, which are involved in processing miRNAs from their precursor genes, demonstrated variation that was associated with increased risk and breast-cancer metastasis in AA women; thus, variation in miRNA-related genes could potentially contribute to breast-cancer etiology and/or disease progression in various groups. Overall findings suggest a role for epigenetic DNA methylation and miRNAs in breast-cancer disparities.

3.10.4 Colorectal Cancer Disparity

In addition to chromosomal instability, aberrant DNA methylation changes have been demonstrated to be a major mechanism underlying colorectal cancer risk. However, very few studies have examined differences in DNA methylation and colorectal cancer risk in AA ad other racial and ethnic groups. Mokarram et al. (2009) analyzed 13 genes associated with colorectal cancer and observed that three genes, namely, CHD5, ICAM5, and GPNMB, very significantly hypermethylated in AA tumors when compared to EA tumors. The CHD5 (helicase binding protein 5) is a member of the SWI/SNF-like/ATPase chromatin remodeling complex with a putative tumor-suppressor function (Fatemi et al. 2014). Methylation of CDH5, a gene involved in histone modification, demonstrates a crosstalk between histone modification and DNA methylation through various physiologic and pathologic conditions that set the transcriptional states of chromatin. Thus, preferential inactivation of CDH5 by DNA methylation may contribute to early colorectal-cancer stages in the AA population. Other reports have observed differences in miRNA expression in AA and EA colorectal cancers. For instance, Li et al. (2014) observed significantly higher expression of mir-182 in AA colorectal cancers in comparison with EA cancers. Transcription factors, FOXO1a and FOXO3a that play a role by interfering with apoptosis and cell-cycle arrest in colon cancer cells, are potential targets for mir-182, and protein-expression analysis demonstrates that these proteins are decreased in AA tumors in comparison to EA tumors (Li et al. 2014). The increased expression of mir-182 and concomitant decreased expression of its targets FOXO1 and FOXO3a suggest that mir-182 may contribute to increased disease incidence and mortality in the AA population by reducing colon-cancer survival and increase metastasis to the liver, as suggested by another report (Huynh et al. 2011).

The few studies that have investigated differential epigenetic alterations in various racial and ethnic groups, in particular AA versus EA, suggest that differential epigenetic changes can alter gene expression and may potentially affect pathogenesis of cancers to create a more aggressive disease milieu in one racial or ethnic group in comparison with the other.

3.11 Genetic Association and Natural Human Variation

Some of the genetic variants in terms of polymorphisms that are associated with disease susceptibility and/or drug response have been consistently linked to DNA methylation known as "methylation quantitative trait loci; (meQTL)". Thus, differential methylation at meQTL sites in populations exposed to different environmental factors with respect to their geographic location can provide insights into the role of environmental exposure and natural human variation and thus provide a link between genetic variation and phenotypic differences.

One genome-wide methylation analysis carried out by Heyn et al. (2013a, b) using samples of lymphoblastoid cell lines derived from EA (96 samples), AA (96 samples), and Han Chinese (96 samples) identified several differentially methylated sites in these populations, with methylated CpG sites scattered throughout the genome. Some of the CpG sites were located in gene-promoter CpG islands, gene bodies or intergenic regions, CpG shores, or island shelves. Other intragenic CpG sites were enriched in insulator genes such as CTCF, which underlies the importance of regulatory elements outside the promoter context for natural human variation, while other CpG sites outside the promoter regions were associated with histone modifications and various transcription factors to suggest a regulatory network that contribute to the variance observed between different populations. Overall, CpG sites with population-specific differential methylation were enriched for genes associated with natural human variation including (GST1, GSTM5, ABCB11, and SPATC1L) genes with functional roles in xenobiotic metabolism and transport, the (ARNTL, PRSS3, CNR2) gene that plays roles in environmental adaptation, or genes involved in immune response (CERK, LCK, CD226, SEPT8), and growth factors (FGFR2) (Heyn et al. 2013a, b).

Other interesting findings from this study were differential methylation of genes that are associated with different disease penetration among various ethnic and racial groups. Notable disease-associated genes included diabetes (HLA-B/C, PRKCZ), Parkinson's disease onset (PM20D1), HIV infection (HIVEP3, HTATIP2, CDK11B), enteropathogenic *Escherichia coli* and measles virus infection (FYN), and hepatitis B virus infection (HLA-DPA1) (Heyn et al. 2013a, b). This study also identified differential DNA methylation for genes under local selective pressure, including immune genes (CERK, CDK11B, HTATIP2), and xenobiotic response factors (GSTT1, SPATC1L) indicating that selection of these genes may have been driven by differences in local pathogen and environmental pressure. For one gene, SPATC1L (Spermatogenesis and centriole associated 1 like), they observed that DNA methylation of the gene promoter was associated with polymorphism in the promoter region, and this was inversely associated with gene expression. This finding demonstrates a crosstalk between DNA methylation changes and genetic variation that may be different in different racial and ethnic groups. Findings from this study indicate that genomic variation in different ethnic and racial population takes place at both the genetic and epigenetic levels, indicating a potential role of epigenetic alterations and natural selection.

To study ancestry and environmental exposure in DNA methylation patterns, one report profiled genes that show ancestry-dependent methylation marks by examining differential CpG sites in neonatal cord-blood samples from AA and EA population in the so-called CANDLE (Conditions Affecting Neurocognitive Development and Learning in Early Childhood) study (Mozhui et al. 2015). To find ancestry-specific differential CpG methylation, this study was replicated using lymphoblastoid cell lines derived from the Yoruba African population versus CEU (Utah residents with European ancestry). Correlation analysis was carried out to find ancestry and maternal-dependent methylation patterns. Overall they observed stable ancestry-dependent methylation for genes with tumor suppressor and cell-cycle regulation function including APC, BRCA1 and MCC. In addition, maternal nutrition, especially folate, appears to shape the methylation pattern of newborn babies, indicating that DNA methylation levels are remarkably stable, and maternal micronutrients can exert an influence on the child's epigenome.

3.12 Summary

Recently, the scientific focus has shifted from genetic studies underlying complex human phenotypes, such as skin pigmentation, hair, weight, and common diseases and disease disparities, to understanding the epigenetic contribution to disease phenotype, especially in areas where genetic variation cannot explain the phenotypic outcome.

While the role of aberrant epigenetic changes in some rare developmental syndromes and cancer is well established, identification of the epigenetic contribution to common diseases and disease disparities is in its infancy. Technological advances in microarray-based and sequencing-based analysis of large-sample-sized profiling of epigenetic marks, in other words the era of epigenome-wide association study (EWAS), has just begun and will undoubtedly lead to elucidating the role of epigenetic changes in health disparities. Many of the disease-associated genetic variations are found in chromosomal regions, such as intergenic or intronic regions of unknown biological significance, thus studies intended to elucidate the roles of both the epigenetic and epigenetic changes in gene regulation would increase our understanding of these connections, which are otherwise hard to explain.

Epigenetics mechanisms are directly influenced by environmental exposures and suggest that novel epigenetic markers can be developed for monitoring the progression of diseases, particularly, diseases with a strong environmental component. In addition, epigenetic changes, such as chromatin modification and DNA methylation changes, are potentially reversible (Ramchandani et al. 1999), even in post-mitotic tissues (Weaver et al. 2004) indicating that epigenetic drugs can be

3.12 Summary

used to modulate gene expression, and epigenetic-based therapeutic targets are currently being explored as alternative approaches, or in conjunction with current therapies, for disease treatment.

References

Adkins, R. M., Krushkal, J., Tylavsky, F. A., & Thomas, F. (2011). Racial differences in gene-specific DNA methylation levels are present at birth. *Birth Defects Research Part A: Clinical and Molecular Teratology, 91*(8), 728–736. Available from: PM:21308978.
Almen, M. S., Jacobsson, J. A., Moschonis, G., Benedict, C., Chrousos, G. P., Fredriksson, R., et al. (2012). Genome wide analysis reveals association of a FTO gene variant with epigenetic changes. *Genomics, 99*(3), 132–137. Available from: PM:22234326.
Alvarez-Garcia, I., & Miska, E. A. (2005). MicroRNA functions in animal development and human disease. *Development, 132*(21), 4653–4662. Available from: PM:16224045.
Ambrosone, C. B., Young, A. C., Sucheston, L. E., Wang, D., Yan, L., Liu, S., et al. (2014). Genome-wide methylation patterns provide insight into differences in breast tumor biology between American women of African and European ancestry. *Oncotarget, 5*(1), 237–248. Available from: PM:24368439.
Amir, R. E., Van den Veyver, I. B., Wan, M., Tran, C. Q., Francke, U., & Zoghbi, H. Y. (1999). Rett syndrome is caused by mutations in X-linked MECP2, encoding methyl-CpG-binding protein 2. *Nature Genetics, 23*(2), 185–188. Available from: PM:10508514.
Anon. (2000). *Obesity: Preventing and managing the global epidemic.* Report of a WHO consultation. World Health Organ Tech Rep Ser 894, 1–253.
Ay, E. (2013). Epigenetics of HIV infection: Promising research areas and implications for therapy.
Ben Zeev, G. B. (2007). Rett syndrome. *Child and Adolescent Psychiatric Clinics of North America, 16*(3), 723–743. Available from: PM:17562589.
Bergmann, A., & Lane, M. E. (2003). HIDden targets of microRNAs for growth control. *Trends in Biochemical Sciences, 28*(9), 461–463. Available from: PM:13678953.
Bibikova, M., Laurent, L. C., Ren, B., Loring, J. F., & Fan, J. B. (2008). Unraveling epigenetic regulation in embryonic stem cells. *Cell Stem Cell, 2*(2), 123–134. Available from: PM:18371433.
Bird, A. (2002). DNA methylation patterns and epigenetic memory. *Genes & Development, 16*, 6–21.
Bomotti, S. M., Smith, J. A., Zagel, A. L., Taylor, J. Y., Turner, S. T., & Kardia, S. L. (2013). Epigenetic markers of renal function in African Americans. *Nursing Research and Practice, 2013*, 687519. Available from: PM:24396594.
Bomsztyk, K., & Denisenko, O. (2013). Epigenetic alterations in acute kidney injury. *Seminars in Nephrology, 33*(4), 327–340. Available from: PM:24011575.
Boyer, L. A., Lee, T. I., Cole, M. F., Johnstone, S. E., Levine, S. S., Zucker, J. P., et al. (2005). Core transcriptional regulatory circuitry in human embryonic stem cells. *Cell, 122*(6), 947–956. Available from: PM:16153702.
Branco, M. R., Oda, M., & Reik, W. (2008). Safeguarding parental identity: Dnmt1 maintains imprints during epigenetic reprogramming in early embryogenesis. *Genes & Development, 22*(12), 1567–1571. Available from: PM:18559472.
Brunet, A. (2014). Epigenetics of aging and aging-related disease.
Carmona, J. J., & Michan, S. (2016). Biology of healthy aging and longevity. *Rev. Invest Clin., 68*(1), 7–16. Available from: PM:27028172.
Catana, C. S., Calin, G. A., & Berindan-Neagoe, I. (2015). Inflamma-miRs in aging and breast cancer: Are they reliable players?. *Frontiers in Medicine (Lausanne), 2*, 85.

Cervoni, N., & Szyf, M. (2001). Demethylase activity is directed by histone acetylation. *Journal of Biological Chemistry*, *276*(44), 40778–40787. Available from: PM:11524416.

Chen, Y., Sharma, R. P., Costa, R. H., Costa, E., & Grayson, D. R. (2002). On the epigenetic regulation of the human reelin promoter. *Nucleic Acids Research*, *30*(13), 2930–2939. Available from: PM:12087179.

Comb, M., & Goodman, H. M. (1990). CpG methylation inhibits proenkephalin gene expression and binding of the transcription factor AP-2. *Nucleic Acids Research*, *18*(13), 3975–3982. Available from: PM:1695733.

Costa, E., Chen, Y., Davis, J., Dong, E., Noh, J. S., Tremolizzo, L., et al. (2002). REELIN and schizophrenia: A disease at the interface of the genome and the epigenome. *Molecular Interventions*, *2*(1), 47–57. Available from: PM:14993361.

De Marzo, A. M., Platz, E. A., Sutcliffe, S., Xu, J., Gronberg, H., Drake, C. G., et al. (2007). Inflammation in prostate carcinogenesis. *Nature Reviews Cancer, 7*(4), 256–269. Available from: PM:17384581.

Demerath, E. W., Guan, W., Grove, M. L., Aslibekyan, S., Mendelson, M., Zhou, Y. H., et al. (2015). Epigenome-wide association study (EWAS) of BMI, BMI change and waist circumference in African American adults identifies multiple replicated loci. *Human Molecular Genetics*, *24*(15), 4464–4479. Available from: PM:25935004.

Devaney, J. M., Wang, S., Furbert-Harris, P., Apprey, V., Ittmann, M., Wang, B. D., et al. (2015). Genome-wide differentially methylated genes in prostate cancer tissues from African-American and Caucasian men. *Epigenetics*, *10*(4), 319–328. Available from: PM:25864488.

Dias, S. J., Zhou, X., Ivanovic, M., Gailey, M. P., Dhar, S., Zhang, L., et al. (2013). Nuclear MTA1 overexpression is associated with aggressive prostate cancer, recurrence and metastasis in African Americans. *Scientific Reports*, *3*, 2331. Available from: PM:23900262.

Dick, K. J., Nelson, C. P., Tsaprouni, L., Sandling, J. K., Aissi, D., Wahl, S., et al. (2014). DNA methylation and body-mass index: A genome-wide analysis. *Lancet*, *383*(9933), 1990–1998. Available from: PM:24630777.

Dogan, M. V., Xiang, J, Beach, S. R., Cutrona, C., Gibbons, F. X., Simons, R. L., et al. (2015). Ethnicity and smoking-associated DNA methylation changes at HIV co-receptor GPR15. *Front Psychiatry*, *132*, 1–11.

Dressler, G. R. (2008). Epigenetics, development, and the kidney. *Journal of the American Society of Nephrology*, *19*(11), 2060–2067. Available from: PM:18715994.

Eckhardt, F., Lewin, J., Cortese, R., Rakyan, V. K., Attwood, J., Burger, M., et al. (2006). DNA methylation profiling of human chromosomes 6, 20 and 22. *Nature Genetics*, *38*(12), 1378–1385. Available from: PM:17072317.

Enokida, H., Shiina, H., Urakami, S., Igawa, M., Ogishima, T., Pookot, D., Li, L. C., et al. (2005). Ethnic group-related differences in CpG hypermethylation of the GSTP1 gene promoter among African-American, Caucasian and Asian patients with prostate cancer. *International Journal of Cancer*, *116*(2), 174–181. Available from: PM:15800905.

Esteller, M. (2005). Aberrant DNA methylation as a cancer-inducing mechanism. *Annual Review of Pharmacology and Toxicology*, *45*, 629–656. Available from: PM:15822191.

Fatemi, M., Paul, T. A., Brodeur, G. M., Shokrani, B., Brim, H., & Ashktorab, H. (2014). Epigenetic silencing of CHD5, a novel tumor-suppressor gene, occurs in early colorectal cancer stages. *Cancer*, *120*(2), 172–180. Available from: PM:24243398.

Feinberg, A. P., Irizarry, R. A., Fradin, D., Aryee, M. J., Murakami, P., Aspelund, T., et al. (2010). Personalized epigenomic signatures that are stable over time and covary with body mass index. *Science Translational Medicine*, *2*(49), 49ra67. Available from: PM:20844285.

Feinberg, A. P., & Tycko, B. (2004). The history of cancer epigenetics. *Nature Reviews Cancer*, *4*(2), 143–153. Available from: PM:14732866.

References

Finch, J. T., Lutter, L. C., Rhodes, D., Brown, R. S., Rushton, B., Levitt, M., et al. (1977). Structure of nucleosome core particles of chromatin. *Nature, 269*(5623), 29–36. Available from: PM:895884.

Fraga, M. F., Ballestar, E., Paz, M. F., Ropero, S., Setien, F., Ballestar, M. L., et al. (2005a). Epigenetic differences arise during the lifetime of monozygotic twins. *Proceedings of the National Academy of Sciences of the United States of America, 102*(30), 10604–10609. Available from: PM:16009939.

Fraga, M. F., Ballestar, E., Paz, M. F., Ropero, S., Setien, F., Ballestar, M. L., et al. (2005b). Epigenetic differences arise during the lifetime of monozygotic twins. *Proceedings of the National Academy of Sciences of the United States of America, 102*(30), 10604–10609. Available from: PM:16009939.

Fuke, C., Shimabukuro, M., Petronis, A., Sugimoto, J., Oda, T., Miura, K., et al. (2004). Age related changes in 5-methylcytosine content in human peripheral leukocytes and placentas: An HPLC-based study. *Annals of Human Genetics, 68*(Pt 3), 196–204. Available from: PM:15180700.

Gentilini, D., Mari, D., Castaldi, D., Remondini, D., Ogliari, G., Ostan, R., et al. (2013). Role of epigenetics in human aging and longevity: genome-wide DNA methylation profile in centenarians and centenarians' offspring. *Age (Dordr.), 35*(5), 1961–1973. Available from: PM:22923132.

Gonzalgo, M. L., Liang, G., Spruck, C. H., III, Zingg, J. M., Rideout, W. M., III, & Jones, P. A. 1997. Identification and characterization of differentially methylated regions of genomic DNA by methylation-sensitive arbitrarily primed PCR. *Cancer Research, 57*(4), 594–599. Available from: PM:9044832.

Haberland, M., Montgomery, R. L., & Olson, E. N. (2009). The many roles of histone deacetylases in development and physiology: Implications for disease and therapy. *Nature Reviews Genetics, 10*(1), 32–42. Available from: PM:19065135.

Hahn, M. A., Hahn, T., Lee, D. H., Esworthy, R. S., Kim, B. W., Riggs, A. D., et al. (2008). Methylation of polycomb target genes in intestinal cancer is mediated by inflammation. *Cancer Research, 68*(24), 10280–10289. Available from: PM:19074896.

Hansen, K. D., Timp, W., Bravo, H. C., Sabunciyan, S., Langmead, B., McDonald, O. G., et al. (2011). Increased methylation variation in epigenetic domains across cancer types. *Nature Genetics, 43*(8), 768–775. Available from: PM:21706001.

Heyn, H., Moran, S., & Esteller, M. (2013a). Aberrant DNA methylation profiles in the premature aging disorders Hutchinson-Gilford Progeria and Werner syndrome. *Epigenetics, 8*(1), 28–33. Available from: PM:23257959.

Heyn, H., Moran, S., Hernando-Herraez, I., Sayols, S., Gomez, A., Sandoval, J., et al. (2013b). DNA methylation contributes to natural human variation. *Genome Research, 23*(9), 1363–1372. Available from: PM:23908385.

Hoffmann, M. J., Engers, R., Florl, A. R., Otte, A. P., Muller, M., & Schulz, W. A. (2007). Expression changes in EZH2, but not in BMI-1, SIRT1, DNMT1 or DNMT3B are associated with DNA methylation changes in prostate cancer. *Cancer Biology & Therapy, 6*(9), 1403–1412. Available from: PM:18637271.

Huang, Y., Myers, S. J., & Dingledine, R. (1999). Transcriptional repression by REST: Recruitment of Sin3A and histone deacetylase to neuronal genes. *Nature Neuroscience, 2*(10), 867–872. Available from: PM:10491605.

Huynh, C., Segura, M. F., Gaziel-Sovran, A., Menendez, S., Darvishian, F., Chiriboga, L., et al. (2011). Efficient in vivo microRNA targeting of liver metastasis. *Oncogene, 30*(12), 1481–1488. Available from: PM:21102518.

Imai, K. (2011). Role of histone modification on transcriptional regulation and HIV-1 gene expression: Possible mechanisms of periodontal diseases in AIDS progression.

Issa, J. P. (2000). CpG-island methylation in aging and cancer. *Current Topics in Microbiology and Immunology, 249*, 101–118. Available from: PM:10802941.

Issa, J. P. (2014). Aging and epigenetic drift: A vicious cycle. *Journal of Clinical Investigation, 124*, 24–29.

Jenuwein, T., & Allis, C. D. (2001). Translating the histone code. *Science, 293*(5532), 1074–1080. Available from: PM:11498575.

Johansson, M., van, G. B., Vollset, S. E., Hultdin, J., Bergh, A., Key, T., et al. (2009). One-carbon metabolism and prostate cancer risk: Prospective investigation of seven circulating B vitamins and metabolites. *Cancer Epidemiology, Biomarkers and Prevention, 18*(5), 1538–1543. Available from: PM:19423531.

Jones, P. A., & Baylin, S. B. (2002). The fundamental role of epigenetic events in cancer. *Nature Reviews Genetics, 3*(6), 415–428. Available from: PM:12042769.

Jones, P. A., & Baylin, S. B. (2007). The epigenomics of cancer. *Cell, 128*(4), 683–692. Available from: PM:17320506.

Kanellopoulou, C., Muljo, S. A., Kung, A. L., Ganesan, S., Drapkin, R., Jenuwein, T., et al. (2005). Dicer-deficient mouse embryonic stem cells are defective in differentiation and centromeric silencing. *Genes & Development, 19*(4), 489–501. Available from: PM:15713842.

Kawakami, K., Yamamura, S., Hirata, H., Ueno, K., Saini, S., Majid, S., et al. (2011). Secreted frizzled-related protein-5 is epigenetically downregulated and functions as a tumor suppressor in kidney cancer. *International Journal of Cancer, 128*(3), 541–550. Available from: PM:20340127.

Kim, Y. I. (2007). Folate and colorectal cancer: An evidence-based critical review. *Molecular Nutrition & Food Research, 51*(3), 267–292. Available from: PM:17295418.

Kuo, M. H., & Allis, C. D. (1998). Roles of histone acetyltransferases and deacetylases in gene regulation. *Bioessays, 20*(8), 615–626. Available from: PM:9780836.

Kwabi-Addo, B. (2007). Age-related DNA methylation changes in normal human prostate tissues.

Kwabi-Addo, B., Chung, W., Shen, L., Ittmann, M., Wheeler, T., Jelinek, J., et al. (2007). Age-related DNA methylation changes in normal human prostate tissues. *Clinical Cancer Research, 13*(13), 3796–3802. Available from: PM:17606710.

Kwabi-Addo, B., Wang, S., Chung, W., Jelinek, J., Patierno, S. R., Wang, B. D., et al. 2010. Identification of differentially methylated genes in normal prostate tissues from African American and Caucasian men. *Clinical Cancer Research, 16*(14), 3539–3547. Available from: PM:20606036.

Lakatta, E. G., & Sollott, S. J. (2002). Perspectives on mammalian cardiovascular aging: Humans to molecules. *Comparative Biochemistry and Physiology Part A: Molecular & Integrative Physiology, 132*(4), 699–721. Available from: PM:12095857.

Lee, D. Y., Hayes, J. J., Pruss, D., & Wolffe, A. P. (1993). A positive role for histone acetylation in transcription factor access to nucleosomal DNA. *Cell, 72*(1), 73–84. Available from: PM:8422685.

Levenson, J. M., Roth, T. L., Lubin, F. D., Miller, C. A., Huang, I. C., Desai, P., et al. (2006). Evidence that DNA (cytosine-5) methyltransferase regulates synaptic plasticity in the hippocampus. *Journal of Biological Chemistry, 281*(23), 15763–15773. Available from: PM:16606618.

Li, E., Ji, P., Ouyang, N., Zhang, Y., Wang, X. Y., Rubin, D. C., et al. (2014). Differential expression of miRNAs in colon cancer between African and Caucasian Americans: Implications for cancer racial health disparities. *International Journal of Oncology, 45*(2), 587–594. Available from: PM:24865442.

Liu, L., & Rando, T. A. (2011). Manifestations and mechanisms of stem cell aging. *Journal of Cell Biology, 193*(2), 257–266. Available from: PM:21502357.

Lorenzen, J. M., Martino, F., & Thum, T. (2012). Epigenetic modifications in cardiovascular disease. *Basic Research in Cardiology, 107*(2), 245. Available from: PM:22234702.

Lu, T., Aron, L., Zullo, J., Pan, Y., Kim, H., Chen, Y., et al. (2014). REST and stress resistance in ageing and Alzheimer's disease. *Nature, 507*(7493), 448–454. Available from: PM:24670762.

Mann, F. G. (2016). Deactivation of the GATA transcription factor ELT-2 is a major driver of normal aging in *C. elegans*.

Mathiyalagan, P., Chang, L., Du, X. J., & El-Osta, A. (2010). Cardiac ventricular chambers are epigenetically distinguishable. *Cell Cycle, 9*(3), 612–617. Available from: PM:20090419.

References

Mayer, W., Niveleau, A., Walter, J., Fundele, R., & Haaf, T. (2000). Demethylation of the zygotic paternal genome. *Nature, 403*(6769), 501–502. Available from: PM:10676950.

Mehrotra, J., Ganpat, M. M., Kanaan, Y., Fackler, M. J., McVeigh, M., Lahti-Domenici, J., et al. (2004). Estrogen receptor/progesterone receptor-negative breast cancers of young African-American women have a higher frequency of methylation of multiple genes than those of Caucasian women. *Clinical Cancer Research, 10*(6), 2052–2057. Available from: PM:15041725.

Mikovits, J. A., Young, H. A., Vertino, P., Issa, J. P., Pitha, P. M., Turcoski-Corrales, S., et al. (1998). Infection with human immunodeficiency virus type 1 upregulates DNA methyltransferase, resulting in de novo methylation of the gamma interferon (IFN-gamma) promoter and subsequent downregulation of IFN-gamma production. *Molecular Cell Biology, 18*(9), 5166–5177. Available from: PM:9710601.

Miller, C. A., & Sweatt, J. D. (2007). Covalent modification of DNA regulates memory formation. *Neuron, 53*(6), 857–869. Available from: PM:17359920.

Miremadi, A., Oestergaard, M. Z., Pharoah, P. D., & Caldas, C. (2007). Cancer genetics of epigenetic genes. *Human Molecular Genetics, 16*(Spec No 1), R28–R49. Available from: PM:17613546.

Mokarram, P., Kumar, K., Brim, H., Naghibalhossaini, F., Saberi-firoozi, M., Nouraie, M., et al. (2009). Distinct high-profile methylated genes in colorectal cancer. *PLoS ONE, 4*(9), e7012. Available from: PM:19750230.

Mozhui, K., Smith, A. K., & Tylavsky, F. A. (2015). Ancestry dependent DNA methylation and influence of maternal nutrition. *PLoS ONE, 10*(3), e0118466. Available from: PM:25742137.

Nagarajan, R. P., Hogart, A. R., Gwye, Y., Martin, M. R., & LaSalle, J. M. (2006). Reduced MeCP2 expression is frequent in autism frontal cortex and correlates with aberrant MECP2 promoter methylation. *Epigenetics, 1*(4), e1–e11. Available from: PM:17486179.

Nan, X., Campoy, F. J., & Bird, A. (1997). MeCP2 is a transcriptional repressor with abundant binding sites in genomic chromatin. *Cell, 88*(4), 471–481. Available from: PM:9038338.

Nelson, W. G., De Marzo, A. M., & Isaacs, W. B. (2003). Prostate cancer. *New England Journal of Medicine, 349*(4), 366–381. Available from: PM:12878745.

Okano, M., Bell, D. W., Haber, D. A., & Li, E. (1999). DNA methyltransferases Dnmt3a and Dnmt3b are essential for de novo methylation and mammalian development. *Cell, 99*(3), 247–257. Available from: PM:10555141.

Patra, S. K., Patra, A., Zhao, H., & Dahiya, R. (2002). DNA methyltransferase and demethylase in human prostate cancer. *Molecular Carcinogenesis, 33*(3), 163–171. Available from: PM:11870882.

Perry, M., & Chalkley, R. 1982. Histone acetylation increases the solubility of chromatin and occurs sequentially over most of the chromatin. A novel model for the biological role of histone acetylation. *Journal of Biological Chemistry, 257*(13), 7336–7347. Available from: PM:7085629.

Picketts, D. J., Higgs, D. R., Bachoo, S., Blake, D. J., Quarrell, O. W., & Gibbons, R. J. (1996). ATRX encodes a novel member of the SNF2 family of proteins: Mutations point to a common mechanism underlying the ATR-X syndrome. *Human Molecular Genetics, 5*(12), 1899–1907. Available from: PM:8968741.

Probst, A. V., Dunleavy, E., & Almouzni, G. (2009). Epigenetic inheritance during the cell cycle. *Nature Reviews Molecular Cell Biology, 10*(3), 192–206. Available from: PM:19234478.

Ramchandani, S., Bhattacharya, S. K., Cervoni, N., & Szyf, M. (1999). DNA methylation is a reversible biological signal. *Proceedings of the National Academy of Sciences of the United States of America, 96*(11), 6107–6112. Available from: PM:10339549.

Razin, A. (1998). CpG methylation, chromatin structure and gene silencing-a three-way connection. *EMBO Journal, 17*(17), 4905–4908. Available from: PM:9724627.

Razin, A., & Shemer, R. (1995). DNA methylation in early development. *Human Molecular Genetics, 4*(Spec No 1), 1751–1755. Available from: PM:8541875.

Riggs, A. D., & Xiong, Z. (2004). Methylation and epigenetic fidelity. *Proceedings of the National Academy of Sciences of the United States of America, 101*(1), 4–5. Available from: PM:14695893.

Rodriguez-Rodero, S., Fernandez-Morera, J. L., Fernandez, A. F., Menendez-Torre, E., & Fraga, M. F. (2010). Epigenetic regulation of aging. *Discovery Medicine, 10*(52), 225–233. Available from: PM:20875344.

Seligson, D. B., Horvath, S., Shi, T., Yu, H., Tze, S., Grunstein, M., et al. (2005). Global histone modification patterns predict risk of prostate cancer recurrence. *Nature, 435*(7046), 1262–1266. Available from: PM:15988529.

Shantikumar, S., Caporali, A., & Emanueli, C. (2012). Role of microRNAs in diabetes and its cardiovascular complications. *Cardiovascular Research, 93*(4), 583–593. Available from: PM:22065734.

Shapira, N. A., Lessig, M. C., He, A. G., James, G. A., Driscoll, D. J., & Liu, Y. (2005). Satiety dysfunction in Prader-Willi syndrome demonstrated by fMRI. *Journal of Neurology, Neurosurgery & Psychiatry, 76*(2), 260–262. Available from: PM:15654046.

Shen, L., Kondo, Y., Guo, Y., Zhang, J., Zhang, L., Ahmed, S., et al. (2007). Genome-wide profiling of DNA methylation reveals a class of normally methylated CpG island promoters. *PLoS Genetics, 3*(10), 2023–2036. Available from: PM:17967063.

Shilatifard, A. (2006). Chromatin modifications by methylation and ubiquitination: implications in the regulation of gene expression. *Annual Review of Biochemistry, 75*, 243–269. Available from: PM:16756492.

Skinner, M. K., Manikkam, M., & Guerrero-Bosagna, C. (2010). Epigenetic transgenerational actions of environmental factors in disease etiology. *Trends in Endocrinology & Metabolism, 21*(4), 214–222. Available from: PM:20074974.

Srivastava, A., Goldberger, H., Dimtchev, A., Ramalinga, M., Chijioke, J., Marian, C., et al. (2013). MicroRNA profiling in prostate cancer—The diagnostic potential of urinary miR-205 and miR-214. *PLoS ONE, 8*(10), e76994. Available from: PM:24167554.

Stein, R. A. (2012). Epigenetics and environmental exposures. *Journal of Epidemiology and Community Health, 66*, 8–13.

Tan, F. L., Moravec, C. S., Li, J., Apperson-Hansen, C., McCarthy, P. M., Young, J. B., et al. (2002). The gene expression fingerprint of human heart failure. *Proceedings of the National Academy of Sciences of the United States of America, 99*(17), 11387–11392. Available from: PM:12177426.

The ARIC Investigators. (1989). The Atherosclerosis Risk in Communities (ARIC) study: Design and objectives. *American Journal of Epidemiology, 129*, 687–702. Ref Type: Generic.

Toperoff, G., Aran, D., Kark, J. D., Rosenberg, M., Dubnikov, T., Nissan, B., et al. (2012). Genome-wide survey reveals predisposing diabetes type 2-related DNA methylation variations in human peripheral blood. *Human Molecular Genetics, 21*(2), 371–383. Available from: PM:21994764.

Toyota, M., Ho, C., Ahuja, N., Jair, K. W., Li, Q., Ohe-Toyota, M., et al. (1999). Identification of differentially methylated sequences in colorectal cancer by methylated CpG island amplification. *Cancer Research, 59*(10), 2307–2312. Available from: PM:10344734.

Valk-Lingbeek, M. E., Bruggeman, S. W., & van Lohuizen, M. (2004). Stem cells and cancer; The polycomb connection. *Cell, 118*(4), 409–418. Available from: PM:15315754.

Vo, Q. N., Geradts, J., Gulley, M. L., Boudreau, D. A., Bravo, J. C., & Schneider, B. G. (2002). Epstein-Barr virus in gastric adenocarcinomas: Association with ethnicity and CDKN2A promoter methylation. *Journal of Clinical Pathology, 55*(9), 669–675. Available from: PM:12194996.

Volkmar, M., Dedeurwaerder, S., Cunha, D. A., Ndlovu, M. N., Defrance, M., Deplus, R., et al. (2012). DNA methylation profiling identifies epigenetic dysregulation in pancreatic islets from type 2 diabetic patients. *EMBO Journal, 31*(6), 1405–1426. Available from: PM:22293752.

Waddington, C. H. (1942). The epigenotype. *Endeavour, 1*, 18–20.

Wang, S., Dorsey, T. H., Terunuma, A., Kittles, R. A., Ambs, S., & Kwabi-Addo, B. (2012). Relationship between tumor DNA methylation status and patient characteristics in

References

African-American and European-American women with breast cancer. *PLoS ONE, 7*(5), e37928. Available from: PM:22701537.
Wang, X., Zhu, H., Snieder, H., Su, S., Munn, D., Harshfield, G., et al. (2010). Obesity related methylation changes in DNA of peripheral blood leukocytes. *BMC Medicine, 8,* 87. Available from: PM:21176133.
Weaver, I. C., Cervoni, N., Champagne, F. A., D'Alessio, A. C., Sharma, S., Seckl, J. R., et al. (2004). Epigenetic programming by maternal behavior. *Nature Neuroscience, 7*(8), 847–854. Available from: PM:15220929.
Widschwendter, M., Fiegl, H., Egle, D., Mueller-Holzner, E., Spizzo, G., Marth, C., et al. (2007). Epigenetic stem cell signature in cancer. *Nature Genetics, 39*(2), 157–158. Available from: PM:17200673.
Wolffe, A. P. (1996). Histone deacetylase: A regulator of transcription. *Science, 272*(5260), 371–372. Available from: PM:8602525.
Woodson, K., Hanson, J., & Tangrea, J. (2004). A survey of gene-specific methylation in human prostate cancer among black and white men. *Cancer Letters, 205*(2), 181–188. Available from: PM:15036650.
Yao, S., Graham, K., Shen, J., Campbell, L. E., Singh, P., Zirpoli, G., et al. (2013). Genetic variants in microRNAs and breast cancer risk in African American and European American women. *Breast Cancer Research and Treatment, 141*(3), 447–459. Available from: PM:24062209.
Zheng, Z., Chen, H., Li, J., Li, T., Zheng, B., Zheng, Y., et al. (2012). Sirtuin 1–mediated cellular metabolic memory of high glucose via the LKB1/AMPK/ROS pathway and therapeutic effects of metformin. *Diabetes, 61,* 217–228. Ref Type: Generic.
Zingg, J. M., & Jones, P. A. (1997). Genetic and epigenetic aspects of DNA methylation on genome expression, evolution, mutation and carcinogenesis. *Carcinogenesis, 18*(5), 869–882. Available from: PM:9163670.

Part II
Non-Genetic Factors

Chapter 4
Economic Factors and Health Disparities

Abstract Income is an important determinant of health, as individuals of low income status, particular minority groups such as African-Americans (AAs), have higher prevalence rates of morbidity and mortality than their European-American (EA) counterparts. This is because individuals of limited economic resources reside in neighborhoods with higher exposure to pollutants and toxic conditions that have adverse effects on their health. They also have limited access to good nutrition and medical care, both preventive and curative, or the information resources about health risk and health care patterns or how to alleviate environmental stresses. On the other hand, educational investments in formal schooling and graduate degree, as well as on-the-job training, are recognized as means to improve health outcomes.

4.1 Introduction

According to the National Health Expenditure Accounts in the USA, the total official estimate for healthcare spending in 2014 accounted for 17.5% of the national Gross Domestic Product (GDP), making healthcare expenditure a significant proportion of the nation's GDP. Research data indicates that individuals, who have access to quality education, are able to obtain gainful employment, have stable homes, become productive citizens, and have better quality of life, suggesting that economic investment in education and training has immense social and economic benefits.

Despite the general recognition of the importance of economic investment in education towards a healthy future in terms of economic returns, reports indicate there are significant differences in economic returns for various racial and ethnic groups, even for those of the same educational status. The summary report of the Secretary's Task Force on Black and Minority Health of the US Department of Health and Human Services, referred to as the "Heckler's Report" (http://minorityhealth.hhs.gov/assets/pdf/checked/1/ANDERSON.pdf) indicated that there are persistent differences in the quality of education, occupational opportunity, and income levels of AAs and other minorities, in comparison with their EA counterparts.

In general, AAs have fewer years of formal education, and those with equivalent education have fewer job opportunities in comparison with their EA counterparts. Adverse economic factors in terms of low income are influenced indirectly by educational resources, childhood circumstances, inadequate housing, environmental pollution, family disruption, violence, delinquency, general disorder, and healthcare. Limited income, in turn, contributes to residential segregation such that AAs and other minority populations are unable to move out of areas plagued by sub-standard educational resources, environmental pollutants, inadequate housing, family disruption, and general disorder. All of these constraints driven by economic hardships have adverse consequences on health outcomes, such as low birth weight, infant mortality, and high morbidity and mortality rates among AAs and other minority adults in comparison to the general population.

It is well known that education is the primary determinant of higher economic income. Racial segregation of AAs within poor neighborhoods with poor quality schools and sub-standard education, as well as discrimination on the job and other facets of their lives, have persisted across generations since slavery times, and this has negatively impacted the wealth of the AA population, as well as investment in the human capital of their family members. Gaskin et al. (2016) argues that slavery and past discrimination due to certain federal, state and local policies have limited the investment opportunities for AAs to improve their economic wealth and accumulate financial resources and human capital for subsequent generations, which has limited their ability to endow current and future generations. As a result, smaller endowments from previous generation have reduced the current generation's life opportunities.

Although policies that restricted past economic opportunities have been relaxed or eliminated, the damage done has not been corrected by providing compensation or reparation that will give parents the ability to invest in the human capital of their children. Some argue against reparation by pointing to the fact that the direct victims of slavery are deceased, there are no claimants to receive compensation/settlements, or that the perpetrators who should pay for the reparations are also deceased. These arguments assume that slavery and past discrimination only affected the generation that lived through it. However, as economists have pointed out and is also discussed in Sect. 4.3, the transfer of wealth from one generation to the next has a direct association with human capital investments. Factors such as racial segregation and the mass incarceration of AA men have limited the opportunities that can afforded the AA population to accumulate wealth.

Health is determined in part by wealth, and wealth is determined in part by health. Wealth determines an individuals' access to housing, nutrition, education, health services, employment, recreation, and other determinants of health. Thus, opportunities for health-stock accumulation also provide opportunities to break the multi-generational cycle of limited wealth transfers. If wealth accumulation does not occur, the ability to maintain and improve health stock becomes compromised, and any compromised health stock and associated negative risk factors are passed on to future generations. The lesser financial wealth of current generation may be traced in part to lower investment in this generation's human capital by previous generations. Policy makers should consider remedies that will limit racial discrimination and reduce the relative cost of human capital investment for racial and ethnic minorities, such as the AA population.

4.2 The Economic Factor

Economic wealth provides a sense of security when there is job loss or another crisis strikes and allows for creating opportunities for the next generation. The economic and social standing of individuals, families, and communities often provide access to important social, emotional, and material resources that help individuals care for themselves and others. Income in any household is therefore essential to satisfy several household needs such as providing food, drinking water, and housing. While the household economy can be a main driving force for the market economy, a significant portion of the household income is spent on health. Therefore, it is important for each household to achieve their maximum economic potential in order to achieve an optimal health outcome and general welfare. Several factors prevent members of minorities from achieving their maximum economic potential, such as race, gender, and income constraints, as well as limited time and resources needed to navigate social and economic environments where opportunities for changing or moving to a higher economic and social level are available.

There is abundant evidence in public-health research to demonstrate an association between income level and health outcomes, with geographic concentrations of low-income households experiencing significantly poorer health outcomes compared to the better health of high-income earners (Lynch and Kaplan 2000). In addition, there is a direct correlation between health and education, with better health leading to more schooling and vice versa. Some of the factors that have been postulated for the causal association between income, education, and health outcomes includes: (1) Access and quality of healthcare, both preventive and curative; (2) Information and resources on health risks and health care; (3) Health risk behaviors (such as smoking, drinking, unhealthy diet, and inadequate exercise); (4) Environmental exposures to poor and toxic housing, unsafe neighborhoods, and occupational hazards; (5) Psychosocial stress and access to resources that mediate the physiological consequences of stress; (6) The ability to control one's environment which gives an individual a sense of security about his/her position in society which in turn helps to adopt effective coping strategies; and (7) The availability of social relationships and support (Goldman 2001). Although it seems that individuals with high incomes have control of their environment and enjoy optimum health and wellbeing, Lachman and Weaver (1998) observed that some low-income individual with a high sense of control and social support demonstrated levels of health and well-being that were comparable to high-income individuals, suggesting that some underlying psychosocial effects are also important in health outcomes.

4.3 Health and Human Capital

Human capital encompasses education, experience, specific training, and knowledge that affect one's market and non-market productivity. An individual stock of health determines the total amount of time spent earning a living. Individuals in good health are able to engage in gainful employment, work more hours, and generate more income. In other words, they are able to maximize their market productivity. On the other hand, people in poor or frail health are not able to work long hours, are more likely to lose jobs than those in good health, and may rely on government assistance, which may affect their income or may even force them to leave the workforce completely, thereby relinquishing all current earnings.

Grossman (1972) developed a human-capital model based in part on his Ph.D. thesis, which suggests that an individual's health capital can be viewed as durable capital stock. The model proposes that every individual inherits an initial stock of health that can decline over time if there is no investment. There are several factors that can determine the stage at which the decline begins and also the rate, such as age, illness or injury, and economic factors, although the decline can be reduced or reversed by investment. This human-capital theory suggests that an increase in a person's stock of knowledge will raise their level of productivity in the economic sector to produce more income. This can only be accomplished if an individual is allocated the necessary resources to invest in formal schooling or on-the-job training. Days of good health allow consumer to generate more income and engage in consumption, whereas sick days equate to an inability to generate income or spend it. This model predicts that an individual's income level will be positively correlated with her/his demand for health and medical care. Also, education will be positively associated with the efficiency with which gross investments in health are produced, such that more education would have a larger optimal stock of health. On the other hand, there will be a negative correlation between education and medical-care expenditures.

4.3.1 Human Capital and Health Disparities

Economists put a value on health because sickness reduces the enjoyment of life and days in good health can be spent on both work and leisure. Thus, medical care is only one of many choices that individuals make in order to maximize satisfaction (utility). Economists have also extended the human-capital framework to provide insights into why parents make investments in child health. Understanding health as human capital also brings insights into how discrimination can drive health disparities. Any discriminatory practices that restrict human-capital accumulation, such as forcing a disenfranchised group to attend sub-standard schools and job and income inequality can ultimately affect health outcomes. Similarly, limiting group access to medical care or providing lower quality care can result in poorer health outcomes. Over time, differences in intergenerational wealth and health transfer, whether or not these are caused by discriminatory practices, can lead to persistent health disparities. Policies and practices that widen income inequity produce long-term health outcomes, and this is a big challenge in current studies on health disparities.

Certain minority populations, in particular AAs, are prevented from maximizing human capital for several reasons: According to the National Association for Advancement of Colored People (NAACP), it is estimated that AAs constitutes one million of the total 2.3 million incarcerated people in the USA and that AAs and Hispanics make up 58% of the US prison population, although these two groups account only for one quarter of the US population (http://www.naacp.org/pages/criminal-justice-fact-sheet). Incarceration of the AA population, in particular AA men, affects the economic strength of the AA families and their communities. In addition, unemployment as a result of incarceration, felony records, or lack of appropriate job skills can contribute to lower economic power in the AA population.

Even for educated AAs, with comparable working skills as their EA counterparts, there is a significant gap in wages. An analysis carried out by Goldsmith et al. (2007) used data collected by the National Survey of Black Americans and the Multicity Study of Urban Inequality on 9000 households and 2400 firms in multiple cities; it found that, when individuals were stratified by education, marital status, and the same age cohort, there were significant differences in wages, not only between EAs and AAs, but they also observed that the wage disparity was gradual, with EAs at the top of the income level and AAs of darker complexion at the bottom. Thus, AAs with darker-skin complexion suffers heavier penalties in wage compensation in comparison with AA counterparts of light-skinned complexion. Other characteristics and traits, including diction, accents, mannerisms, hair texture, and clothing, may influence the wage disparity, but using skin color alone as a proxy was able to correlate significantly with the disparity in income level. Reaction to skin shade in the AA population has a long history of attitude and treatment in both EA and AA populations, which has persisted since slavery times, even though, under Title VII of the Civil Rights Act of 1964, discrimination in employment on the basis of color (also race, religion, gender, and national origin) is prohibited. There is a long history of employment bias based on skin complexion. For instance, light-skinned complexioned AAs who were often the offspring of EA slave masters and enslaved Africans obtained preferential assignment in households compared to dark- skinned African slaves. Similarly, one study by Hersch (2011) suggests that recent darker complexioned immigrants to the USA earn less (a differential estimated at 16–23%) than their lighter-skinned counterparts from the same countries, after controlling for years of legal residence, education, and proficiency in the English language. There are no signs of the skin-color penalty diminishing with time, indicating that skin-color discrimination is a persistent problem. As already stated, there is abundant scientific evidence to indicate that low incomes or inadequate resources to cover basic needs is associated with poor health outcomes. A study in the AA population determined that lifetime financial hardships (defined as how income fails to cover needs) on adults are linked to increased incidence of disability, depression, inability to access healthcare, and overall poor health outcomes in comparison with individuals who are well off (Szanton et al. 2010). Furthermore, this study suggested that persistent financial strain is more deleterious to health than episodic financial strain.

According to the 2014 US Census Bureau data on income and poverty among US ethnic and racial groups (www.census.gov/content/dam/Census/library/publications/2015/demo/p60-252.pdf), AAs have the lowest medium income, as well as the highest poverty rate in comparison with all the other ethnic and racial groups in the USA (Fig. 4.1). Household income is measured by earnings, unemployment compensation, social security, supplementary security, public assistance,

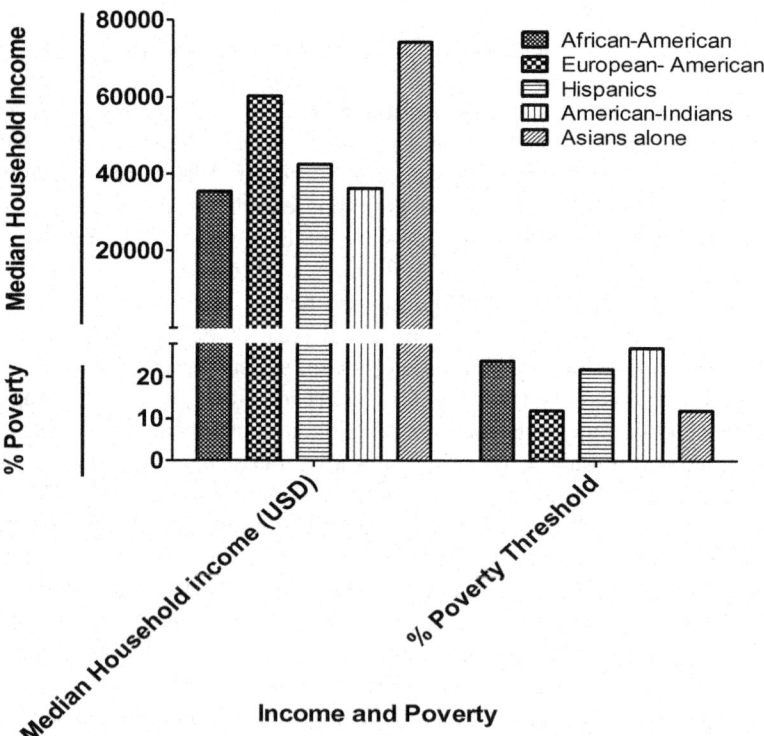

Fig. 4.1 Median Household Income and % Poverty Threshold. Data used in generating graph is obtained from the 2014 US Consensus Bureau data on median household income and % poverty threshold for USA African-American, European-American, Hispanics, American-Indians and Asians

veterans' payment, and pension and retirement income or interest dividends on investments. Therefore intervention that helps alleviate adult financial hardships within minority populations, in particular in the AA population, can compensate for some of these adverse health outcomes.

4.4 Economic Investment in the Intrauterine Environment

There is abundant data in the literature to demonstrate the fetal origins of several diseases including cardiovascular disease, cancer, asthma, hypertension, diabetes, and obesity, and this is independent of adult-lifestyle risk factors that are associated with these diseases, such as smoking, alcohol consumption, socioeconomic status, and sedentary lifestyle (Frankel et al. 1996; Martyn et al. 1996). The accumulating evidence clearly indicates that the time spent in the intrauterine environment constitutes a very important period in an individual's development, with consequential life-long effects on future health outcomes.

Nobel prize-winning economist Amartya Sen co-authored a paper entitled "The hidden penalties of gender inequality: fetal origins of ill-health" that addressed undernourishment of pregnant mothers, the adverse effects this has on the fetus, and long-term consequences on childhood and adult susceptibility to diseases (Osmani and Sen 2003).

More than a decade prior to the Osmani and Sen's report, British physician David Barker made a landmark observation of an odd correlation between low birth weights and increased rates of heart disease in middle-aged individuals. Low birth weight as defined by WHO as birth weight below 2500 g Barker made this observation based on an epidemiological analysis of 16,000 individuals who had heart disease and had been of low birth weight (Barker and Fall 1993). Barker concluded that low birth weight can be caused by intrauterine growth restrictions, such as that undernutrition of pregnant mothers would force a fetus to divert nutrients to its most important organ, the brain, at the cost of starvation to other organs, and this would contribute to future adverse health outcomes including CVDs. Other supporting observations of studies of intrauterine conditions and future health outcomes were reported for the Dutch famine of 1944–1945 and the Chinese famine of 1959–1961. These studies contained remarkable agreement that individuals born to pregnant women who suffered malnutrition during either famine period were twice as likely to develop schizophrenia as those gestated at other times (Neugebauer 2005).

The growing fetus shares the exposures that the pregnant mother encounters, such as food, drink, environmental and chemical pollutants, and even her emotional well-being. Maternal malnutrition may disrupt the development of the fetal neurons and other organs, and this has been demonstrated to have long-term adverse health effects over the life span of an individual. A potential epigenetic mechanism for prenatal folate deficiency in diet and neuronal development is discussed in Chaps. 3 and 10. On the other extreme are the observational studies on both animals and humans that found that maternal obesity is linked to increased birth weight, which leads to increased risk of overweight and obesity in childhood and adulthood (Drake and Reynolds 2010). In the case of obesity caused by an abundance of nutrition, this can give rise to metabolic dysfunction that offsets glucose/insulin hemostasis and pancreatic function which has later-in-life health consequences, including not only obesity but is also associated with co-morbidities such as CVD and hypertension, as well as psychiatric disorders or mood swings and cognitive function. There are reports to indicate that managing maternal weight through weight-loss surgery can reduce the likelihood of obesity in the children as compared to siblings born while the mother was overweight (Paul 2010).

The observation that higher risk of heart disease is associated with low birth weight led Barker to hypothesize the fetal origins of adult disease, noting that the first nine months of life have consequences for future health outcomes. There are other literature references that indicate that low birth-weight infants have fewer nephrons at birth, in comparison with normal birth-weight infants (Manalich et al. 2000), and fewer nephrons is associated with hypertension (Keller et al. 2003) and, subsequently, higher blood pressure in adults (Yiu et al. 1999). Fetal undernutrition and lower birth weight have also been linked to fewer beta cells within the pancreas at birth (Hales and Barker 1992), predisposing for insulin resistance and type 2 diabetes, as well as obesity. One report indicate that fetuses living in low-glucose environments approximately adapt by increasing insulin resistance (Leger et al. 1997), thus maintaining adequate serum-glucose concentrations for the developing brain at the expense of other tissues. These observations led Hales and Barker to propose their hypothesis known as the "thrifty phenotype" whereby a fetus can program its developmental growth by adapting to an environment of chronic food shortage, such as low glucose, whereas, an environment of abundant glucose supply could lead to abnormal metabolic conditions that are associated with higher risk of type II diabetes in later life (Hales and Barker 1992). Interestingly, infants of high birth weight are also at risk of developing metabolic diseases, such as diabetes and obesity.

Although this study did not take into account confounding factors, such as genetic predisposition and social behavior and was greeted with much skepticism, other independent reports have replicated these observations linking smaller birth size with several future adverse health outcomes, including higher blood pressure (Adair and Dahly 2005), insulin resistance and diabetes (Yajnik 2004), and an elevated risk of suffering or dying from CVD (Huxley et al. 2007). Since the first nine months of individuals set the trajectory of their health, investments in human capital should start in the "womb" by examining the lifestyles of pregnant mothers to ensure the quality of health of the fetus and subsequently reduce susceptibility to diseases such as CVD, diabetes, and cancer, which create huge public-health burdens.

Overall, the intrauterine conditions affect health and mortality. In particular, during certain critical period of fetal development, exposure to adverse environmental conditions can induce certain damages in the growing fetus that may manifest themselves later in life as increased susceptibility to diseases (Barker 1998). These observations made by Barker and others suggest that in utero conditions influence not only physical well-being but also intelligence, sanity, and even temperament. Thus interventions, including reducing environmental pollution by using clean-air technologies for vehicles, providing pregnant women with adequate food resources, especially minority women such as those in underserved communities, and intervention in maternal weight loss, will have positive economic impact for the public-health sector. Health policy that encourages prenatal checkups, in particular among minority population, would help to ensure good health of the growing fetus.

4.5 Infant Mortality

Infant mortality, as defined by the Center for Disease Control and Prevention, is the death of an infant before his or her first birthday (http://www.cdc.gov/reproductivehealth/maternalinfanthealth/infantmortality.htm). The infant-mortality rate (IMR) measures mortality per 1000 live births. Trends in child health and IMR over the past century have seen astounding improvements in childhood health and declines in mortality rates. In the early 1900s, US infant mortality was estimated to be as high as 140 per 1000 live births (Anon 1975). This high infant-mortality rate coincided with chronic urban poverty, child labor, chronic disease, and contagious illness, as well as poor nutrition. About this same time, there began widespread social activism and political reforms that dealt with child labor by enacting laws against child labor in 1920. The decades of the 1920s through the 1940s welcomed the era of scientific advancements in nutrition and greater understanding of the causes of infectious disease, which led to the discovery of sulfonamides, antibacterial/antimicrobial agents, that have been especially effective against common infectious diseases. Furthermore, significant advancement in pediatric therapy in the 1950–1960s has led to widespread vaccination that coincided with the development of antibodies against infectious diseases. By the 1960s and 1970s, efficacious antibiotics and vaccines had the significant impact of decreasing infectious diseases. During this era, pediatricians began collaborating with others in the community to prevent disease, promote health, and encourage national and global childhood vaccination (Haggerty et al. 1975).

Globally, vaccination is now widely regarded as an effective and inexpensive tool for improving the health of not only of children but also of the general population and is heralded as one of the global public-health success stories. For instance, smallpox used to kill two-million people per year until the late 1960s, after which it was completely wiped through a major worldwide immunization campaign (Bloom 2011). Globally, childhood mortality to measles has dropped from six million to less than one million per year, and is considered to be eradicated in the USA.

There has likely been an economic impact from widespread vaccination in the USA and globally as large numbers of illnesses, hospitalization, and deaths have been prevented by childhood immunization. According to the CDC assessment of the benefits of childhood vaccination, in the period 1994–2013 (https://www.cdc.gov/mmwr/preview/mmwrhtml/mm6316a4.htm), the US tax payers were saved US $107 billion and US$121 billion in direct and societal costs, respectively, as a result of routine children immunization. This equates to US$10 in societal savings from each US$1 invested in immunization. Despite the success story with vaccination, routine vaccination faces obstacles from well-organized movements that attribute diseases such as autism as side effects of vaccination.

In the period of the 1970s–1990s, there were advancements in child development supporting healthy psychosocial development, lower morbidities, and high-technology care. As a result, infant mortality has been on the decline, and, in 2000, the rate was 6.9 per 1000, indicating tremendous progress in reducing infant mortality in the USA. Despite the substantial progress made over the past 50 years in reducing IMR, there is still a persistent disparity in infant mortality rates in various racial and ethnic groups in the USA. The infant death rate among AAs has persistently remained twice as high as among their EA counterparts for many years. The most affected geographical area is the southern US states. Some of the risk factors associated with disparities in infant mortality include AA women having increased prevalence of premature births, low birth-weight and consequently high infant-mortality rates in comparison with EA women. AA infants are two to three times more likely than EA infants to be born prematurely and/or have low birth weight (Martin et al. 2003, 2010). Some of the underlying causes associated with premature birth and low birth weights include biological, environmental, and psychosocial exposures, as well as complex interactions of these with each other.

There was however a brief period in the 1960s that witnessed the greatest reduction in IMRs for AAs, one comparable to their EA counterparts. This period coincided with social policies that led to infant health improvements (e.g., Title VI of the 1964 Civil Rights Act and expansions of the maternal and infant care component of Title V of the 1935 Social Security Act) with long-run and intergenerational health benefits.

4.6 Economic Investment in Childhood

"A true measure of a nation's standing is how well it attends to its children—their health and safety, their material security, their education, socialization and their sense of being loved, valued and included in the families and societies in which they were born"... "By creating safe and nurturing environments for today's youth-environments that focus on young people's assets and minimize chances for engaging in health-risk behaviors—we can help ensure that tomorrow's adults will be healthy and productive"—UNICEF

4.6.1 Breastfeeding of Infants

There is overwhelming scientific evidence to suggest that breast-feeding children has better health benefits for the individual and is associated with decreases in risks to many diseases, including severe lower-respiratory-tract infection, asthma, obesity, types 1 and 2 diabetes, childhood leukemia and sudden-infant-death syndrome, ear infections, respiratory illness, gastrointestinal infections, and many allergy-related problems (Ip et al. 2007). These benefits extend beyond childhood because children, who were breast-fed as infants, are at reduced risk of childhood cancer, the development of juvenile-onset diabetes, and having high cholesterol levels as adults.

One study that examined the association between breast feeding and several indicators of physical, emotional, and cognitive health was a longitudinal analysis of 16,903 adolescents, including 2734 sibling pairs, comparing those who were breast-fed and not during infancy. Overall, the study found that children who were breast-fed had better health and cognitive outcomes in comparison with children that are not breast-fed (Evenhouse and Reilly 2005). Breast-fed infants, children, and adolescent score higher on IQ tests which reflects higher cognitive ability (Evenhouse and Reilly 2005), and mothers who breast-feed appear to be protected against type 2 diabetes and breast and ovarian cancers (Zheng et al. 2001).

There is disparity among women in various racial and ethnic populations with regards to breast-feeding their children. AA women are less likely to initiate breast-feeding compared to mothers belonging to other racial and ethnic groups. Some of the factors for the reduced breast-feeding practices in AA women are the pain and discomfort associated with breast feeding, concerns about breast- feeding in public, and potential interference of breast-feeding with gainful employment and other activities, as well as a lack of social support. Adolescent mothers are also less likely than older women to breast-feed their children. Because there is a high prevalence of adolescent pregnancies in the AA and Hispanic populations, these age-related disparities may be yet another source of inequality in breast–feeding rates. Some of the reasons for worse health outcomes among children from low-income family, young, less–educated, and AA mothers may be linked to lower rates of breast-feeding. From an economic perspective, breast-feeding is relatively inexpensive and also has important health benefits for both the mother and child.

4.6.2 Childhood Poverty

According to the U.S. Census Bureau, in 2014 (the most recent year for which data are available), the poverty threshold as defined for a family of four is an annual income of $24,203. Based on this definition, the childhood poverty rate for US children is 21% (http://www.census.gov/topics/income-poverty/poverty.html). There is variance in the poverty-level rate. Overall, the childhood poverty level is lowest for a married-parent household, followed by a single-parent household with male head (no spouse), and then a single-parent household with a female head (no spouse). Nationally, childhood poverty was more persistent in rural than urban areas in the USA. Childhood poverty is significantly higher in the AA population than other racial and ethnic groups in the US. Childhood poverty is associated with several adherent health outcomes, including low birth weight, learning disabilities, mental health problems, iron-deficiency anemia, burns and injuries, obesity, and hospitalization in comparison with children from affluent families. Poor children are more likely to experience adverse health outcomes than their richer peers. In one study, 38% of children from poor families reported less than very good or excellent health in comparison with only 10% of children from wealthier families that made the same assessments about their health status (Blackwell and Tonthat 2003). Childhood poverty is associated with chronic health conditions that may become more pronounced as they reach adulthood and may also result in youths with high-risk health behaviors. Income therefore plays a very important role in the health of individuals even at the childhood stage. Income offers a protective effect in wealthier families that mitigates the impact of chronic health conditions. On the other hand, children from low-income families may have poorer health, which may affect their economic power and the ability for intergenerational transmission of wealth (Case et al. 2001).

The many risk factors associated with poor childhood health outcomes among minorities include: (1) low income and inadequate insurance coverage that often reduce access to appropriate medical care; (2) preexisting disease conditions; (3) poor nutrition; (4) poor housing and crowded living conditions; (5) limited maternal education; (6) stressful work environments; (7) disrupted family lives and lack of social supports; and (8) lack of transportation and child-care services. All these risk factors are more prevalent among poor and minority women. Furthermore, child-bearing patterns are related both to pregnancy outcome and ethnicity. Populations with worse pregnancy outcomes tend to include more teenage mothers, more unmarried mothers, and more unintended births. Young women should be educated about the importance of personal reproductive responsibility.

Childhood poverty is also reflected in the environmental or community exposure, in particular, housing conditions during childhood can adversely affect heath in later life. Barker et al. (1990) found a link between domestic, over-crowding living conditions during childhood and high mortality rates from stomach cancer in later years. Other studies on military veterans, who were exposed to certain diseases during their childhood and during military services found that exposure to infectious disease was linked to increased mortality rates, whereas reduced rates of infectious disease in early life may account for increased longevity (Costa Dora 2000). Similarly, a recent Penn State study using the National Longitudinal Study of Older Men found that, after accounting for demographic differences, men's mortality is affected by their childhood conditions (Hayward and Gorman 2001).

Squalid living and typically unhygienic conditions may promote the transmission of viruses and bacteria, such as *Helicobacter pylori*, among poor children, which may lead to adverse health effects later in life. Identifying all the risk factors and tackling these adverse effects through government and local policies, such as improving the living conditions of under-privileged children and proper schools, will support the reduction of childhood health disparities over time and across generations.

The health sequelae of childhood poverty are pervasive and persistent. Many of the early poverty and low-socioeconomic status (SES) linkages to adult health outcomes persist even when one incorporates adult SES into the model. It is also known that early childhood deprivation has grave consequences for cognitive development and academic achievement. How does early experience with financial hardship get into the body and apparently stay there for such a long time? Are there potential linkages between the biological and cognitive influences of childhood deprivation? We are not at a point to answer these questions, but knowledge is expanding rapidly on biological pathways, including both brain developments and epigenetic effects that raise intriguing possibilities.

Children who fall behind economically may never catch up, therefore there should be social policies in place regarding early childhood intervention. Mastery of skills early in life is essential for economic success. The foundation for acquisition of these skills occurs very early in life, when there is gene-environment interaction in the development of cognitive skills. In addition to cognitive skills, non-cognitive skills such as motivation, perseverance and tenacity are all important for success in life. Numerous reports indicate that early-life interventions, such as providing effective nutrition, targeted towards children has substantial economic returns (Alderman et al. 2014).

4.7 Investing in Child and Adolescent Health

Racial disparities in adolescent mortality statistics are stark: AA male youths are 15 times more likely to die from homicide in comparison with EAs of the same age (Anon 2004). Childhood and adolescent health is a wise investment to prevent or delay future morbidity. A life-course perspective makes sense for research and policy to preempt diseases, promote early prevention, and design preventive measures. There is a shift in the disease trends among children and adolescent from mainly infectious-disease epidemics to new epidemics of morbidity or "millennial-morbidity" epidemics as a result of enormous changes in lifestyle. Currently, obesity, drugs, and the violence of family stress, behavioral disorders, and mental illness are the prevailing trends in adverse health. While our forbearers often cared for children with too little to eat, children and youth today are offered an excess of available calories with readily available, high-energy, dense fast food.

This new trend in disease epidemics ties in with technological advances (e.g., enhanced food production, television, automobiles, oral contraception, computers, and the internet). Many of the new technological developments have positive benefits for the health and wellbeing of children and youth, such as the scientific advancements in medicine, surgery, and pharmacology. However the benefits are not equally spread: the ever-widening gap between rich and poor has produced large differences in child health outcomes by class and race. Social policies that include job training, tuition subsidies, and rewards for attending school, as well as convict rehabilitation, can improve the economic outcomes of children and adolescents. However, studies show that early interventions targeted towards disadvantaged children have much higher returns than later interventions (Heckman 2006). If we create a safe and nurturing environment for today's kids, we can help ensure healthy and productive future adults.

4.8 Investing in Adult Health

Education and, in particular college education is essential for economic success that can leads to greater lifetime income and wealth creation. However, the chances for AAs and other minority populations to obtain college-level education are hampered by several factors. Neighborhood segregation and lower- income families, which predominate in the AA population, are afforded only lower-quality schools that are less competitive academically so less likely to prepare them well to go to college. The high cost of university education and student-debt issues puts AA students in a very vulnerable position, making some AA college students less likely to complete a college degree and force them to drop out in search of a steady income. It is estimated that 83% of children from low-income families are at risk for not graduating from college with a degree, cutting their earning power in half. It is estimated that the cost of a student dropping out of college is $260,000 to tax payers, whereas there is economic gain for every student who successfully completes a undergraduate program.

According to US labor-force statistics on unemployment rates for 2016, AAs are at an approximately two-fold higher rate of being unemployed in comparison with EAs and Asians, although the gap in unemployment rate is similar to that of Hispanics (http://www.bls.gov/web/empsit/cpsee_e16.htm). In addition, AAs occupy lower paying jobs or do jobs that are less likely to have employer-based retirement plans and other benefits, which makes it had for AAs to save and build wealth. Another factor that is a barrier for wealth building in the AA community is inheritance. As already mentioned above, AAs are less likely to receive a family inheritance in comparison with EAs, who are able additionally to increase their wealth portfolio with the inheritance obtain from family members.

4.9 Summary

The USA is becoming increasingly diverse. The US Census Bureau estimates that, by 2050, half of the US population will be minorities—therefore the higher burden of disease and mortality among minorities has profound economic implications for

4.9 Summary

the entire population. On the other hand, reducing health disparities could reduce the economic burden. Slavery, racial segregation, and discrimination have reduced the positive life chances of AAs. These experiences have led to irreparable injury to the adults of the current generation. Whether that irreparable injury will continue into future generations depends on the quantity and quality of additional investments in health and other forms of human capital on behalf of AA children. Government could enact enhanced policies to promote health and wealth accumulation in AA communities. For example, government could improve the quality of housing and education available to AAs and other minority communities. In general, policies that reduce the relative costs of investment in human capital for AA adults and children would be a move in the right direction.

Public policies can play a role in creating more equitable society—policies that help the AA middle class to build wealth through college loans, preferential house ownership, and retirement tax policies, as well as Medicare and social security that protects wealth. More policies likely to produce the desired effect include: raising the minimum wage; enforcing equal pay provisions, and employment-based retirement plans; and investing in affordable high-quality childcare and early-child development to prepare children for schools. At the same time, it is important to provide support for minorities to attend and get college educations, while adopting policies which does not leave students strapped with huge debt or reasons to drop out of college. Some of these policies have been initiated in the past before, and also during President Obama's administration; there has been the push to increase the minimum wage and to impose the requirement of employers to provide health benefits to alleviate some of the economic hardships associated with adverse health outcomes in AA and other minority populations.

References

Adair, L., & Dahly, D. (2005). Developmental determinants of blood pressure in adults. *Annual Review of Nutrition, 25,* 407–434 (available from: PM:16011473).

Alderman, H., Behrman, J. R., Grantham-McGregor, S., Lopez-Boo, F., & Urzua, S. (2014). Economic perspectives on integrating early child stimulation with nutritional interventions. *Annals of New York Academy of Sciences, 1308,* 129–138. Available from: PM:24405371.

Anon. (1975). US Department of Commerce, Bureau of the Census. Infant mortality rates for Massachusetts, 1851–1970. In: Historical Statistics of the United States: Colonial Times to 1970. Part 1. Bicentennial ed.

Anon. (2004). National SAFE KIDS Campaign. Injury facts: childhood injury. National SAFE KIDS Campaign. www.safekids.org/tier3_cd.cfm?content_item_id. Accessed October 28, 2004.

Barker, D. J. (1998). *Mothers, babies and health in later life.* Edinburgh: Churchill Livingstone.

Barker, D. J., Coggon, D., Osmond, C., & Wickham, C. (1990). Poor housing in childhood and high rates of stomach cancer in England and Wales. *British Journal of Cancer, 61*(4), 575–578.

Barker, D. J. & Fall, C. H. (1993). Fetal and infant origins of cardiovascular disease. *Archives of Disease in Childhood, 68*(6), 797–799. Available from: PM:8333778.

Blackwell, D. L., & Tonthat, L. (2003). Summary health statistics for U.S. children: National Health Interview Survey 1999. National Center for Health Statistics. *Vital Health Statistics 10* [2010].

Bloom, D. E. (2011). The value of vaccination. *Advances in Experimental Medicine and Biology, 697*, 1–8. Available from: PM:21120715.

Case, A., Lubotsky, D., & Paxson, C. (2001). Economic status and health in childhood: The origins of the gradient. *NBER Working Paper No. 8344.*

Costa Dora, L. (2000). Understanding mid-life and older age mortality declines: Evidence from Union Army Veterans. *NBER Working Paper No.8000.*

Drake, A. J., & Reynolds, R. M. (2010). Impact of maternal obesity on offspring obesity and cardiometabolic disease risk. *Reproduction, 140*(3), 387–398. Available from: PM:20562299.

Evenhouse, E., & Reilly, S. (2005). Improved estimates of the benefits of breastfeeding using sibling comparisons to reduce selection bias. *Health Services Research Journal, 40*(6 Pt 1), 1781–1802. Available from: PM:16336548.

Frankel, S., Elwood, P., Sweetnam, P., Yarnell, J., & Smith, G. D. (1996). Birthweight, body-mass index in middle age, and incident coronary heart disease. *Lancet, 348*(9040), 1478–1480. Available from: PM:8942776.

Gaskin, D. J., Headen, A. E., & White-Means, S. I. (2016). Racial disparities in health and wealth: The effects of slavery and past discrimination. *The Review of Black Political Economy, 32*, 95–110.

Goldman, N. (2001). Social inequalities in health disentangling the underlying mechanisms. *Annals of the New York Academy of Sciences, 954*, 118–139. Available from: PM:11797854.

Goldsmith, A. H., Hamilton, D., & Darity, W. (2007). From dark to light skin color and wages among African-Americans. *The Journal of Human Resources, 4*, 701–738.

Grossman, M. (1972). On the concept of health capital and the demand for health. *The Journal of Political Economy, 80*, 223–255.

Haggerty, R. J, Roghmann, K. J., & Pless, I. B. (1975). *Child health and the community*. New York: Wiley.

Hales, C. N., & Barker, D. J. (1992). Type 2 (non-insulin-dependent) diabetes mellitus: The thrifty phenotype hypothesis. *Diabetologia, 35*(7), 595–601. Available from: PM:1644236.

Hayward, M. D., & Gorman, B. K. (2001). The long arm of childhood: The influence of early life social conditions on men's mortality. *Population Research Institute Working Paper No.1–4. 2001. The Pennsylvania State University.*

Heckman, J. J. (2006). Skill formation and the economics of investing in disadvantaged children. *Science, 312*(5782), 1900–1902. Available from: PM:16809525.

Hersch, J. (2011). The persistence of skin color discrimination for immigrants. *Social Science Research, 40*, 1337–1349.

Huxley, R., Owen, C. G., Whincup, P. H., Cook, D. G., Rich-Edwards, J., Smith, G. D., et al. (2007). Is birth weight a risk factor for ischemic heart disease in later life? *The American Journal of Clinical Nutrition, 85*(5), 1244–1250. Available from: PM:17490959.

Ip, S., Chung, M., Raman, G., Chew, P., & Magula, N. (2007). Breastfeeding and maternal and infant health outcomes in developed countries. *Evidence Report Technology Assessment, 153*, 1–186.

Keller, G., Zimmer, G., Mall, G., Ritz, E., & Amann, K. (2003). Nephron number in patients with primary hypertension. *The New England Journal of Medicine, 348*(2), 101–108. Available from: PM:12519920.

Lachman, M. E., & Weaver, S. L. (1998). The sense of control as a moderator of social class differences in health and well-being. *Journal of Personality and Social Psychology, 74*(3), 763–773. Available from: PM:9523418.

Leger, J., Levy-Marchal, C., Bloch, J., Pinet, A., Chevenne, D., Porquet, D., et al. (1997). Reduced final height and indications for insulin resistance in 20 year olds born small for gestational age: regional cohort study. *BMJ, 315*(7104), 341–347. Available from: PM:9270455.

Lynch, J. W., Kaplan, G. A. (2000). Socioeconomic position. In L. F. Berkman & I. Kawachi (Eds.), *Social epidemiology* (pp. 3–35). New York: Oxford University Press.

Manalich, R., Reyes, L., Herrera, M., Melendi, C., & Fundora, I. (2000). Relationship between weight at birth and the number and size of renal glomeruli in humans: a histomorphometric study. *Kidney International, 58*(2), 770–773. Available from: PM:10916101.

Martin, J. A., Hamilton, B. E., Sutton, P. D., Ventura, S. J., Mathews, T. J., & Osterman, M. J. (2010). Births: Final data for 2008. *National Vital Statistics Report, 59*(1), 1, 3-1, 71. Available from: PM:22145497.

Martin, J. A., Hamilton, B. E., Sutton, P. D., Ventura, S. J., Menacker, F., & Munson, M. L. (2003). Births: final data for 2002. *National Vital Statistics Report, 52*(10), 1–113. Available from: PM:14717305.

Martyn, C. N., Barker, D. J., & Osmond, C. (1996). Mothers' pelvic size, fetal growth, and death from stroke and coronary heart disease in men in the UK. *Lancet, 348*(9037), 1264–1268. Available from: PM:8909378.

Neugebauer, R. (2005). Accumulating evidence for prenatal nutritional origins of mental disorders. *JAMA, 294*(5), 621–623. Available from: PM:16077059.

Osmani, S. & Sen, A. (2003). The hidden penalties of gender inequality: Fetal origins of ill-health. *Economics & Human Biology, 1*(1), 105–121. Available from: PM:15463967.

Paul, A. M. (2010). The womb. Your mother. Yourself. *Time, 176*(14), 50–55. Available from: PM:20928973.

Szanton, S. L., Thorpe, R. J., & Whitfield, K. (2010). Life-course financial strain and health in African-Americans. *Social Science and Medicine, 71*(2), 259–265. Available from: PM:20452712.

Yajnik, C. S. (2004). Early life origins of insulin resistance and type 2 diabetes in India and other Asian countries. *Journal of Nutrition, 134*(1), 205–210. Available from: PM:14704320.

Yiu, V., Buka, S., Zurakowski, D., McCormick, M., Brenner, B., & Jabs, K. (1999). Relationship between birthweight and blood pressure in childhood. *American Journal of Kidney Diseases, 33*(2), 253–260. Available from: PM:10023635.

Zheng, T., Holford, T. R., Mayne, S. T., Owens, P. H., Zhang, Y., Zhang, B., et al. (2001). Lactation and breast cancer risk: a case-control study in Connecticut. *British Journal of Cancer, 84*(11), 1472–1476. Available from: PM:11384096.

Chapter 5
Social Determinants and Health Disparities

Abstract Social determinants and the underlying socioeconomic status as measured by employment, education, environment, housing, government, public health, psychosocial elements, and behavior, as well as their complex interplay, influences health disparities. There is a strong association between higher levels of socioeconomic status and good health. Conversely, individuals of lower socioeconomic status (SES) have increased exposure to stress, psychological distress, and negative behavioral effects, which in turn increases the risk for many diseases. There is therefore a need to gain more insight into the socioeconomic context within which individuals, families, and/or communities work and play and the consequential impact on health outcomes in order to devise interventions that would improve adverse health outcomes.

5.1 Introduction: The Non-Genetic Factors that Affect Our Health

There have been abundant epidemiological studies into the relationship between socioeconomic status (SES) and health outcomes. The history of the relationship between SES and health outcomes dates back to the period of migration of people from rural areas into the cities of Europe, which coincided with industrialization. Scientific observations have reported an association between socioeconomic status, such as poor living conditions due to poverty, and poor health outcome.

Socioeconomic status is a multifaceted concept that can be measured at the individual, family, and/or community level. The differences in SES in individuals belonging to the same ethnic and racial groups or belonging to different groups as it relates to education, living/working environments, behavior, or healthcare access is directly correlated with health disparities. We commonly associate declines in physical health or increases in disease risks with age, gender, and the genetic factors that we inherit from our parents. Most people realize that health is also affected by lifestyle choices, exercise, diet, and unhealthy habits like smoking and excessive alcohol consumption. However, these factors are only a small part of what affects our health. There is a plethora of interacting factors including education, employment status, income, social relationships with friends and family, the work environment, disability, and early-life exposures, all of which can act independently or interact with each other to influence our health outcomes (Fig. 5.1).

There is interest in studying how social factors influence health, for instance, how environmental stress or diet can influence the vasculature of the heart and blood vessels and contribute to heart disease. Several of these studies have focused on individual risk factors such as the content of food choice (such as high caloric or high-cholesterol diets) or a sedentary lifestyle. However, food choice itself is influenced by financial resources, as well as access and availability. For instance, hamburger is cheaper than fresh fruits and vegetables and is readily available in the so called "food deserts" of low-income communities, where there is less access to fresh fruits and vegetables. In turn, income level itself is influenced by other social determinants like education, which means individuals in low-paying jobs are at a higher risk of adverse health outcomes, such as higher susceptibility to heart disease. However, dietary habits, in addition to being influenced by income level, are also shaped by family influences during early life and can be reshaped by friends later on in life, habits that maybe difficult to break.

Employment status can also influence health outcomes through many various pathways. Unemployment or a low-paying job can increase stress levels, causing poor sleeping patterns and poor physical health. In addition, some workplace conditions, such as long working hours, and hazardous working conditions can cause stress and other adverse effects on health. Many of these complex social factors are connected with each other and make it difficult to identify individual social factors and their effects on adverse health outcomes.

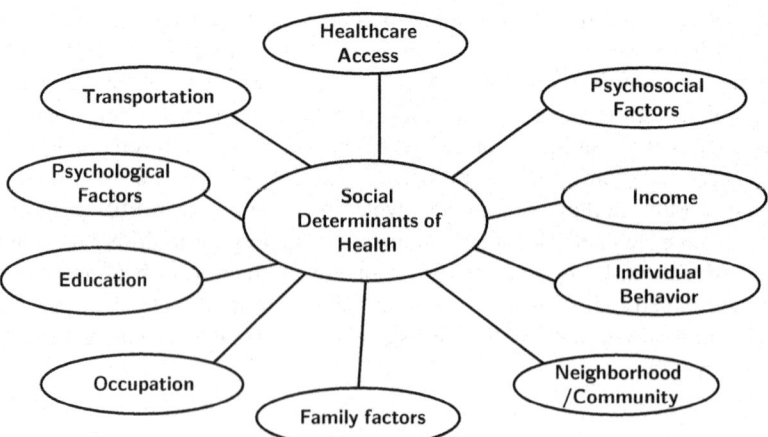

Fig. 5.1 Some of the social, political, and environmental factors that constituents the social determinats of health

Public-health research commonly measure SES by education, income, and occupation. While each factor represents specific SES information, there are correlations among these factors to suggest that they are interrelated, but not completely overlapping with each other. There is sufficient evidence to demonstrate that people of higher socioeconomic status and more socially integrated have lower morbidity and mortality in comparison with poor or low-income individuals (Adler and Ostrove 1999). For instance, landmark studies in Britain in the nineteenth century, known as the Whitehall Studies, were undertaken to understand the risk factors associated with health disparities with a focus on social-class-based differences in mortality rates. The results from the Whitehall Studies demonstrated a direct association between good health and socioeconomic-status hierarchy. Thus individuals of high SES were healthier and at a lower risk of dying at a young age. In contrast, individuals of low SES were reported to be in poor health condition and more susceptible to die at a younger age. The conclusion from this study was that high poverty and adverse lifestyle factors in the low SES population, particularly among the poorer working class, were responsible for the high mortality rates in this population (Macintyre 1997).

This study was carried out in Britain, a country with a homogenous Caucasian population. According to the 2011 census on population, over 87% of the British population is Caucasian, with ethnic and minority groups making up the remaining 13% (http://www.ons.gov.uk/peoplepopulationandcommunity/populationandmigration/populationestimates). The general conclusion based on this study was that social class is a predictor of health disparities and the challenges of racial and ethnic differences in health outcome. However, when analyses similar to the Whitehall Study are carried out and stratified by racial and ethnic groups, there are clear differences in the health disparities in the different ethnic and racial populations, even when economic status are accounted for, suggesting that other factors besides social class must account for health disparities.

Socioeconomic status plays a central role in health determinants and health disparities, and it conceptualize an individual's class, status, and power in society (Galobardes et al. 2006). However, SES is more than income level or educational attainment, which are often used as indicators for SES. Rather, SES encompasses a lifetime of access to knowledge, skill, resources and opportunities. Thus, the influence of SES on health outcomes begins early in life, perhaps even in the prenatal state (discussed in Chap. 4) and continues throughout the entire lifespan of the individual. The following sections discuss the various social determinant factors and their association with health disparities.

5.2 Education as a Social Determinant of Health

Basic education is designed to instruct and equip individuals with knowledge and skills for reasoning and critical thinking. In addition, basic education is designed to equip individuals with socio-emotional awareness and the ability to have self-control, as well as to acquire the social skills that will enable individuals to grow, become productive, creative, and independent members of society. The process of education occurs at home and in schools, religious establishments, and other community settings. Thus there are many opportunities for education outside the school context. Regardless of the educational setting, the strong relationship between health and education is well established. First, health is a pre-requisite for education because a sick child's ability to learn may be hindered by risk factors such as hearing impairment, attention deficit, or hunger. Secondly, knowledge about health can be taught in schools and in many public-health settings, and finally physical education in schools combines information about the importance of physical activity and good health while promoting such activity (Hahn and Truman 2015).

Education is therefore an essential component and a major contributing factor to health, which makes it an important public-health concern because it is an area where intervention can disrupt the cycle of poverty and adverse health, as well as health disparities. However, education is a relatively crude indicator of health, with few categories, and does not include information about the quality of the education (Matthews and Gallo 2011). Researchers studying the educational context and health have generally used the percent of the adult population not completing high school as an indicator. Such analysis has consistently reported positive correlation of individuals who have not completed high school with all-cause mortality, including homicide, motor-vehicle deaths, coronary heart disease, smoking, severe pediatric injury, and elevated serum cholesterol (Bosma et al. 2001; Cubbin et al. 2000; Diez-Roux et al. 1997, 2001).

Overall, there are several studies in support of strong association between education and health outcomes. Self-assessment reports on health and educational attainment found that individuals with less than a high- school-level education are likely to report having poor health. Similarly, most health conditions, such as diabetes and several psychological symptoms (such as loneliness or depression, which is discussed in more detail in Chap. 6) are reported at higher rates among individuals with lower levels of education. One study by Matthews et al. (2008) investigated educational standards and stress levels in a cohort of middle-aged women without a high-school diploma. The objective of this study was to test emotional distress among individuals and reserve capacity, which is a measure of optimism, self-esteem, and social support. The result from this study was that middle-aged women with less than a high-school education had increased metabolic syndrome, which is linked to chronic stress. Based on the reserve-capacity model, a potential mechanism linking lower educational achievement and increased risk of metabolic syndrome is a combined lack of optimism, self-esteem, and social supports. In this particular study and contrary to the tenets of the reserve-capacity model, stress was not the primary driving force linking educational attainment (a measurement of SES) and metabolic syndrome. However, stress was directly related to the development of the metabolic syndrome in another analysis performed on this sample (Raikkonen et al. 2007).

Another study that investigated the difference in daily stressors in well-educated individuals in comparison with less well-educated individuals observed that well-educated individuals reported fewer physical symptoms and less psychological distress. However, well-educated individuals reported more daily stressors that could be related to their role on the job, such as higher expectations, meeting targets, and engagement in key roles. There is at least one report which suggests that high education attainment may be linked to certain adverse health outcomes, such as the high incidence of prostate cancer among the well-educated (Zeigler-Johnson et al. 2015). However, the prevailing evidence supports a strong association between high educational attainment and good health, as well as increased life expectancy. On the other hand, poorly educated individuals reported more severe stressors, suggesting that poorly educated individuals and low-income individuals are disproportionally more vulnerable to stress (Grzywacz et al. 2004). Additional studies are required in order to elucidate the signaling pathway linking stress as an underlying mechanism for SES and health disparities. This report, while it does not undermine the role of stress in physical health, indicates that it may not be the primary mediator of SES–physical-health association (Cohen et al. 2007). Currently, in the USA, a man with less than a high-school education could be expected to live to an age of 69.2 years, whereas a man with a graduate degree can be expected to live for an additional 15 years. Similarly, a woman with less than a high-school education can be expected to live to 74.9, whereas a woman with a graduate degree lives for 11 more years on average.

The mechanism through which education can improve health can be summed up in three main pathways. First, knowledge and problem-solving skills, as well as emotional awareness and self-control, in addition to the development of psycho-social skills and awareness of social support, can equip individuals to maintain better health. Second, through education, individuals can obtain work with higher incomes and satisfaction that allows the affordability of life's essentials, and, third, healthy behavior through education can help protect against health risks.

5.3 Income as a Social Determinant of Health

Economic income or family wealth is another widely-used indicator of SES. Income level and inequality in income distribution, wealth, poverty, and the geographic concentration of poverty show significant association with health status (Kennedy et al. 1998; Yen and Kaplan 1999), as discussed in Chap. 4. There are several well-documented reports for the correlation between higher levels of economic resources and better health (Lynch and Kaplan 2000).

Income is not directly related to health outcomes but is closely associated with health-related resources and provides access to health-related resources, including housing and transportation that are necessary for good health outcomes. For instance, African-American (AA) individuals of low-income, who predominantly live in segregated neighborhoods with poor environmental conditions, are more likely to be exposed to increased levels of environmental hazards. Individuals with low income may also live far away from supermarkets and, without the necessary transportation, may be unable to get access to fresh fruits and vegetables or attend medical check-ups or routine screening. Consequently, low-income individuals are more prone to poorer health outcomes. However, income alone fails to address deep-rooted social inequities but must to be put into a broader concept of social determinants in addressing health disparities.

5.4 Occupation as a Social Determinant of Health

Occupation provides the opportunity to acquire material resources via salary and employment benefits. Hierarchical categorization of occupation is linked to prestige and social standing and controls how we spend most of our waking hours, either doing mental or manual labor in order to earn money. According to the 2011 US Bureau of Labor Statistics (http://www.bls.gov/opub/ted/2012/ted_20121026.htm), AAs and other minority groups such as Hispanics are over-represented in lower-paid jobs, such as production, transportation, and material moving jobs compared to European Americans (EAs) and Asians who hold positions in high-paying jobs, including management, business, and financial-operation jobs. Even for the same job qualification, discriminatory hiring practices, albeit illegal, mean that AAs are more likely to be paid less than their EA counterparts. In addition, AAs are disproportionately represented in hazardous employment and so are at a higher risk of work-related injuries. Furthermore, the AA population is the only racial or ethnic group where women represent a higher percentage of the employed work force than do men; this is in part due to the high incarceration rate of AA men.

One study of work-related health disparities in Michigan found a high incidence of silicosis in AA men compared to EAs because of the environmental exposure of AAs to high-risk hazardous industrial conditions and fewer safety interventions (Stanbury and Rosenman 2014). These hazardous occupational exposures can directly affect health. However, if there are occupational safety regulations and policies in place, this can protect against work-related injuries (McQuiston et al. 1998). The work environment can also adversely affect health because working in a hostile environment can create stress and stress-related illness. There are reports to indicate that individuals who are engaged in low-income occupations experience more social conflict or hostile working environment during a typical workday in comparison with people who hold high-status occupations (Gallo et al. 2005; Matthews et al. 2000). Moreover, several desirable aspects of the job, including wage equity, family-friendly policies and safety can reduce job-related stress and its sequalae (Cheng et al. 2000). The establishment of labor unions also leads to the creation of better working conditions and higher employee compensation (Hirsch and Macpherson 2001).

5.4 Occupation as a Social Determinant of Health

Unemployment and fewer job opportunities are significantly associated with adverse health outcomes in all US racial and ethnic groups and adverse health outcomes have also been found to be positively associated with communities where there are high levels of unemployment (LeClere et al. 1998). However, this is especially more severe in the AA population where the average unemployment rate is more than twice that of their EA counterparts. Lower incomes and the lack of family wealth means that there are fewer resources to buffer against times of employment downturns in comparison with their EA counterparts (Strully 2009). Measurement of health outcomes in economically depressed communities with high unemployment rates are frequently combined with other social determinants, such as low income, inadequate education level, lack of car ownership, and overcrowded housing (Carstairs and Morris 1989). Thus, occupational health disparities, as well as education and income, are rooted in basic social structures, which are all reflected in the broader sense of the social determinants of health. AAs and other minority populations, including Hispanics, have relatively lower rates of higher education, disproportionally earn lower mean hourly incomes, and are also represented disproportionally employed at lower frequencies in the US labor force in comparison with EA and Asian populations (Fig. 5.2); thus overall, AAs have lower SES in comparison with their EA counterparts.

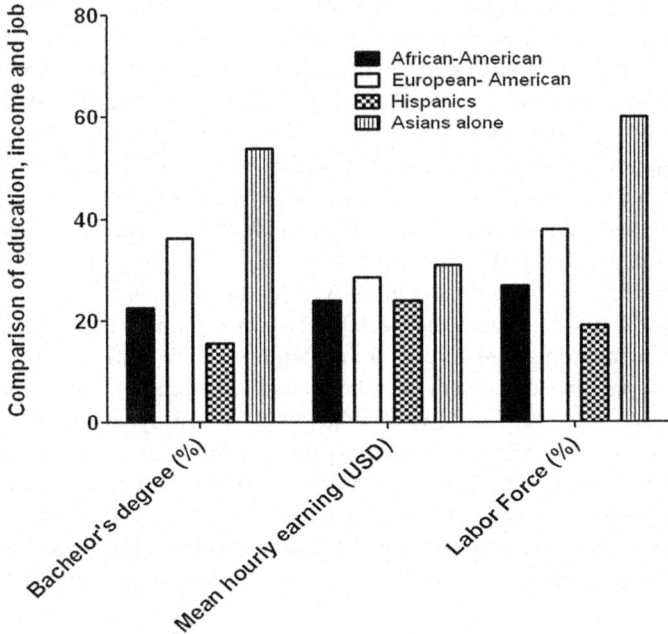

Fig. 5.2 Comparsion of education (degree level), mean hourly income, and labor among over 25-year-olds in US ethnic and racial groups. Data used in generating graph is obtained from the 2014 US Census Bureau and US Labor Department

5.5 Socioeconomic Status (SES) and Family Factors

The SES of individual families is one of the nested factors associated with health disparities. Several reports suggest a strong association between childhood SES and adult SES, as well as childhood health and adult health. Other factors, such as family dynamics (conflict, relationships) and psychological well-being have reciprocal effects on each other, creating feedback loops that accentuate the effects any one factor can have on health.

The past hundred years have seen tremendous changes in childhood health and illness. In the early 1900s, high infant mortality was associated with malnutrition and infectious or communicable diseases. As discussed in Chap. 4, medical advances, including the development of antibiotics and vaccines coupled with technological advances in food production over the past 50 years, have been successful in eradicating most infectious diseases and consequently causing a significant decline in overall childhood mortality. Yet there is a persistent disparity in childhood mortality between AA and EA infants; AA infants are more likely to be born premature and with low birth weight compared to EA infants. As discussed throughout this book, prematurity and low birth weight are significantly associated with adverse health, as well as increased mortality rates.

Studies have found that 30–68% of the racial differences in asthma could be explained by low birth weight (Joseph et al. 2002). Some of the factors that have been attributed to differences in birth weight are maternal behavior, includes smoking and undernourishment (David and Collins 1997). It is reported that cigarette smoking accounts for at least 15% of preterm births and 33% of intrauterine growth restriction (Wickstrom 2007). However, AA women who did not smoke during pregnancy still have high infant mortality or give birth to infants with low birth weight in comparison with EA mothers, even when other factors such as SES, prenatal care, and educational factors are accounted for, suggesting that multiple factors account for the birth outcomes in various racial and ethnic groups. For instance, low SES and low birth weight in AAs has been found to be a risk factor for asthma. Several findings have also established that family dynamics, including parent-child interaction, child care, and the stability of the home environment, can have impacts on physical health and behavioral outcomes in subsequent years (Wadsworth and Kuh 1997). However, the psychosocial dynamics of a family is strongly associated with SES, demonstrating that the conditions in which "people are born, grow, live, work and age, including the health system are influenced by distribution of money, power and resources both at the global, national and local levels, which are themselves influenced by policy choices, thus the social determinants of health are mostly responsible for health inequities" (Marmot 2005).

5.5.1 Parenting

Early-childhood training is a critical period that forms the lasting foundation for later health outcomes. The health of the parents is a determining factor for the well-being of their children such that the adverse health of a parent due to low SES is often considered a negative risk factor for children. Children may learn behaviors that affect their parents: if a parent develops unhealthy attitudes due to societal racism, children may retain similar behaviors even in a race-friendly environment.

Although low SES parents face many challenges, quality parenting, which involves establishing clear standards and limits in addition to positive discipline, is associated with high self-esteem, positive social behavior, and acceptance and overall better social skills in children (Bolar et al. 2016). Poor parenting, on the other hand, regardless of SES, is often observed in young teenage parents who lack parental skills and the knowledge required to be fully present or engaged in a child's welfare. Teenage parents may also lack the social support or may be pre-occupied with other things that contribute to a lack of parental supervision and children's general well-being. The lack of proper parental supervision presents itself as children being sent to school even though sick, not dressed appropriately in poor weather condition, and not getting enough food or sleep. These are all associated with poor health outcomes for children (Bolar et al. 2016). Studies suggests that parents, who neglect proper parental responsibility and supervision, are a predictor for increased risk of obesity in later years in life as young adults (Lissau and Sorensen 1994).

5.5.2 Family Conflict

Low-SES families face financial hardship that can take its toll on the quality of family relationships. Low-SES parents often face multiple, competing demands that drain their energy and patience, making family conflict more likely. For instance, low-SES parents work at low skill paying jobs and often have to do multiple jobs at odd hours and undesirable shifts. In addition, they may have to commute farther to work each day, compared to high-SES parents, who often own their businesses and can even afford to work from home. Low-SES parents are often faced with issues around the house on a regular basis (including plumbing leaks or electrical problems) because their housing is either old or not as high quality. In addition, low-SES parents have old vehicles which often break down or public transportation may be a significant chunk of their income and time because they have to commute far from their place of residence.

Such financial hardship causes low-SES parents to experience emotional distress and poor-quality interactions with their children and other family members. This increases the chances that low-SES parents are distant and irritable with their children and use harsh disciplinary techniques, as well as lack family-typical daily routines (Conger and Donnellan 2007). Parents are also less available for their children, which affects families' day-to-day routines. Because low-SES parents may work multiple jobs at odd hours and undesirable shifts, they have less time to spend at home with their children (Bradley et al. 2001). Low-SES parents are also often less well-educated and may not even be able to help their children with school work

(McLoyd 1990), and, even when there is time, parents have less mental energy because of the toll of life's demands on them. Low-SES parents may even have health issues, such as psychological problems on their own (Conger and Elder 1994), making them less available to provide the emotional support when children need help (Dodge et al. 1994).

The multiple demands that parents face, and the reduced time and energy they have for their children, increase the likelihood of conflicts. Parents of low SES also have inconsistent approaches to parenting; punishing one time but not another for the same offense (Conger and Donnellan 2007). Such approaches could stem from stress associated with juggling competing demands, which makes it difficult for the parents to even have the time to explain the choice of punishments or to apply the punishment consistently across multiple situations (McLoyd 1990).

Family relationships, including conflicts and functional interactions, have established associations with health outcomes (Repetti et al. 2002; Troxel and Matthews 2004). An analysis of the effect of marital conflict, whose underlying cause is often due to financial insecurity, revealed that this causes disruption of the family environment and is associated with poor health in children (Troxel and Matthews 2004). This demonstrates that parental conflict can lead to absence of family warmth and affection, decreased monitoring of children, and inconsistent communication and discipline style. Well-functioning families are associated with positive health outcomes. On the other hand, negative family relationships associated with low SES, such as family conflict, are also predictive of increased smoking and drinking in both youths and adults (Kristjansson et al. 2009). Thus, family conflicts are associated with adverse health outcome in youths (Sweeting and West 1995). One report indicates that great amounts of family conflict are predictive of the onset of diseases such as asthma (Klinnert et al. 2001) and of metabolic disorders in youth with diabetes (Miller-Johnson et al. 1994). One retrospective study observed that dysfunctional families and conflicts within families during the formative years of childhood were a predictor of future adult illness and mortality (Lundberg 1993).

Children from low-SES families face greater unpredictability with regards to day-to-day routines (Evans 2004), such that, when an emergency occurs or unanticipated demands arise, low-SES families may not have the resources to address them, an effect that can spill over to children. For instance, a low-SES parent missing a bus ride can end up in the parent being late for work and having to make up for the lost/missed hour(s), causing sudden changes in caretaking arrangements for the child. Such experiences can create chaos in the family environment (Evans et al. 2005) with children experiencing the stress in parent's lives through the impact on their own day-to-day schedules.

Inconsistencies in family patterns of daily routines in low-SES families can also have adverse impact on childhood health. For instance, low-SES families have difficulty in establishing regular family routines such as cleaning, laundry, and finding time to eat together. One study noticed increased incidences of youth who are overweight in families which eat together less frequently (Taveras et al. 2005). In turn, these individuals, who grew up in homes that eat together less frequently, were also less likely to consume diets rich in fruits and vegetables (Larson et al. 2007). Furthermore, youths from families with irregular mealtime routines are more likely to drink or smoke (Compan et al. 2002). On the other hand, clearly defined family routines have been shown to have inverse correlation with disease manifestation: Clearly defined routines within the family structure are related to youths having fewer asthma symptoms (Sawyer et al. 2000), greater adherence to asthma medication, and less need for emergency inhalers (Fiese et al. 2005). Similarly, consistency in family patterns are associated with better adherence to treatment recommendations among youths with type 1 diabetes (Greening et al. 2007).

5.5.3 Adverse Childhood Experiences

Adverse childhood experiences (ACE) is a phrase used to conceptualize much of the research associated with negative childhood experiences. According to the CDC, behavior risk factors in ACE can be categorized into two main groups: abuse and household challenges (www.cdc.gov/ace/index.htm). Abuse includes physical, emotional and sexual abuse, whereas household challenges include intimate-partner abuse, household substance abuse, household mental illness, parental separation or divorce, and an incarcerated family member. Adverse childhood experiences especially among low-SES individuals in the AA and other ethnic minority populations, who grew up in environments involving abusive parenting, have been associated with several adverse health conditions. Several reports suggests that, compared with people who experienced no ACE, those who experienced four or more ACEs are more likely to smoke and become alcoholics and/or drug addicts (Dong et al. 2005). Furthermore, individuals who experience four or more ACEs are more likely to experiment with sex before the age of 15, attempt suicide, or to be diagnosed with coronary heart disease (Dong et al. 2004) and to die prematurely (Anda et al. 2009).

Other findings suggests that for individuals who experience multiple ACEs and did not smoke, drink, or became overweight, these individuals were still predisposed to high risk of heart disease in comparison with individuals who experiences no ACEs. On the other hand, children who grew up in a loving home with warm nurturing parents had reduced risk to chronic diseases, such as coronary artery disease and hypertension 35 years later (Russek and Schwartz 1997). These observations suggest that various risk factors for poor adult health are embedded in ACE. Regardless if social class changes from childhood to adulthood, childhood ACE gets biologically programmed into future health outcomes. Overall, traumatic ACE is associated with a life course of progressive health disparities linked to adverse social, economic, and health outcomes, including school failure and teen pregnancy, obesity, elevated blood pressure, depression, coronary heart problem, premature aging, and memory loss.

5.6 SES and Neighborhood Factors

Currently, there is appreciation of the need to understand the effects of community or neighborhood exposures on individual health outcomes. For instance, certain physical features of a neighborhood, such as abandoned buildings, litter, graffiti on walls, and other physical decay, is associated with unsafe or violent neighborhoods and undesirable places to live, whereas neighborhoods of strong social cohesion and a higher level of exchange of help and information are linked to reduced risk of depression and stress (Diez-Roux and Mair 2010). A large body of scientific findings suggests that neighborhood SES is a better indicator of overall health than individual SES (Pickett and Pearl 2001).

Low-SES individuals, in particular AAs and other minority groups, are segregated to reside in neighborhoods of poor municipal services (transportation, police, fire, garbage), and lack of access to medical care (primary care, hospitals, pharmacies). There is racial segregation even among the low-SES population, such that low-SES AAs live in poorer neighborhoods in comparison with low-SES EA, who live in much better neighborhoods. Low-SES individuals living in poor neighborhoods are more likely to witness or be the victim of violence (Buka et al. 2001). Low-SES individuals reside in environments with high concentrations of pollutions, including hazardous waste, such as heavy metals, lead poisoning (Johnson 1997), allergens, pesticides (Blindauer et al. 1999), air pollutants (Pope et al. 1995), water pollutants (Griffith et al. 1989), suboptimal housing, and excessive noise, which are known to have adverse effects on health. In addition, low-SES people resides in neighborhoods with poor schools or high rates of school dropout and high unemployment rates.

Overall, segregation by race or ethnicity has been associated with adverse health outcomes among AAs, as well as among EAs in some cases (Williams and Collins 2001). Residential segregation does not only have adverse effect on the health of low-SES AAs but also middle-class AAs. This is because middle-class AAs with similar income levels as their EA counterparts frequently reside in poorer low-income neighborhoods (Williams and Jackson 2005). Statistical analysis shows that, of the 171 largest cities in the USA, not one of them demonstrates equal residential-living standards in terms of poverty rates or rates of single parenthood between AA and EA populations. Overall, urban residential areas regarded as worse for the health and well-being of the EA population are generally considerably better than the residential-living standards for minorities such as AAs.

5.6.1 Neighborhood Housing

Certain physical features of housing have been linked to adverse health outcomes. For instance, long-term exposure to mold and dampness has been associated with increased risk of respiratory and other illnesses, particularly in children (Packer et al. 1994), whereas dilapidated and abandoned housing in residential neighborhoods increases the risk of accidental injury among residents (Gielen et al. 1995) and is associated with increased emotional stress (Ellaway et al. 2000). In addition, overcrowding provides opportunities for contracting, and the spread of, infectious diseases, as well as an increased chance of injury (Acevedo-Garcia 2000). Low-SES individuals live in areas close to industrial sites with greater exposure to toxicants, pollutants, and other hazards both in their primary residence and in the community at large. Homelessness is known to be associated with differentially poorer health outcomes (Hwang 2001), whereas home ownership, on the other hand, which is typically viewed as a marker for general material well-being, has been associated with reduced morbidity and mortality risk (O'Campo et al. 1997).

5.6.2 Neighborhood Violence

A study indicates an inverse correlation between household-income level and the likelihood of experiencing or witnessing violence (Crouch et al. 2000), as evidenced by the high level of crime and violence in low-SES neighborhoods, where over 50% children are reported to have witnessed or are the victims of violence (e.g., shootings or stabbings) (Margolin and Gordis 2000). The exposure to neighborhood violence and its associated stresses is significantly linked to adverse health outcomes, such as a high incidence of chronic pain (Coker et al. 2000) in comparison with neighborhoods where there is less violence. In addition, neighborhood violence is linked to more frequent asthma symptoms, especially among children and youth (Sternthal et al. 2010; Wright et al. 2004) and greater risk of cardiovascular disease (Sundquist et al. 2006b). Low-SES neighborhoods are often referred to as "food deserts" which means there is less access to fresh farm produce, such as fruits and vegetables, and can also be unsafe for exercise because of the threat of violence. Diet and exercise are two important factors associated with healthy living, so individuals in low-SES neighborhoods with less access to healthy foods and an inability to exercise are clearly at a disadvantage with regards to healthy living (Lovasi et al. 2009).

Neighborhood violence can also affect the dynamics of the social relationship between residents, such that individuals may be less likely to venture outside their homes and may not get to know neighbors well. In low-SES neighborhoods where violence is common, studies suggests that neighbors are less likely to trust each other and less likely to help each other. In addition, neighbors are more likely to take advantage of others if given the opportunity arises (Sampson et al. 1997). Thus, the lack of trust and an unfriendly neighborhood existence means that neighbors are less likely to contribute to a common neighborhood goal, such as the informal social control that enforces order by regulating undesirable behavior, e.g., confronting individuals engaged in deviant behaviors (Coleman 1988). These neighborhood factors feed into each other and create a cycle whereby low levels of social control facilitate neighborhood violence and vice versa (Sampson et al. 1997). On the other hand, neighborhoods that have higher social trust and cohesion are linked to better health outcomes (Kawachi et al. 1999) including reduced incidence of myocardial infarctions and cardiovascular disease (Chaix et al. 2008; Sundquist et al. 2006a).

5.7 SES, Interaction of Family Values, and Neighborhood Norms

The social norms in low-SES neighborhoods can affect or influence family behaviors. For instance, neighborhood violence can shape parenting patterns such that parents living in low-SES areas, who would normally encourage independence in the lives of children, would rather keep children indoors. This restricts their children's social interactions in the neighborhoods and, because of fear of bad influence in the neighborhood, the parents are more likely to use harsh and punitive parenting strategies and exert excessive control (Jarrett 1997). Such clashes of neighborhood and family features in turn have adverse effects on child mental and physical health. Children in dangerous neighborhoods are less likely to go out and engage in physical activities, such as walking, playing in parks, or riding bicycles (Carver et al. 2008). Instead, they engage in a sedentary lifestyle by spending too much time in front of a television set, which can contribute to increased risk of obesity. While there are many reasons why this is adaptive in the context of more dangerous neighborhood environments (e.g., it is better to be harsh and controlling than to have your child be a victim of violence), such excessive and harsh parental treatments are typically labeled as negative and associated with poor child outcomes (Repetti et al. 2002).

There are various philosophies as to what is the best way to raise your own child in the context of one's life circumstances. Whereas high-SES parents often want to encourage independent thinking and questioning, low-SES parents often see obedience as critical (Kohn 1977; McLoyd 1990). Obedience helps insure that children do not stray into bad behaviors or fall under the influence of delinquent peers. Thus it is important to understand how differences in parenting styles can stem from the broader neighborhood contexts in which low-SES families are situated. Neighborhood social norms also shape the behaviors of individuals, even if they come from homes with good behavioral ethics. For instance, individuals living in neighborhoods where deviant behavior, such as smoking among peers, is rampant and are exposed to such behaviors are more likely to smoke (Alexander et al. 2001).

5.8 SES and Health Behaviors

Social, physical, and cultural behavior in association with SES is one pathway that can impact health status. For instance, low SES in association with poor health behaviors is significantly linked to increased morbidity and mortality (Pampel et al. 2010).

5.8 SES and Health Behaviors

Individuals who live in poor neighborhoods have a high prevalence of poor health behaviors. The presence of tobacco and alcohol outlets and fast-food chains, instead of access to healthy foods and coupled with neighborhood violence, financial stress, or other family conflict, makes it easy for individuals to adopt poor health behaviors. Lack of recreational facilities, such as swimming pools or safe playing environments, increases the chance for physical inactivity that can impact overall health outcomes and premature mortality among low-SES populations (Krueger and Chang 2008), and these behaviors have long-term health consequences.

Youths who are less engaged in physical activity are at greater risk to become overweight and obese (Patrick et al. 2004). In addition, the adoption of unhealthy diets is also related to increased risk of becoming overweight and obese among youths (Delva et al. 2007). Over time, individuals, who are engaged in unhealthy lifestyle behaviors including smoking, a sedentary lifestyle, and poor diet, alcohol and illicit-drug use and violence, are disproportionately affected by premature morbidity and mortality due to cardiovascular diseases, cancer, diabetes, and other diseases (Heidemann et al. 2008). Another adverse health outcome is linked to sexual behavior and birth outcomes in low SES pregnancy, in particular, teenage pregnancy. Infants born to low-SES mothers with poor education, especially if the mothers are teenagers, are more likely to experience intrauterine growth restriction, to be born prematurely, and to have a low birth weight (Kramer et al. 2000). This sets trajectories of poorer health and lower adult SES because, as childhood illness affects academics, it leads to determining adult SES. The role of behavior in health disparities is discussed in Chap. 6.

5.9 SES and Transportation

Individuals of low SES and who reside in poor neighborhoods often have to work far away from their place of residence. Many of these individuals do not have their own transportation, and the lack of convenient and affordable public transportation and lengthy travel times can add additional stress to the health of these individuals. In addition, transportation difficulties mean such individuals may not be able to access the healthcare that they need, are more likely to miss their doctor's appointment, or be unable to attend health checkups, such as routine mammogram screening for breast cancer. Access to healthcare may work synergistically with the other SES factors to shape health disparities.

5.10 SES and Access to Health Care

Medical care encompasses a range of health-care services, including primary care, specialty care, emergency services, home healthcare, emergency services, mental health services, long-term care, oral health care, and alternate care, which are all aspects of medical-care services generally considered to impact health care (Andrulis 1998). Abolishing inequalities in access to healthcare alone does not seem to address health disparities, as evidenced by the universal health-care system in the UK. Although the UK's national healthcare system was created to abolish inequalities in access to healthcare, there are still gross inequalities in health. This is because other social inequalities have not been addressed, such as housing, employment, neighborhood conditions, and psycho-social behaviors. What good does it do to treat people's illnesses and send them back to conditions that made them sick in the first place?

Clearly, eliminating the disparity associated with the quality and access to healthcare alone will not solve health-disparities issues. However, and as other chapters in this book deal with the various factors associated with health disparities, access to healthcare works synergistically with improved social conditions, such as safe neighborhoods for minority groups, to produce better health outcomes. To overcome the issue with access to healthcare in the USA, the Affordable Care Act (universal health coverage) was instituted to help every person in the USA afford the much needed health insurance for medical care. Yet, countries such as Great Britain with similar universal health coverage still show persistent health disparities. The disparities in health observed in Great Britain demonstrate an inverse association between SES and health outcomes, although the association is less steep in comparison with other countries without the universal health care, suggesting that differential access to care is not the primary explanation for SES disparities (Adler et al. 1993).

There is a pervasive and striking disparity in emergency-room visitation in hospitals between low-SES and high-SES populations. For example, individuals from low-SES groups are 2.5-times more likely to have repeated emergency room visits and 2.7-times more likely to have repeat hospitalizations during a one-year period compared to those from high-SES groups (www.cdc.gov/nchs/data/hus/hus10.pdf). In addition, individuals from low-SES groups are also 3.5-times more likely to suffer high morbidity due to adverse health in comparison with high-SES individuals (Braveman et al. 2010).

There is also disparity in the number and quality of hospital in low-SES neighborhoods in comparison to high-SES neighborhood. Hospitals in low-SES neighborhoods are sub-standard in comparison with hospitals in high-income neighborhoods and are often more likely to close. The standard of care is equally sub-optimal, as AAs and other minorities are more often seen by physicians who are not board certified and who are less able to provide high-quality care and referral to specialty care. Often, specialty and board-certified physicians are not attracted to the low-SES neighborhood hospitals that participate in Medicaid services. Thus AAs and other minority populations are faced with multiple barriers to receiving high-quality healthcare service. In addition, pharmacies in low-SES districts are also less likely to have adequate supplies of medications.

Differences in access and the quality of health care are important determinants for health disparities in the USA and, for the right reasons, have received much scientific attention. One report indicated that patients with hypertension, regardless of SES, when monitored for their condition and provided with comparable follow-up program care, had the disparities associated with death from hypertension eliminated. However, provision of health insurance will not eliminate disparities. For one thing, insurance coverage alone will not ensure equal access to, and use of, medical care.

5.11 SES and Psychosocial Factors

Family SES directly impacts the psychosocial factors in the life course of individual members in the family and can have adverse health outcomes, particularly emotional behavior and social competence. Several reports have demonstrated that, in low-SES families, economic pressures, such as the lack of financial resources to purchase basic necessities like adequate food and medical supplies, can affect parent-child interaction, and this can spill over into psychosocial outcomes. In addition, the lack of parental emotional support and nurturing can adversely affects a child's emotional health. Furthermore, family conflicts as a result of financial hardship can manifest in emotions, such as displaced anger and aggression by parents, and this too can adversely affect a child's health. One report demonstrates the generational consequences of marital conflict, noting that it is a predictor for later adolescent-depression that in turn predicts subsequent marital conflicts (Cui et al. 2007). Hence, psychological states of individual family members can feed into negative family behaviors that create cyclical and escalating patterns over time (Patterson et al. 1989).

Other studies that have examined social variables such as social support and integration in a social group found that anger and hostility in marital relationships make individuals psychosocially vulnerable because hostility erodes the quality of close associations and is linked to increase risk of CVD and premature deaths, whereas optimism and a sense of mastery or being in control with underlying family or social support is significantly associated with positive physical health (Rasmussen et al. 2009; Uchino 2006). Other reports have studied not only the effect of psychosocial factors such as violence and poverty but their interaction with other environmental exposure (e.g., air and industrial pollution) in low-SES neighborhoods and how these risk factors are interconnected to adversely affect health (Clougherty and Kubzansky 2010).

5.12 SES and Psychological Characteristics

The relationship between psychological factor and SES on health disparities has a long scientific history. Epidemiological studies into the role of psychological factors and health outcomes coincided with industrialization and the migration of people from rural areas into urban areas in Europe. Many of these studies that compared disease risk and living conditions observed that low SES is a reliable indicator of poor physical health. Some of the underlying risk factors are stress and its associated distress and psychological effects at the individual or family level or community at large. The role of psychology on health disparities is covered in Chap. 9.

5.13 Summary

While the scientific community has made significant progress in understanding the risk factors associated with health disparities, the plethora of social determinants that act alone or in combination with each other have significant impact on health and health disparities (summarized in Fig. 5.1). The plethora of social determinants indicates that efforts to reduce health disparities would require interventions at multiple levels. While several studies have investigated social determinants across the life course of an individual and its' associated combined or cumulative effect on health outcomes, overall the observations indicate that adverse social determinants in childhood stages, and in some cases prenatal stages, are most critical for the health outcome of the individual, suggesting that interventions should focus at the critical stages of development. Although SES differences among racial groups account for a substantial fraction of the racial disparities in health, adjustment for SES rarely eliminates the differences, suggesting that a range of initiatives that address social determinants and individual behaviors are needed in order to reduce the associated health disparities in the USA.

References

Acevedo-Garcia, D. (2000). Residential segregation and the epidemiology of infectious diseases. *Social Science and Medicine, 51,* 1143–1161. Ref Type: Generic.

Adler, N. E., Boyce, W. T., Chesney, M. A., Folkman, S., & Syme, S. L. (1993). Socioeconomic inequalities in health. No easy solution. *JAMA, 269*(24), 3140–3145. Available from: PM:8505817.

Adler, N. E., & Ostrove, J. M. (1999). Socioeconomic status and health: What we know and what we don't. *Annals of the New York Academy of Sciences, 896,* 3–15. Available from: PM:10681884.

Alexander, C., Piazza, M., Mekos, D., & Valente, T. (2001). Peers, schools, and adolescent cigarette smoking. *Journal of Adolescent Health, 29*(1), 22–30. Available from: PM:11429302.

Anda, R. F., Dong, M., Brown, D. W., Felitti, V. J., Giles, W. H., Perry, G. S., et al. (2009). The relationship of adverse childhood experiences to a history of premature death of family members. *BMC Public Health, 9,* 106. Available from: PM:19371414.

Andrulis, D. P. (1998). Access to care is the centerpiece in the elimination of socioeconomic disparities in health. *Annals of Internal Medicine, 129*(5), 412–416. Available from: PM:9735070.

Blindauer, K. M., Jackson, R. J., McGeehin, M., Pertowski, C., & Rubin, C. (1999). Environmental pesticide illness and injury: The need for a national surveillance system. *Journal of Environmental Health, 61*(10), 9–13. Ref Type: Generic.

Bolar, C. L., Hernandez, N., Akintobi, T. H., McAllister, C., Ferguson, A. S., Rollins, L., et al. (2016). Context matters: A community-based study of urban minority parents' views on child health. *Journal of the Georgia Public Health Association, 5*(3), 212–219. Available from: PM:27275021.

Bosma, H., van de Mheen, H. D., Borsboom, G. J., & Mackenbach, J. P. (2001). Neighborhood socioeconomic status and all-cause mortality. *American Journal of Epidemiology, 153*(4), 363–371. Available from: PM:11207154.

Bradley, R. H., Corwyn, R. F., McAdoo, H. P., & Coll, C. G. (2001). The home environments of children in the United States part I: Variations by age, ethnicity, and poverty status. *Child Development, 72*(6), 1844–1867. Available from: PM:11768149.

Braveman, P. A., Cubbin, C., Egerter, S., Williams, D. R., & Pamuk, E. (2010). Socioeconomic disparities in health in the United States: What the patterns tell us. *American Journal of Public Health, 100*(Suppl 1), S186–S196. Available from: PM:20147693.

Buka, S. L., Stichick, T. L., Birdthistle, I., & Earls, F. J. (2001). Youth exposure to violence: Prevalence, risks, and consequences. *American Journal of Orthopsychiatry, 71*(3), 298–310. Available from: PM:11495332.

Carstairs, V., & Morris, R. (1989). Deprivation: Explaining differences in mortality between Scotland and England and Wales. *BMJ, 299*(6704), 886–889. Available from: PM:2510878.

Carver, A., Timperio, A., & Crawford, D. (2008). Playing it safe: The influence of neighbourhood safety on children's physical activity. A review. *Health Place, 14*(2), 217–227. Available from: PM:17662638.

Chaix, B., Lindstrom, M., Rosvall, M., & Merlo, J. (2008). Neighbourhood social interactions and risk of acute myocardial infarction. *Journal of Epidemiology and Community Health, 62*(1), 62–68. Available from: PM:18079335.

Cheng, Y., Kawachi, I., Coakley, E. H., Schwartz, J., & Colditz, G. (2000). Association between psychosocial work characteristics and health functioning in American women: Prospective study. *British Medical Journal, 320*(7247), 1432–1436.

Clougherty, J. E., & Kubzansky, L. D. (2010). A framework for examining social stress and susceptibility to air pollution in respiratory health. *Ciência and Saúde Coletiva, 15*(4), 2059–2074. Available from: PM:20694328.

Cohen, S., Janicki-Deverts, D., & Miller, G. E. (2007). Psychological stress and disease. *JAMA, 298*(14), 1685–1687. Available from: PM:17925521.

Coker, A. L., Smith, P. H., Bethea, L., King, M. R., & McKeown, R. E. (2000). Physical health consequences of physical and psychological intimate partner violence. *Archives of Family Medicine, 9*(5), 451–457. Available from: PM:10810951.

Coleman, J. S. (1988). Social capital in the creation of human capital. *American Journal of Sociology, 94*, S95–S120.

Compan, E., Moreno, J., Ruiz, M. T., & Pascual, E. (2002). Doing things together: Adolescent health and family rituals. *Journal of Epidemiology and Community Health, 56*(2), 89–94. Available from: PM:11812805.

Conger, R. D., & Donnellan, M. B. (2007). An interactionist perspective on the socioeconomic context of human development. *Annual Review of Psychology, 58*, 175–199. Available from: PM:16903807.

Conger, R. D., & Elder, G. H. (1994). *Families in troubled times*. Hawthorne, NY: Aldine de Gruyter.

Crouch, J. L., Hanson, R. F., Saunders, B. E., Kilpatrick, D. G., & Resnick, H. S. (2000). Income, race/ethnicity, and exposure to violence in youth: Results from the National survey of adolescents. *Journal of Community Psychology, 28*, 625–641.

Cubbin, C., LeClere, F. B., & Smith, G. S. (2000). Socioeconomic status and injury mortality: Individual and neighbourhood determinants. *Journal of Epidemiology and Community Health, 54*(7), 517–524. Available from: PM:10846194.

Cui, M., Donnellan, M. B., & Conger, R. D. (2007). Reciprocal influences between parents' marital problems and adolescent internalizing and externalizing behavior. *Developmental Psychology, 43*(6), 1544–1552. Available from: PM:18020831.

David, R. J., & Collins, J. W., Jr. (1997). Differing birth weight among infants of U.S.-born blacks, African-born blacks, and U.S.-born whites. *New England Journal of Medicine, 337*(17), 1209–1214. Available from: PM:9337381.

Delva, J., Johnston, L. D., & O'Malley, P. M. (2007). The epidemiology of overweight and related lifestyle behaviors: Racial/ethnic and socioeconomic status differences among American youth. *American Journal of Preventive Medicine, 33*(4 Suppl), S178–S186. Available from: PM:17884566.

Diez-Roux, A. V., & Mair, C. (2010). Neighborhoods and health. *Annals of the New York Academy of Sciences, 1186,* 125–145. Available from: PM:20201871.

Diez-Roux, A. V., Merkin, S. S., Arnett, D., Chambless, L., Massing, M., Nieto, F. J., et al. (2001). Neighborhood of residence and incidence of coronary heart disease. *New England Journal of Medicine, 345*(2), 99–106. Available from: PM:11450679.

Diez-Roux, A. V., Nieto, F. J., Muntaner, C., Tyroler, H. A., Comstock, G. W., Shahar, E., et al. (1997). Neighborhood environments and coronary heart disease: A multilevel analysis. *American Journal of Epidemiology, 146*(1), 48–63. Available from: PM:9215223.

Dodge, K. A., Pettit, G. S., & Bates, J. E. (1994). Socialization mediators of the relation between socioeconomic status and child conduct problems. *Child Development, 65*(2 Spec No), 649–665. Available from: PM:8013245.

Dong, M., Anda, R. F., Felitti, V. J., Williamson, D. F., Dube, S. R., Brown, D. W., et al. (2005). Childhood residential mobility and multiple health risks during adolescence and adulthood: The hidden role of adverse childhood experiences. *Archives of Pediatrics and Adolescent Medicine, 159*(12), 1104–1110. Available from: PM:16330731.

Dong, M., Giles, W. H., Felitti, V. J., Dube, S. R., Williams, J. E., Chapman, D. P., et al. (2004). Insights into causal pathways for ischemic heart disease: Adverse childhood experiences study. *Circulation, 110*(13), 1761–1766. Available from: PM:15381652.

Ellaway, A., Macintyre, S., & Fairley, A. (2000). Mums on prozac, kids on inhalers: The need for research on the potential for improving health through housing interventions. *Health Bulletin, 58*(4), 336–339.

Evans, G. W. (2004). The environment of childhood poverty. *American Psychologist, 59*(2), 77–92. Available from: PM:14992634.

Evans, G. W., Gonnella, C., Marcynyszyn, L. A., Gentile, L., & Salpekar, N. (2005). The role of chaos in poverty and children's socioemotional adjustment. *Psychological Science, 16*(7), 560–565. Available from: PM:16008790.

Fiese, B. H., Wamboldt, F. S., & Anbar, R. D. (2005). Family asthma management routines: Connections to medical adherence and quality of life. *Journal of Pediatrics, 146*(2), 171–176. Available from: PM:15689901.

Gallo, L. C., Bogart, L. M., Vranceanu, A. M., & Matthews, K. A. (2005). Socioeconomic status, resources, psychological experiences, and emotional responses: A test of the reserve capacity model. *Journal of Personality and Social Psychology, 88*(2), 386–399. Available from: PM:15841865.

Galobardes, B., Shaw, M., Lawlor, D. A., Lynch, J. W., & Davey, S. G. (2006). Indicators of socioeconomic position (part 1). *Journal of Epidemiology and Community Health, 60*(1), 7–12. Available from: PM:16361448.

Gielen, A. C., Wilson, M. E., Faden, R. R., Wissow, L., & Harvilchuck, J. D. (1995). In-home injury prevention practices for infants and toddlers: The role of parental beliefs, barriers, and housing quality. *Health Education Quarterly, 22*(1), 85–95.

Greening, L., Stoppelbein, L., Konishi, C., Jordan, S. S., & Moll, G. (2007). Child routines and youths' adherence to treatment for type 1 diabetes. *Journal of Pediatric Psychology, 32*(4), 437–447. Available from: PM:17030526.

Griffith, J., Duncan, R. C., Riggan, W. B., & Pellom, A. C. (1989). Cancer mortality in U.S. counties with hazardous waste sites and ground water pollution. *Archives of Environmental Health, 44,* 69–74.

Grzywacz, J. G., Almeida, D. M., Neupert, S. D., & Ettner, S. L. (2004). Socioeconomic status and health: A micro-level analysis of exposure and vulnerability to daily stressors. *Journal of Health and Social Behavior, 45*(1), 1–16. Available from: PM:15179904.

Hahn, R. A., & Truman, B. I. (2015). Education improves public health and promotes health equity. *International Journal of Health Services, 45*(4), 657–678. Available from: PM:25995305.

Heidemann, C., Schulze, M. B., Franco, O. H., van Dam, R. M., Mantzoros, C. S., & Hu, F. B. (2008). Dietary patterns and risk of mortality from cardiovascular disease, cancer, and all causes in a prospective cohort of women. *Circulation, 118*(3), 230–237. Available from: PM:18574045.

Hirsch, B. T., & Macpherson, D. A. (2001). *Union membership and earnings data book: Compilations from the current population survey.* Washington, DC: Bureau of National Affairs.

Hwang, S. (2001). Homelessness and health. *Canadian Medical Association Journal, 164*(2), 229–233.

Jarrett, R. L. (1997). Bringing families back in: Neighborhoods' effect on child development. In J. Brooks-Gunn, G. J. Duncan, & J. L. Aber (Eds.), *Neighborhood poverty* (Vol. 2, pp. 48–64). Policy implications in studying neighborhoods New York: Sage Found.

Johnson, B. L. (1997). Hazardous waste: Human health effects. *Toxicology and Industrial Health, 13*(2–3), 121–143. Available from: PM:9200784.

Joseph, C. L., Ownby, D. R., Peterson, E. L., & Johnson, C. C. (2002). Does low birth weight help to explain the increased prevalence of asthma among African-Americans? *Annals of Allergy, Asthma & Immunology, 88*(5), 507–512. Available from: PM:12027073.

Kawachi, I., Kennedy, B. P., & Glass, R. (1999). Social capital and self-rated health: A contextual analysis. *American Journal of Public Health, 89*(8), 1187–1193. Available from: PM:10432904.

Kennedy, B. P., Kawachi, I., Glass, R., & Prothrow-Stith, D. (1998). Income distribution, socioeconomic status, and self rated health in the United States: multilevel analysis. *BMJ, 317* (7163), 917–921. Available from: PM:9756809.

Klinnert, M. D., Nelson, H. S., Price, M. R., Adinoff, A. D., Leung, D. Y., & Mrazek, D. A. (2001). Onset and persistence of childhood asthma: Predictors from infancy. *Pediatrics, 108* (4), E69. Available from: PM:11581477.

Kohn, M. L. (1977). *Social class and conformity.* Chicago, IL: University of Chicago Press.

Kramer, M. S., Seguin, L., Lydon, J., & Goulet, L. (2000). Socio-economic disparities in pregnancy outcome: Why do the poor fare so poorly? *Paediatric and Perinatal Epidemiology, 14*(3), 194–210. Available from: PM:10949211.

Kristjansson, A. L., Sigfusdottir, I. D., Allegrante, J. P., & Helgason, A. R. (2009). Parental divorce and adolescent cigarette smoking and alcohol use: Assessing the importance of family conflict. *Acta Paediatrica, 98*(3), 537–542. Available from: PM:19021591.

Krueger, P. M., & Chang, V. W. (2008). Being poor and coping with stress: Health behaviors and the risk of death. *American Journal of Public Health, 98*(5), 889–896. Available from: PM:18382003.

Larson, N. I., Neumark-Sztainer, D., Hannan, P. J., & Story, M. (2007). Family meals during adolescence are associated with higher diet quality and healthful meal patterns during young adulthood. *Journal of the American Dietetic Association, 107*(9), 1502–1510. Available from: PM:17761227.

LeClere, F. B., Rogers, R. G., & Peters, K. (1998). Neighborhood social context and racial differences in women's heart disease mortality. *Journal of Health and Social Behavior, 39*(2), 91–107. Available from: PM:9642901.

Lissau, I., & Sorensen, T. I. (1994). Parental neglect during childhood and increased risk of obesity in young adulthood. *Lancet, 343*(8893), 324–327. Available from: PM:7905145.

Lovasi, G. S., Hutson, M. A., Guerra, M., & Neckerman, K. M. (2009). Built environments and obesity in disadvantaged populations. *Epidemiologic Reviews, 31,* 7–20. Available from: PM:19589839.

Lundberg, O. (1993). The impact of childhood living conditions on illness and mortality in adulthood. *Social Science and Medicine, 36,* 1047–1052.

Lynch, J. W., & Kaplan, G. A. (2000). Socioeconomic position. In L. F. Berkman & I. Kawachi (Eds.), *Social epidemiology* (pp. 13–35). New York: Oxford University Press.

Macintyre, S. (1997). The black report and beyond: What are the issues? *Social Science and Medicine, 44*(6), 723–745. Available from: PM:9080558.

Margolin, G., & Gordis, E. B. (2000). The effects of family and community violence on children. *Annual Review of Psychology, 51,* 445–479. Available from: PM:10751978.

Marmot, M. (2005). Social determinants of health inequalities. *Lancet, 365*(9464), 1099–1104. Available from: PM:15781105.

Matthews, K. A., & Gallo, L. C. (2011). Psychological perspectives on pathways linking socioeconomic status and physical health. *Annual Review of Psychology, 62,* 501–530. Available from: PM:20636127.

Matthews, K. A., Raikkonen, K., Everson, S. A., Flory, J. D., Marco, C. A., Owens, J. F., et al. (2000). Do the daily experiences of healthy men and women vary according to occupational prestige and work strain? *Psychosomatic Medicine, 62*(3), 346–353. Available from: PM:10845348.

Matthews, K. A., Raikkonen, K., Gallo, L., & Kuller, L. H. (2008). Association between socioeconomic status and metabolic syndrome in women: testing the reserve capacity model. *Health Psychology, 27*(5), 576–583. Available from: PM:18823184.

McLoyd, V. C. (1990). The impact of economic hardship on black families and children: psychological distress, parenting, and socioemotional development. *Child Development, 61*(2), 311–346. Available from: PM:2188806.

McQuiston, T. H., Zakocs, R. C., & Loomis, D. (1998). The case for stronger OSHA enforcement–evidence from evaluation research. *American Journal of Public Health, 88*(7), 1022–1024. Available from: PM:9663147.

Miller-Johnson, S., Emery, R. E., Marvin, R. S., Clarke, W., Lovinger, R., & Martin, M. (1994). Parent-child relationships and the management of insulin-dependent diabetes mellitus. *Journal of Consulting and Clinical Psychology, 62*(3), 603–610. Available from: PM:8063987.

O'Campo, P., Xue, X., Wang, M. C., & Caughy, M. (1997). Neighborhood risk factors for low birthweight in Baltimore: A multilevel analysis. *American Journal of Public Health, 87*(7), 1113–1118. Available from: PM:9240099.

Packer, C. N., Stewart-Brown, S., & Fowle, S. E. (1994). Damp housing and adult health: Results from a lifestyle study in Worcester, England. *Journal of Epidemiology and Community Health, 48,* 555–559.

Pampel, F. C., Krueger, P. M., & Denney, J. T. (2010). Socioeconomic disparities in health behaviors. *Annual Review of Sociology, 36,* 349–370. Available from: PM:21909182.

Patrick, K., Norman, G. J., Calfas, K. J., Sallis, J. F., Zabinski, M. F., Rupp, J., et al. (2004). Diet, physical activity, and sedentary behaviors as risk factors for overweight in adolescence. *Archives of Pediatrics and Adolescent Medicine, 158*(4), 385–390. Available from: PM:15066880.

Patterson, G. R., Debaryshe, B. D., & Ramsey, E. (1989). A developmental perspective on antisocial behavior. *American Psychologist, 44*(2), 329–335. Available from: PM:2653143.

Pickett, K. E., & Pearl, M. (2001). Multilevel analyses of neighbourhood socioeconomic context and health outcomes: A critical review. *Journal of Epidemiology and Community Health, 55*(2), 111–122. Available from: PM:11154250.

Pope, C. A., 3rd, Bates, D. V., & Raizenne, M. E. (1995). Health effects of particulate air pollution: Time for reassessment? *Environmental Health Perspectives, 103*(5), 472–480. Ref Type: Generic.

Raikkonen, K., Matthews, K. A., & Kuller, L. H. (2007). Depressive symptoms and stressful life events predict metabolic syndrome among middle-aged women: A comparison of world health organization, adult treatment panel III, and international diabetes foundation definitions. *Diabetes Care, 30*(4), 872–877. Available from: PM:17392548.

Rasmussen, H. N., Scheier, M. F., & Greenhouse, J. B. (2009). Optimism and physical health: A meta-analytic review. *Annals of Behavioral Medicine, 37*(3), 239–256. Available from: PM:19711142.
Repetti, R. L., Taylor, S. E., & Seeman, T. E. (2002). Risky families: Family social environments and the mental and physical health of offspring. *Psychological Bulletin, 128*(2), 330–366. Available from: PM:11931522.
Russek, L. G., & Schwartz, G. E. (1997). Perceptions of parental caring predict health status in midlife: A 35-year follow-up of the Harvard mastery of stress study. *Psychosomatic Medicine, 59*(2), 144–149. Available from: PM:9088050.
Sampson, R. J., Raudenbush, S. W., & Earls, F. (1997). Neighborhoods and violent crime: A multilevel study of collective efficacy. *Science, 277*(5328), 918–924. Available from: PM:9252316.
Sawyer, M. G., Spurrier, N., Whaites, L., Kennedy, D., Martin, A. J., & Baghurst, P. (2000). The relationship between asthma severity, family functioning and the health-related quality of life of children with asthma. *Quality of Life Research, 9*(10), 1105–1115. Available from: PM:11401043.
Stanbury, M., & Rosenman, K. D. (2014). Occupational health disparities: A state public health-based approach. *American Journal of Industrial Medicine, 57*(5), 596–604. Available from: PM:24375809.
Sternthal, M. J., Jun, H. J., Earls, F., & Wright, R. J. (2010). Community violence and urban childhood asthma: A multilevel analysis. *European Respiratory Journal, 36*(6), 1400–1409. Available from: PM:20413538.
Strully, K. (2009). Racial-ethnic disparities in health and the labor market: Losing and leaving jobs. *Social Science and Medicine, 69*(5), 768–776. Available from: PM:19615805.
Sundquist, J., Johansson, S. E., Yang, M., & Sundquist, K. (2006a). Low linking social capital as a predictor of coronary heart disease in Sweden: A cohort study of 2.8 million people. *Social Science and Medicine, 62*(4), 954–963. Available from: PM:16081195.
Sundquist, K., Theobald, H., Yang, M., Li, X., Johansson, S. E., & Sundquist, J. (2006b). Neighborhood violent crime and unemployment increase the risk of coronary heart disease: A multilevel study in an urban setting. *Social Science and Medicine, 62*(8), 2061–2071. Available from: PM:16203075.
Sweeting, H., & West, P. (1995). Family life and health in adolescence: A role for culture in the health inequalities debate? *Social Science and Medicine, 40*(2), 163–175. Available from: PM:7899929.
Taveras, E. M., Rifas-Shiman, S. L., Berkey, C. S., Rockett, H. R., Field, A. E., Frazier, A. L., et al. (2005). Family dinner and adolescent overweight. *Obesity Research, 13*(5), 900–906. Available from: PM:15919844.
Troxel, W. M., & Matthews, K. A. (2004). What are the costs of marital conflict and dissolution to children's physical health? *Clinical Child and Family Psychology Review, 7*(1), 29–57. Available from: PM:15119687.
Uchino, B. N. (2006). Social support and health: A review of physiological processes potentially underlying links to disease outcomes. *Journal of Behavioral Medicine, 29*(4), 377–387. Available from: PM:16758315.
Wadsworth, M. E., & Kuh, D. J. (1997). Childhood influences on adult health: A review of recent work from the British 1946 national birth cohort study, the MRC national survey of health and development. *Paediatric and Perinatal Epidemiology, 11*(1), 2–20. Available from: PM:9018723.
Wickstrom, R. (2007). Effects of nicotine during pregnancy: Human and experimental evidence. *Current Neuropharmacology, 5*(3), 213–222. Available from: PM:19305804.
Williams, D. R., & Collins, C. (2001). Racial residential segregation: A fundamental cause of racial disparities in health. *Public Health Reports, 116*, 404–416.
Williams, D. R., & Jackson, P. B. (2005). Social sources of racial disparities in health. *Health Affairs (Millwood), 24*(2), 325–334. svailable from: PM:15757915.

Wright, R. J., Mitchell, H., Visness, C. M., Cohen, S., Stout, J., Evans, R., et al. (2004). Community violence and asthma morbidity: The Inner-City Asthma study. *American Journal of Public Health, 94*(4), 625–632. Available from: PM:15054016.

Yen, I. H., & Kaplan, G. A. (1999). Poverty area residence and changes in depression and perceived health status: Evidence from the Alameda County Study. *International Journal of Epidemiology, 28*(1), 90–94. Available from: PM:10195670.

Zeigler-Johnson, C., Morales, K. H., Glanz, K., Spangler, E., Mitchell, J., & Rebbeck, T. R. (2015). Individual- and neighborhood-level education influences the effect of obesity on prostate cancer treatment failure after prostatectomy. *Cancer Causes and Control, 26*(9), 1329–1337. Available from: PM:26169299.

Chapter 6
Behavior and Health Disparities

Abstract The roles of diet, physical activity, tobacco use, and alcohol consumption are widely recognized as determinants for poor health outcomes. However, some of the choices are themselves determined by availability such that heavy marketing of unhealthy foods, alcohol, and cigarettes, especially targeting children, is commonplace in low-income neighborhoods along with limited access to stores selling healthy foods. Many of the behavioral factors are complicated by psychological and emotional issues, such as depression. Behavioral intervention is one option to reduce health disparities.

6.1 Introduction

The association between individual behavior and health is formidable. According to the US Office of Behavioral Health Equity, there are significant differences in behavior and health outcomes related to mental illness, substance-use disorders, suicidal rates, poverty, domestic violence, and tobacco use, as well as other drugs of addiction in various racial and ethnic groups (http://www.samhsa.gov/behavioral-health-equity). Behavioral activity and patterns play crucial roles in the development, prevention, treatment, and management of preventable diseases and health conditions, including heart disease, cancer, stroke, obesity, and HIV/AIDs. These are diseases for which the African-American (AA) population and other minority groups show significantly higher incidence and mortality rates in comparison with the European-American (EA) population. In addition, behavior is important for the improvement of health and treatment of chronic diseases, as well as the quality of life and overall mortality rates.

The link between behavior and health is well established. A recent review by Fisher et al. (2011) documented the important role of behavior in association with four disease-risk factors, namely, tobacco use, excessive alcohol consumption, sedentary lifestyle, and poor diet. These four disease-risk factors are collectively linked to major diseases such as CVD, HIV/AIDs, diabetes, and cancer. Furthermore, they are also modifiable life-style-related behavioral factors, which together are estimated to account for 36.8% of all mortality in the USA (Mokdad et al. 2004), a percentage that is increasing. Unhealthy life-style-related behaviors are particularly prevalent among low socioeconomic status (SES) groups, such as the AA population and other minority groups. For instance, smoking rates are higher among those with low SES in the majority of developed countries (Cavelaars et al. 2000; Marcus et al. 1989). In the USA for example, less than 20% of those at or above the poverty level smoke, whereas more than 30% of those below the poverty level smoke (Dube 2008).

There is abundant evidence in support of healthy behaviors (e.g., smoking cessation and increased physical activity), as well as the widespread awareness of the importance of healthy behaviors at least among the middle class or high-SES groups and good health outcomes. The central role of behavior in health, health care, and prevention has recently been recognized in the 2010 annual status report of the National Prevention, Health Promotion, and Public Health Council (Fisher et al. 2011). However, there are significant barriers to behavioral changes, including health literacy, emotional distress, and social and economic factors and systems, as well as policy factors at the local community, state, and national levels. These barriers are particularly prominent among the low-SES AA population and other minority groups. The following sections will discuss some of the behavioral choices associated with health disparities.

6.2 Dietary Behavior

The consumption of high-energy, dense foods, such as processed foods, red meat (hamburger), fried foods, and high-energy (sugary) drinks, are significantly associated with poor health. Poor diets that are rich in salt, fat, and sugars are implicated in many diseases, including diabetes, hypertension, hyperlipidemia, cardiovascular diseases (CVDs), and cancer. Some reports indicate that a diet rich in saturated fat, such as red meat, is associated with increased risk of prostate cancer (Lee et al. 2001; Liu et al. 2000). Poor diet, in combination with sedentary lifestyle, is significantly associated with weight gain and obesity, as well as obesity co-morbidities (Hayman et al. 2007; Lloyd-Jones et al. 2010; Williams et al. 2002). On the other hand, good dietary behaviors, such as the consumption of less saturated fat and more fruit, whole grain or unprocessed cereals, vegetables, legumes, and fresh fish, and the low- meat consumption that typifies a Mediterranean diet, are associated with good health. Furthermore, the high consumption of foods rich in fiber and vegetables, in combination with physical exercise, is associated with reduced risk of breast and colon cancers (Hill 2003) and coronary artery disease (Roberts and Barnard 2005).

However, the choice of foods is influenced by several factors that can be personal, practical, economic, and social. Availability and accessibility are the external constraining factors for expressing individual choice, as well as cost and convenience. Individuals of low SES, in particular the AA population and other minorities, reside in areas with limited access to fresh fruits and vegetables, whereas there are many fast-food shops that are cheaper and more convenient than nutritious home-prepared meals. Time constraints may not permit the opportunities for meal preparation in AA homes. For instance, low-income SES adults may have to work multiple jobs and, because of busy schedules, are less likely to have time to prepare nutritious and healthy foods, whereas unhealthy foods are more convenient to obtain. In turn, the choice of foods is influenced by family and/or cultural behavior, as well as socio-economic factors.

Like most families, when AA families get together, their typical social interactions are centered on food. The stereotypical AA cuisine, derived from cultural influence and necessity, which has come to be known as "soul food," is composed of fried foods and lots of fatty meats that are prepared in energy-rich gravies. A typical cuisine includes fried chicken, pig's feet, pork entrails, barbecued pork ribs, ham hocks, collard greens, cornbread, biscuits and gravy, and corn fritters, and the dessert delicacy is sweet-potato pie (Solomons 2003). In comparison, Africans on the native African continent typically cook their own foods of corn, black-eyed peas, rice, yams, and okra, which are much healthier than what is eaten in the diaspora. These foods are influenced by the dominant Western diets, which consist of high amounts of fat and salt and meat instead of vegetables. Unfortunately, because the typical soul food contains large amounts of meat, fat, sugar, and salt, this is not a healthy diet. AA individuals who consume this type of food on a regular basis are more likely to become obese and have increased susceptibility to hypertension and heart disease.

The dietary choices of the AA population have a strong cultural influence, so a good approach to encouraging healthier eating habits would be to educate the AA population to cook a healthier, modified version of soul food by baking, roasting, or broiling meats instead of frying them. The National Cancer Institute's (NCI) released a 5-A-Day report in 2002 that indicated a link between poor diet and life-threatening diseases in AA men, suggests that eating five to nine servings of fruits and vegetable a day can reduce the risk of many diseases that disproportionally affect the AA population. Making fruits and vegetables accessible, as well as affordable, will encourage healthy eating. Food markets in AA neighborhoods should supply vegetables that AA are already used to and are also rich in vitamins and nutrients, such as okra, collard greens, sweet potatoes, and coleslaw.

6.3 Physical Activity

According to the World Health Organization (WHO), physical inactivity or a sedentary lifestyle is one of the leading causes of global deaths (http://www.who.int/mediacentre/factsheets/fs385/en/) and is significantly associated with increased risk of type 2 diabetes (T2D), ischemic heart disease, and colorectal cancer. With urbanization in various parts of the world and changes in lifestyle patterns that contribute to more sedentary lifestyle, as well as the increase in the adoption of high-energy diets, these diseases are becoming more common, as well as impacting the younger generation. As mentioned in Sect. 6.1, unhealthy diets, in combination with a lack of physical activity, substantially contribute to increased disease risk and progression. On the other hand, increased physical activity and healthy diet are associated with reduced risks of coronary artery disease and colon cancer.

There is abundant scientific evidence of the benefits of physical activity in general health and well-being. Physical activity may benefit various parts of the human body, including the heart, skeletal muscles, bones, immune and nervous systems, and blood (e.g., cholesterol level) and is associated with the reduction of risks of many non-communicable diseases as described below (Penedo and Dahn 2005). Because of the many benefits of physical exercise to health, the American College of Sports Medicine recommends that, to promote and maintain good health, all healthy adults aged 18–65 should engage in moderate-intensity aerobic exercise for a minimum of 30 min per day for five days a week, or vigorous-intensity aerobic physical exercise for a minimum of 20 min for three days per week, however, exceeding this minimum recommendation has added benefits for reducing the risk of chronic diseases, such as diabetes and preventing unhealthy weight gain (Haskell et al. 2007). Walking is one of the best forms of exercise because of its low impact on the body joints, improvement of bone density, and its contribution to reducing weight through the process on burning calories.

In support of these recommendations, several studies have provided scientific proof for the benefits of physical activity. One study of 4672 men and women aged 25–74 found reduced risk of CVDs and cancer mortality in individuals who engaged in work, household activity, and total physical activity, suggesting that these exercises may be protective against premature deaths (Autenrieth et al. 2011). Obesity and diabetes are two conditions that are directly associated with physical inactivity. Abdominal obesity is associated with insulin resistance, hyperinsulinemia, hyperglycemia, dyslipidemia, hyperglycemia, and hypertension, whereas diabetes is associated with hyperglycemia. These conditions are often referred to as the metabolic syndrome. Obesity and diabetes are also associated with long-term complications, such as damage to kidneys, eyes, nerves, the heart, and blood vessels. Regular exercise in non-diabetic individuals has been correlated with beneficial effects in all aspects of metabolic symptoms, including that exercise reduced glycemic control as represented by reduced glycosylated hemoglobin (HbA_{Ic}) (Boule et al. 2001).

Other limited reports suggests that physical activity can also improve mental health, as demonstrated by improved educational attainment in children, as well as reduced incidence of obesity in children who engage in physical activity (Penedo and Dahn 2005). Similarly, among adults who engaged in physical activity, the same Penedo and Dahn study demonstrated that there was an overall improvement in mental agility and mobility, as well as longevity.

Given the importance of increased physical activity to good health, promoting the message of physical activity should focus on those who need it most, such as the low-income, low-SES, AA population. Unfortunately, health-promoting messages are often most effective with those who are socially integrated and have high-income SES. Individuals of low SES, including the AA population and other minorities, often reside in poor neighborhoods where streets are less safe for walking or cycling because of traffic and perceived fear of criminal activity, and these factors present real barriers to physical activities. In addition, poor neighborhoods do not have safe, green spaces or infrastructures, such as gymnasiums for physical activities. Thus, health campaigns, while having the right effect of improving the health of the general population, will have little to no impact in low-SES and economically deprived areas. To improve the physical activity among those of low SES, policies are needed at the local/state/governmental levels and additional philanthropic organizations to make changes to their communities and neighborhoods, such as providing safe areas and infrastructures needed for physical activity to specifically target those of low SES.

6.4 Tobacco Use

Twenty-eight various surgeon-general's reports on tobacco use and its impact on health since 1964 have unequivocally concluded that tobacco use is a leading risk factor for cancer, CVD, and pulmonary disease and remains the leading cause of preventable deaths by several other diseases (http://www.cdc.gov/tobacco/data_statistics/sgr/2004/pdfs/28reports.pdf). Smoking harms nearly every organ in the human body, and, as such, has a negative health impact on people at all stages of their lives: it harms unborn babies, infants, children, adolescent, adults, and senior citizens. According to a WHO report, tobacco smoke is the second major cause of mortality globally, and it is estimated that half of the 1.3 million people who smoke will eventually succumb to tobacco-related diseases (http://www.who.int/mediacentre/factsheets/fs339/en/).

Globally, the smoking rates among the socially and economically disadvantaged population in most developed nations can be as high as 60%, which is four times higher in comparison with the most affluent segments of the population (Sharma et al. 2010). There is scientific data to demonstrate that individuals of low-SES status have the highest rates of smoking behavior, although this behavior is not ubiquitous in the various ethnic and racial groups. The US Hispanic and Asian-American populations smoke less than EAs, whereas Native Americans have the highest smoking rates of any ethnic and racial groups in the USA, with the rate among AAs being comparable to that of EAs (Warner 2011). However AA youth in middle and high schools smoke at far lower rates than their EA counterparts, indicating that there are differences in the initiation and cessation rates of smoke behavior in various populations. Although the AA population overall has low smoking rates in comparison with EAs, they have higher incidence of tobacco-related diseases, such as lung cancer, and greater tobacco dependence in comparison with their EA counterparts.

The risk to tobacco use is multifactorial, including genetic influence, multiple environmental factors, social norms and pressures, and familial, marketing, and policy influences. There are scientific reports from twin and adoption studies to show that smoking initiation, as well as cessation, is influenced by genetic and environmental factors. Studies carried out using data from a twin-smoking questionnaire that examined lifetime or current use of tobacco products observed a strong correlation for smoking in monozygotic twins raised apart or reared together and substantial correlations in the smoking patterns between biological parents and offspring that extended to three generations, but not between adoptive parents and their adoptive offspring, indicating a strong genetic component in smoking behavior (Maes et al. 2006). In addition, there was a strong association between shared environmental factors and smoking behavior, as well as increased risk of smoking uptake when children or youths have friends that smoke (Maes et al. 2006). However, these studies were carried out in EA populations and may not necessarily reflect the smoking pattern in other ethnic and racial groups.

Numerous reports demonstrate that smoking is strongly correlated with income level, educational attainment, and employment status. The pattern of parental smoking that is related to SES has been shown to be a predictor of smoking uptake in young people (Amos 2009). This reflects a mixture of influences that includes parental role modeling, social norms, and access to cigarettes/tobacco in the home. One report found a high incidence of smoking behavior in low-income neighborhoods characterized by single-parent households in rented accommodations (Sharma et al. 2010). In this report, the pattern of high smoking behavior was also linked to communities with little social support, high unemployment rates, or individuals with few employment skills, limited transportation options, as well as individuals who spend a large amount of time watching television and are significantly concentrated in minority communities, such as those dominated by racial and ethnic groups. Youths and adolescents of low SES and/or with poor educational performance may feel peer pressure to smoke, even though they have lower awareness and understanding of tobacco's harm and behavioral problems. Overall, the consequences and variations in tobacco-smoking prevalence in various ethnic and racial groups most likely account for a significant proportion of disparities in health outcomes.

Since AAs have the highest incidence of, and mortality rates from, smoking-related lung cancer, studies to investigate the genetic factors associated with smoking behavior are important. This is because the AA population on average initiates smoking at a later age and smokes fewer cigarettes per day in comparison with their EA counterpart and yet is less successful in quitting smoking. Several GWAS have identified genetic variants on chromosome 15q25 to harbor genetic variants that are associated with smoking frequencies in both AA and EA populations (David et al. 2012), although these variances may explain a small proportion of addiction to tobacco smoke. As mentioned earlier, the AA population on average smokes fewer cigarettes per day in comparison with the EA population. However, the AA population appears to take in higher levels of nicotine and carcinogens per cigarette smoked, and there appears to be differences in clearance of nicotine, cotinine, and other tobacco metabolites (Benowitz et al. 2011). Genetic analysis indicates that the molecular mechanisms whereby the AA population takes in high levels of nicotine and has lower clearances of nicotine and tobacco metabolites is in part mediated by differences in genetic variants in the carcinogen detoxifier cytochrome p450 2A6 gene in AAs compared with the EA population, and this could potentially contribute to the observed differences in rates of tobacco consumption.

The AA population and other US minority groups, including Hispanics, carry a disproportionate burden of tobacco-related diseases including cancer and CVDs, despite having generally lower to intermediate frequencies of smoking patterns in comparison with the EA population. One reason for the increased risk of tobacco-related diseases in the AA and Hispanic populations, even though they smoke less frequently, is that they are less likely to quit tobacco smoking (Trinidad et al. 2011) and have low will power to quit, as well as that they experience stronger addiction to tobacco smoke. Furthermore, AAs and other minorities typically reside in neighborhoods where there is reduced social support for quitting (Hiscock et al. 2012). Individuals of low SES, particularly AAs and other minority populations that are socially disadvantaged, also cite tobacco smoking as a coping mechanism for dealing with environmental stresses and psychological challenges; this makes it difficult to quit tobacco smoking for fear of becoming nervous/restless or depressed and may be the reason for relapsing at higher rates than high-SES smokers (Pisinger et al. 2011).

Another challenge faced in low-SES neighborhoods is that tobacco companies deliberately manipulate and target various minority groups, including the AA population with low-education levels, using marketing and advertisement alleging menthol cigarettes are healthier than non-menthol cigarettes to the young and AA populations who might otherwise quit smoking (Anderson 2011). In addition to marketing, tobacco companies have also built relationships with working-class/blue-collar trade unions through financial support for the tobacco industry's position (Balbach et al. 2005) to promote tobacco use. The tobacco companies also use price promotions and discount vouchers as lures, knowing very well the relevance of cost to disadvantaged smokers, thus further reducing the success of tobacco-cessation initiatives (Murphy et al. 2010). Thus, it appears that the tobacco industry is aware of psychosocial impacts of income on the low-SES populations and exploits these effects in their marketing campaigns.

Given the widespread global smoking rates, particularly among those of low SES, such as the long-term unemployed, single parents, ethnic minorities, and immigrants, as well as the homeless, mentally ill, and prisoners, (Bryant et al. 2011), and the debilitating health effects of tobacco-related health risks and health disparities, concerted efforts in tobacco prevention programs designed to promote smoking cessation are crucial. Tobacco-cessation programs should be designed and tailored specifically for low-SES- neighborhood youths and adults with strict enforcement. Government policies can also help to prevent the tobacco companies from targeting low-SES neighborhoods with their ads and financial incentives. Other smoking-control interventions should target the perception of smoking as "cool" or the norm and provide help and support for people who are trying to quit smoking, as well as establishing smoke-free policies in public areas. Early intervention programs through education about tobacco harms may help prevent the low-SES population from developing dependence on, or lessen the influences of, tobacco smoke. Raising tobacco prices may be an intervention strategy with the most potential to reduce health inequalities from tobacco (Hiscock et al. 2012).

Anti-smoking public-health campaigns and government legislation have been successful in reducing tobacco smoking in work places and, secondly, exposure to tobacco toxicity, as well as public-health awareness of tobacco's harmful effects by the general public. While these have resulted in decreased tobacco smoking in the general public in Western societies, including USA, Canada and some European countries, the incidence of tobacco smoking is on the rise in other parts of the world, such as China and India, where government policies are relaxed towards the tobacco industry.

6.5 Excessive Alcohol Consumption

Excessive alcohol consumption is significantly associated with motor-vehicle accidents, intentional injuries, homicides, suicides, falls, drownings, and poisonings. In addition, excessive alcohol consumption is a risk factor for numerous diseases, including fetal alcohol syndrome (a leading cause of preventable mental retardation), gastrointestinal diseases, liver diseases, cardiovascular diseases, diabetes and infectious diseases, e.g., pneumonia, tuberculosis, HIV/AIDs, and certain forms of cancer (esophageal, pancreatic, and liver). Excessive alcohol drinking or binge and heavy drinking as defined by the National Institute on Alcohol Abuse and Alcoholism's (NIAAA) is consuming more than four standard drinks per day (or more than 14 per week) for men, and more than three per day (or more than seven per week) for women (https://www.niaaa.nih.gov/alcohol-health/overview). The NIAAA estimates that, in 2012, there were 11.2 million men and 5.7 million women and an estimated 855,000 adolescent's aged 12–17, who had some form of alcohol-related disorder in the USA.

If the US population is stratified by ethnic and racial groups, there are significant disparities in alcohol-related problems among the various ethnic and racial groups. European-Americans and Native Americans have the highest rates of alcohol use relative to other ethnic groups (http://pubs.niaaa.nih.gov/publications/arh40/152-160.htm). However, AAs and Hispanics are more likely to report alcohol-dependence symptoms than EAs, as well as suffering having significantly greater consequences from alcohol consumption. The AA population and Hispanics have greater risks of developing alcohol-related morbidity and mortality, as they relate to injury, motor-vehicle accidents, cirrhosis, homicide, and certain alcohol-linked cancers (Keyes et al. 2012). Overall, Native Americans have the highest prevalence in the national estimates of alcohol-related motor-vehicle accidents and alcohol-related suicides.

Factors that contribute to ethnic differences in alcohol-related problems are social and cultural, as well as biological factors. Minority groups such as AA and Hispanic populations typically are socially disadvantaged, as characterized by lower-SES, poor neighborhoods with greater availability of alcohol outlets, which lead to a high incidence of alcohol-related violence and morbidity, violent assaults, and high-risk sexual behaviors and other problems (McKinney et al. 2012). Acculturation and the availability of alcohol are also risk factors for alcohol dependency among certain minority groups. For instance, comparison of Mexican-born and natural-born Mexican Americans indicates that being born in the USA was identified as a risk factor for alcohol dependence (Alegria et al. 2008), suggesting that availability of alcohol in US poor neighborhoods may be a contributing factor for alcohol dependence among these recent immigrants.

There are biological factors that contribute to the disparities associated with alcohol dependence. For instance, among the Asian (Chinese, Korean, and Japanese) populations, genetic variants in genes that encode for enzymes responsible for converting alcohol to acetaldehyde (alcohol dehydrogenase or ADH1, 2, or 3), or the breakdown of acetaldehyde to carbon dioxide and water (acetaldehyde dehydrogenase or ALDH1 and 2) are linked to reduced rates of alcohol dependence (Eng 2007). In the AA population, genetic variants in ALDH2 (ALDH2*2 allele) have also been reported to have a protective effect against alcohol dependence. Similarly, variants in alleles ALDH1 A1 *2 and ALDH1A1 *3 may be associated with more-rapid breakdown and reduced risk of alcoholism in AAs and certain Native-American Indian tribes (Scott and Taylor 2007). On the other hand, among Mexican-Americans, genetic variants in alcohol dehydrogenase 3 (ADH3), ADH3*2 allele and cytochrome P450 2E1 (CYP2E1), CYP2E1 c2/C allele might be independently associated with increased risk of alcohol dependence and alcoholism in Mexican-American men (Konishi et al. 2003).

Given that excessive alcohol consumption is the third leading cause of preventable death in the USA and a risk factor for many health and societal problems, interventions that can reduce the access and availability of alcohol would go a long way to alleviate some of the public-health burden of alcohol-related health issues. Some measures such as increasing taxes on alcohol have been found to be associated with less drinking of alcohol by youths and regulation of alcohol-distribution outlets. Generally, increased outlet density was associated with increases in alcohol-related harms. Thus, limiting the number of days and hours of alcohol sales may be beneficial, as studies have shown that removing these restrictions was associated with increased alcohol-related hazards, such as vehicular crashes, assaults and injuries, and increases in violent crime (http://www.thecommunityguide.org/alcohol/limitinghourssale.html).

6.6 Behavioral Intervention and Health Disparities

This chapter has focused on some of the factors associated with unhealthy behavior, such as personal choice, social and cultural influences, and biological factors, as well as governmental policies, all of which can either independently or collectively influence health behavior for good or bad. The prevailing data demonstrates that ethnic minority groups including the AA population have adverse health behaviors, thus behavioral intervention is one option for reducing health disparities. Since the overarching goals of Healthy People 2020 are to improve the quality of life for Americans and to eliminate health disparities, it should have a focus on behavioral interventions tailored towards ethnic and minority groups.

Behavioral intervention as a mechanism for disease prevention and improving overall health makes sense. While there may be many challenges in implementing behavioral-intervention programs, this option presents opportunities to prevent unnecessary pain and suffering and to improve the overall quality of life. According to the former surgeon general David Satcher (Satcher 2006), over 90% of the national health budget goes towards treating diseases and its complication, whereas prevention only accounts for 2–3% of the total budget. Given this evidence, allocating more resources for implementing behavioral interventions would greatly benefit our healthcare system.

6.6.1 Can We Afford Behavioral Interventions?

A 2007 review on the database of medical and economics of behavioral interventions for smoking, physical inactivity, poor diet and alcohol abuse (Gordon et al. 2007) showed an overall favorable cost effectiveness for multiple behavioral interventions. Evidence indicates that the greatest return on investment will come from interventions that simultaneously target multiple risk behaviors in various populations (Gordon et al. 2007). Also interventions targeted at high-risk groups may achieve efficiency through the greater available risk to be reduced. For instance, interventions to diet change were found to be especially cost effective when applied to groups with 3–4 combined risk factors, such as smoking, hypertension, and elevated LDL cholesterol (Krumholz et al. 2002).

A landmark behavioral intervention study named the Diabetes Prevention Program (DPP) was established with the overarching objective to reduce diabetes' risk. The goals set out in the DPP was the total reduction of body weight by 7% and a minimum of 150 min of physical activity per week (Diabetes Prevention Program 2002a, b). The study involved 27-center randomized clinical trial of 1079 participants that were made up of 55% EAs and 45% racial and ethnic minorities. The study used dietary modification focused on reducing total fat and a minimum of 150 min' walk (similar to brisk walk) and equivalent to 700 K Cal/week of total calorie expenditure, with participants instructed to self-monitor fat and calorie intake. In a parallel DPP medication intervention study, individuals received the oral diabetic drug metformin to decrease glucose production, inhibit glucose intolerance, and to prevent T2D. At the end of a six-month study period, these strategies resulted in a 58% reduction in the incidence of diabetes relative to placebo control, whereas the metformin intervention reduced incidence by 31% over a period of 2.8 years. Moreover, group differences were sustained over a total of ten years of observation. The success and the efficacy in the DPP means that lifestyle intervention is now the preferred approach for preventing and managing type 2 diabetes among US young people (Nassis et al. 2005), with increasing incidence of T2D as a result of increasing childhood obesity (McGavock et al. 2007). It is estimated that the routine use of the behavioral and medication interventions would cost a modest $13,200 and $14,300, respectively, over a period of three years (Burnet et al. 2006), when compared to the three-fold higher cost of medical treatment for diabetes.

Similar success stories have been reported for behavioral intervention in smoking cessation that offers benefits to smokers at about a tenth of the cost of surgical rescue for those unable to quit (Hoogendoorn et al. 2010). In the future, cost-effective and state-of-the-art methods of behavioral interventions would save taxpayers money in comparison with other medical approaches to healthcare (Gold 1996). It is estimated that 13.8 million deaths annually can be prevented by implementing interventions for tobacco smoking and salt reduction, globally (Asaria et al. 2007).

6.6.2 Individual and Community Behavioral Interventions

Unhealthy diet and limited physical activity in the AA population and other minority groups are significantly associated with disproportional health disparities in preventable chronic diseases. Therefore, behavioral interventions based on physical activity and healthy diet would alleviate some of these health disparities. A systematic review article on physical activity and nutritional intervention by Lemacks et al. (2013) has demonstrated that educational information and community-based programs about healthy lifestyle choices, with regards to nutrition and physical activity interventions, were significantly associated with reduced risk of chronic diseases as measured by improved clinically relevant outcomes, including weight loss, reduced waist circumference, and reduced body fat, as well as blood lipids. One report indicates that, in addition to providing educational resources, improved interactions with healthcare providers aimed at increasing uptake and compliance of pharmacological intervention was associated with tobacco-smoking cessation in minority groups (Liu et al. 2012).

In addition, because the AA population and other minorities reside in low-income neighborhoods that have large numbers of fast-food outlets, alcohol outlets, and tobacco smoking, intervention strategies at the individual level, therefore, may not be enough. Instead, progress may require community-level intervention strategies, such as limiting the number of alcohol and tobacco outlets in the communities, as well as improving the environment by creating safe and green environment to exercise. In addition, communities should provide access to fresh fruits and vegetables through neighborhood supermarkets and government-subsidized farmers markets. Therefore, striking a balance between individuals and their environment is critical when it comes to behavioral intervention and health (Minkler 1999). Healthcare reforms need to incorporate a "national culture of wellness" (Baucus 2009), which is tailored specifically to various cultures and ethnic settings and balances individual and community-level interventions, as well as the implementation of state and government policies with emphasis on behavior, which is an essential base for all preventive and clinical services.

6.6.3 Government Policies

Successful and widespread implementation of behavioral interventions will require policies at the governmental and local, as well as community, levels to meet the challenges associated with behavioral interventions for chronic diseases that are prevalent in the general population, as well as minority groups, including obesity and diabetes.

6.6.4 Behavioral Intervention for Obesity

Obesity is related to the development of a number of diseases, making it now the second leading cause of preventable disease and death in the USA. A 2005 estimate indicates that it costs the healthcare system in excess of US$190-billion dollars to treat obesity and obesity-related conditions per year, and this number is now likely higher with the increase incidence of obesity nationwide. As stated in Chaps. 2 and 3, racial and ethnic minority groups, such as the AA population, and, in particular, women are at disproportional risk of obesity. The goal of Healthy People 2010 in reducing the prevalence of obesity in adults and children (Ogden et al. 2008) was not achieved but is of continued importance for the goal in health disparities of Healthy People 2020.

Lifestyle-intervention strategies, such as healthy diet and improved physical activity targeted towards weight loss, as well as reducing energy intake and or increasing energy expenditure, has proven successful in the DPP discussed in Sect. 6.6.1 and can be applied to obesity intervention as well (Harvey and Ogden 2014). However, few weight-loss trials in the USA have involved low-income minority groups, including AAs or Hispanics, and several challenges has been cited for this: lack of access, transportation, resources, limited literacy, and a language barrier. One way to address a number of these barriers is to use internet-based behavioral intervention, whereby intervention materials can be delivered in multiple languages at various literacy levels, although there are still some disparities in digital access among high- and low-income populations (Harvey and Ogden 2014). Since it is believed that low-income individuals do not have the same level of motivation that high-income individuals have to recognize unhealthy states and do something about them, some modest financial incentives can also improve behavior regarding responding to intervention regimes.

6.7 Behavior in the Post-Genome Era

The era of post-genomics refers to the period after the completion of the human-genome sequencing. This landmark accomplishment, since the identification of DNA as the genetic material for all eukaryotic organisms, has revolutionized our understanding of the role of DNA sequences in health and disease as well as the disparities associated with diseases. Some current thinking is that genes can explain the underlying causes of diseases, eliminating the roles of behavior and environmental factors. While this may be true for the few diseases that are caused by genetic factors, such as cystic fibrosis and other diseases discussed in Chap. 2, most diseases are caused by the interaction of genetics and environmental and behavioral factors.

Diabetes among Pima Indians provides a good example. Ample evidence links genetics and T2D in the Pima population. Yet, there are significant differences in diabetes risk in this population by geographical regions: For instance, Pima Indians living in Mexico have a relatively low diabetes incidence compared to Pima Indians living in the USA and who have adopted the Western dietary lifestyle. This provides clear evidence that the environment, as well as behavioral changes, is associated with diabetes risk. While there is scientific evidence to demonstrate a genetic component in the high prevalence of T2D in the Pima Indian population, the prevailing observations would indicate that the genetic variants associated with disease risk have little effect in disease incidence in the absence of unhealthy behaviors, such as high-energy or high-fat diets, as well as a sedentary lifestyle (Fisher et al. 2011). Thus, behavioral intervention would have a major impact in reducing T2D incidence among the Pima Indians in the USA.

Similarly, behavioral intervention has a broad and central role in several other major diseases and disease disparities of huge public-health concern in the USA and globally, as summarized in the review by Fisher et al. (2011). For instance, environmental stresses, diet, smoking, and low physical activity are associated with cardiovascular diseases, diabetes, and cancer. Moreover, other behavioral and lifestyle choices, such as high-risk sexual behavior, are significantly associated with HIV/AIDs. Effective interventions such as tobacco-smoking cessation, increased physical activity, and proper diet, as well as behavioral interventions that focus on the psychological factors associated with high-risk behaviors, would have a huge impact on reducing adverse health outcomes and health disparities.

6.8 Summary

The role of behavior in health encompasses a broad spectrum, from lifestyle to diseases, e.g., tobacco and excessive alcohol use, poor diet, physical inactivity, cardiovascular disease, diabetes, and cancer. It is estimated that individual behavior accounts for 40% of the determinants of premature death in the USA, whereas 20% is due to social and environmental factors, 10% due to health care, and the remaining 30% attributed to genetic determinants, see Fig. 6.1 (Schroeder 2007). There is overwhelming evidence that suggests efficacious behavioral intervention can reduce disease risk, as demonstrated by the successful public-health campaigns against tobacco smoking, which now parallels declines in mortality rates of certain types of cancer (e.g., lung) that is associated with tobacco smoking. It took several decades for the successful, broad and multilevel public-health campaign, begun after the first surgeon general's report in 1964, for the public to recognize the dangerous effects of tobacco smoking on health. Similar public-health campaigns based on the tobacco-cessation model should be implemented to foster the wide-range forces that determine diet, alcohol consumption, and physical activity, and this will require interventions addressing multiple layers of influence (Economos et al. 2007; Kumanyika 2008; Story et al. 2008). Unlike the surgeon general's report on the dangers of tobacco smoke that was first published in 1964, the surgeon general's report on physical activity and nutrition was published as recently as 20 years ago, in 1996. At least among the US high-income and well-educated population, predominantly the EA population, there is widespread awareness of the importance of health behaviors, such as decreased consumption of high-fat foods and physical exercise, and this needs to reach low-SES minorities.

Despite the overwhelming evidence in favor of healthy behavior, such as smoking cessation, there is a failure of universal adoption of healthy behaviors,

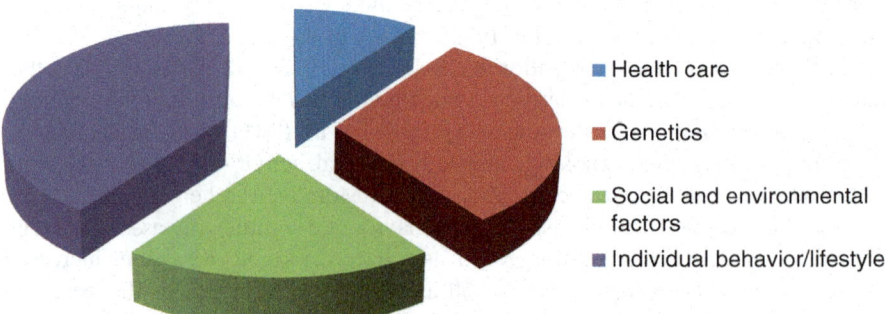

Fig. 6.1 Pie chart depicting the fractions of risk factors associated with premature deaths. Data used for constructing the pie chart was obtained from the Schroeder (2007) and NRJM 357; 1221–1228

particularly among ethnic minority groups, including the AA population. Some of barriers to change include health literacy (low-educational attainment), bad behavior as a stress-controlling mechanism, social and economic factors, and lack of minority advocates for social issues in government and local policy-making bodies. Environmental barriers such as safe neighborhoods are important for low-SES groups to adopt healthy behaviors, such as exercise and recreation. Education and specific approaches to adopting healthy behaviors that are tailored specifically to low-income populations are important to address some of these burdens. Such interventions focused on smoking cessation and T2D diabetes have been effective in high-risk populations, as already discussed in this chapter. One of the overarching aims of Healthy People 2020 is to improve the quality of life for all Americans, and this would have to take into consideration preventive measures that look at behaviors at individual, community, and society levels. With the advent of the Universal Care Act, the opportunity may be upon us to act.

References

Alegria, M., Canino, G., Shrout, P. E., Woo, M., Duan, N., Vila, D., et al. (2008). Prevalence of mental illness in immigrant and non-immigrant U.S. Latino groups. *American Journal of Psychiatry, 165*(3), 359–369. Available from: PM:18245178.

Amos, A. A. K. F. J. A. H. G. (2009). A review of young people and smoking in England. New York: Public Health Research Consortium.

Anderson, S. J. (2011). Marketing of menthol cigarettes and consumer perceptions: A review of tobacco industry documents. *Tobacco Control, 20*(2), ii20–ii28. Available from: PM:21504928.

Asaria, P., Chisholm, D., Mathers, C., Ezzati, M., & Beaglehole, R. (2007). Chronic disease prevention: Health effects and financial costs of strategies to reduce salt intake and control tobacco use. *Lancet, 370*(9604), 2044–2053. Available from: PM:18063027.

Autenrieth, C. S., Baumert, J., Baumeister, S. E., Fischer, B., Peters, A., Doring, A., et al. (2011). Association between domains of physical activity and all-cause, cardiovascular and cancer mortality. *European Journal of Epidemiology, 26*(2), 91–99. Available from: PM:21153912.

Balbach, E. D., Barbeau, E. M., Manteufel, V., & Pan, J. (2005). Political coalitions for mutual advantage: the case of the Tobacco Institute's Labor Management Committee. *American Journal of Public Health, 95*(6), 985–993. Available from: PM:15914820.

Baucus, M. (2009). *Call to action: Health reform 2009*. Washington, D.C: U.S. Senate Finance Committee.

Benowitz, N. L., Dains, K. M., Dempsey, D., Wilson, M., & Jacob, P. (2011). Racial differences in the relationship between number of cigarettes smoked and nicotine and carcinogen exposure. *Nicotine Tobacco Research, 13*(9), 772–783. Available from: PM:21546441.

Boule, N. G., Haddad, E., Kenny, G. P., Wells, G. A., & Sigal, R. J. (2001). Effects of exercise on glycemic control and body mass in type 2 diabetes mellitus: A meta-analysis of controlled clinical trials. *JAMA, 286*(10), 1218–1227. Available from: PM:11559268.

Bryant, J., Bonevski, B., Paul, C., McElduff, P., & Attia, J. (2011). A systematic review and meta-analysis of the effectiveness of behavioural smoking cessation interventions in selected disadvantaged groups. *Addiction, 106*(9), 1568–1585. Available from: PM:21489007.

Burnet, D. L., Elliott, L. D., Quinn, M. T., Plaut, A. J., Schwartz, M. A., & Chin, M. H. (2006). Preventing diabetes in the clinical setting. *Journal of General Internal Medicine, 21*(1), 84–93. Available from: PM:16423130.

Cavelaars, A. E., Kunst, A. E., Geurts, J. J., Crialesi, R., Grotvedt, L., Helmert, U., et al. (2000). Educational differences in smoking: International comparison. *BMJ, 320*(7242), 1102–1107. Available from: PM:10775217.

David, S. P., Hamidovic, A., Chen, G. K., Bergen, A. W., Wessel, J., et al. (2012). Genome-wide meta-analyses of smoking behaviors in African Americans. *Translational Psychiatry, 2*, e119. Available from: PM:22832964.

Diabetes Prevention Program. (2002). The diabetes prevention program. *Diabetes Care, 25*, 2165–2171.

Diabetes Prevention Program Research Group. (2002). Reduction of the incidence of type 2 diabetes with lifestyle intervention or metformin. *New England Journal of Medicine, 346*, 393–403.

Dube, S. R. A. K. M. A. C. R. (2009). Cigarette smoking among adults and trends in smoking cessation-U.S., 2008. *Morbidity and Mortality Weekly Reports, 58*(44), 1227–1232.

Economos, C. D., Hyatt, R. R., Goldberg, J. P., Must, A., Naumova, E. N., Collins, J. J., et al. (2007). A community intervention reduces BMI z-score in children: Shape up somerville first year results. *Obesity (Silver Spring), 15*(5), 1325–1336. Available from: PM:17495210.

Eng, M. Y. L. S. W. T. (2007). ALDH2, ADH1B, and ADH1C genotypes in Asians: A literature review. *Alcohol Research Health, 30*, 22–27.

Fisher, E. B., Fitzgibbon, M. L., Glasgow, R. E., Haire-Joshu, D., Hayman, L. L., Kaplan, R. M., et al. (2011). Behavior matters. *American Journal Preventive Medicine, 40*(5), e15–e30. Available from: PM:21496745.

Gold, M. L. S. J. R. L. W. M. C. (1996). *Cost-effectiveness in health and medicine: The report of the panel on cost-effectiveness in health and medicine*. New York: Oxford University Press.

Gordon, L., Graves, N., Hawkes, A., & Eakin, E. (2007). A review of the cost-effectiveness of face-to-face behavioural interventions for smoking, physical activity, diet and alcohol. *Chronic Illness, 3*(2), 101–129. Available from: PM:18083667.

Harvey, J. R., & Ogden, D. E. (2014). Obesity treatment in disadvantaged population groups: Where do we stand and what can we do? *Preventive Medicine, 68*, 71–75. Available from: PM:24878585.

Haskell, W. L., Lee, I. M., Pate, R. R., Powell, K. E., Blair, S. N., Franklin, B. A., et al. (2007). Physical activity and public health: Updated recommendation for adults from the American College of Sports Medicine and the American Heart Association. *Circulation, 116*(9). 1081–1093. Available from: PM:17671237.

Hayman, L. L., Meininger, J. C., Daniels, S. R., McCrindle, B. W., Helden, L., Ross, J., et al. (2007). Primary prevention of cardiovascular disease in nursing practice: Focus on children and youth: A scientific statement from the American Heart Association Committee on Atherosclerosis, Hypertension, and Obesity in Youth of the Council on Cardiovascular Disease in the Young, Council on Cardiovascular Nursing, Council on Epidemiology and Prevention, and Council on Nutrition, Physical Activity, and Metabolism. *Circulation, 116*(3), 344–357. Available from: PM:17592077.

Hill, M. (2003). Dietary fibre and colon cancer: Where do we go from here? *Proceddings Nutrition Society, 62*(1), 63–65.

Hiscock, R., Bauld, L., Amos, A., Fidler, J. A., & Munafo, M. (2012). Socioeconomic status and smoking: A review. *Annals of the New York Academy Sciences, 1248*, 107–123. Available from: PM:22092035.

Hoogendoorn, M., Feenstra, T. L., Hoogenveen, R. T., & Rutten-van Molken, M. P. (2010). Long-term effectiveness and cost-effectiveness of smoking cessation interventions in patients with COPD. *Thorax, 65*(8), 711–718. Available from: PM:20685746.

Keyes, K. M., Liu, X. C., & Cerda, M. (2012). The role of race/ethnicity in alcohol-attributable injury in the United States. *Epidemiology Reviews, 34*, 89–102. Available from: PM:21930592.

Konishi, T., Calvillo, M., Leng, A. S., Feng, J., Lee, T., Lee, H., et al. (2003). The ADH3*2 and CYP2E1 c2 alleles increase the risk of alcoholism in Mexican American men. *Experimental and Molecular Pathology, 74*(2), 183–189. Available from: PM:12710951.

Krumholz, H. M., Weintraub, W. S., Bradford, W. D., Heidenreich, P. A., Mark, D. B., & Paltiel, A. D. (2002). Task force #2–the cost of prevention: Can we afford it? Can we afford not to do

References

it? 33rd Bethesda Conference. *Journal* of the *American College* of *Cardiology, 40*(4) 603–615. Available from: PM:12204490.

Kumanyika, S. K. (2008). Environmental influences on childhood obesity: Ethnic and cultural influences in context. *Physiology Behavior, 94*(1), 61–70. Available from: PM:18158165.

Lee, I. M., Sesso, H. D., Chen, J. J., & Paffenbarger, R. S., Jr. (2001). Does physical activity play a role in the prevention of prostate cancer? *Epidemiology Reviews, 23*(1), 132–137. Available from: PM:11588837.

Lemacks, J., Wells, B. A., Ilich, J. Z., & Ralston, P. A. (2013). Interventions for improving nutrition and physical activity behaviors in adult African American populations: A systematic review, January 2000 through December 2011. *Preventing Chronic Disease, 10*, E99. Available from: PM:23786910.

Liu, J., Davidson, E., Bhopal, R., White, M., Johnson, M., Netto, G., et al. (2012). Adapting health promotion interventions to meet the needs of ethnic minority groups: Mixed-methods evidence synthesis. *Health Technology Assessment, 16*(44), 1–469. Available from: PM:23158845.

Liu, S., Lee, I. M., Linson, P., Ajani, U., Buring, J. E., & Hennekens, C. H. (2000). A prospective study of physical activity and risk of prostate cancer in US physicians. *International Journal of Epidemiology, 29*(1), 29–35. Available from: PM:10750600.

Lloyd-Jones, D. M., Hong, Y., Labarthe, D., Mozaffarian, D., Appel, L. J., Van, H. L. (2010). Defining and setting national goals for cardiovascular health promotion and disease reduction: The American Heart Association's strategic Impact Goal through 2020 and beyond. *Circulation, 121*(4), 586–613. Available from: PM:20089546.

Maes, H. H., Neale, M. C., Kendler, K. S., Martin, N. G., Heath, A. C., & Eaves, L. J. (2006). Genetic and cultural transmission of smoking initiation: An extended twin kinship model. *Behavior Genetics, 36*(6), 795–808. Available from: PM:16810566.

Marcus, A. C., Shopland, D. R., Crane, L. A., & Lynn, W. R. (1989). Prevalence of cigarette smoking in the United States: Estimates from the 1985 current population survey. *Journal of the* National Cancer Institute, *81*(6), 409–414. Available from: PM:2783978.

McGavock, J., Sellers, E., & Dean, H. (2007). Physical activity for the prevention and management of youth-onset type 2 diabetes mellitus: Focus on cardiovascular complications. *Diabetes Vascular Disease Research, 4*(4), 305–310. Available from: PM:18158700.

McKinney, C. M., Chartier, K. G., Caetano, R., & Harris, T. R. (2012). Alcohol availability and neighborhood poverty and their relationship to binge drinking and related problems among drinkers in committed relationships. *Journal of* Interpersonal Violence, *27*(13), 2703–2727. Available from: PM:22890980.

Minkler, M. (1999). Personal responsibility for health? A review of the arguments and the evidence at century's end. *Health Education & Behavior, 26*(1), 121–140. Available from: PM:9952056.

Mokdad, A. H., Marks, J. S., Stroup, D. F., & Gerberding, J. L. (2004). Actual causes of death in the United States, 2000. *JAMA, 291*(10), 1238–1245. Available from: PM:15010446.

Murphy, J. M., de Moreno, S. L., Cummings, K. M., Hyland, A., & Mahoney, M. C. (2010). Changes in cigarette smoking, purchase patterns, and cessation-related behaviors among low-income smokers in New York State from 2002 to 2005. *Journal of Public Health Management Practice, 16*(4), 277–284. Available from: PM:20520365.

Nassis, G. P., Papantakou, K., Skenderi, K., Triandafillopoulou, M., Kavouras, S. A., Yannakoulia, M., et al. (2005). Aerobic exercise training improves insulin sensitivity without changes in body weight, body fat, adiponectin, and inflammatory markers in overweight and obese girls. *Metabolism, 54*(11), 1472–1479. Available from: PM:16253636.

National Prevention Health Promotion and Public Health Council. (2010). Annual status report of the national prevention. Health Promotion, and Public Health Council.

Ogden, C. L., Carroll, M. D., & Flegal, K. M. (2008). High body mass index for age among US children and adolescents, 2003–2006. *JAMA, 299*(20), 2401–2405. Available from: PM:18505949.

Penedo, F. J. & Dahn, J. R. (2005). Exercise and well-being: A review of mental and physical health benefits associated with physical activity. *Current Opinion Psychiatry, 18*(2), 189–193. Available from: PM:16639173.

Pisinger, C., Aadahl, M., Toft, U., & Jorgensen, T. (2011). Motives to quit smoking and reasons to relapse differ by socioeconomic status. *Preventive Medicine, 52*(1), 48–52. Available from: PM:21047525.

Roberts, C. K. & Barnard, R. J. (2005). Effects of exercise and diet on chronic disease. *The Journal of Applied Physiology (1985), 98*(1), 3–30. Available from: PM:15591300.

Satcher, D. (2006). The prevention challenge and opportunity. *Health Affairs (Millwood), 25*(4), 1009–1011. Available from: PM:16835179.

Schroeder, S. A. (2007). Shattuck lecture. We can do better–improving the health of the American people. *The New England Journal of Medicine, 357*(12), 1221–1228. Available from: PM:17881753.

Scott, D. M. & Taylor, R. E. (2007). Health-related effects of genetic variations of alcohol-metabolizing enzymes in African Americans. *Alcohol Research Health, 30*(1), 18–21. Available from: PM:17718396.

Sharma, A., Lewis, S., & Szatkowski, L. (2010). Insights into social disparities in smoking prevalence using Mosaic, a novel measure of socioeconomic status: An analysis using a large primary care dataset. *BMC Public Health, 10*, 755. Available from: PM:21138555.

Solomons, N. W. (2003). Diet and long-term health: An African Diaspora perspective. *Asia Pacific Journal of Clinical Nutrition, 12*(3), 313–330. Available from: PM:14505996.

Story, M., Kaphingst, K. M., Robinson-O'Brien, R., & Glanz, K. (2008). Creating healthy food and eating environments: Policy and environmental approaches. *Annual Reviews of Public Health, 29*, 253–272. Available from: PM:18031223.

Trinidad, D. R., Perez-Stable, E. J., White, M. M., Emery, S. L., & Messer, K. (2011). A nationwide analysis of US racial/ethnic disparities in smoking behaviors, smoking cessation, and cessation-related factors. *American Journal of Public Health, 101*(4), 699–706. Available from: PM:21330593.

USDHH. (2010). Healthy people 2010: Understanding and improving health (Vol. 2). Washington, DC: U.S. Goverment Printing Office 2000.

Warner, K. E. (2011). Disparities in smoking are complicated and consequential. What to do about them? *American Journal of Health Promotion, 25*(5 Suppl), S5–S7. Available from: PM:21510786.

Williams, C. L., Hayman, L. L., Daniels, S. R., Robinson, T. N., Steinberger, J., Paridon, S., et al. (2002). Cardiovascular health in childhood: A statement for health professionals from the Committee on Atherosclerosis, Hypertension, and Obesity in the Young (AHOY) of the Council on Cardiovascular Disease in the Young, American Heart Association. *Circulation, 106*(1), 143–160. Available from: PM:12093785.

Chapter 7
Health Literacy Deficits

Health literacy is defined as "the degree to which individuals have the capacity to obtain, process and understand basic health information and services needed to make appropriate health decisions." Inherent to this concept are the attributes of the health care system; how to access information and understand prevention, screening and self-management of conditions, and participation in clinical trials. Limited health literacy disproportionately affects lower socioeconomic and racial/ethnic minority groups and contributes to health disparities.

7.1 Introduction

The US Department of Health and Human Services definition of health literacy "… is the degree to which individuals have the capacity to obtain, process, and understand basic health information and services needed to make appropriate health decision" http://health.gov/communication/literacy/.

The history of research into health literacy in the USA, with a focus on how adults are able to use written materials in everyday life to accomplish everyday tasks, goes back to the early 1990s, when the National Adult Literacy Survey (NALS) carried out a nationwide survey profiling the literacy skills of the English language of more than 26,000 American adult. The study found that half of all adults interviewed had limited or low literacy skills as measured by the rate of subjects scoring at an inadequate level comparable to the sixth-grade level or below (Paasche-Orlow and Parker 2005). More recently, attention re-focused on the concept of health literacy when the Office of the Surgeon General of the US Department of Health and Human Services considered health literacy as one of four public-health priorities (Cutilli 2007). In a review by Paasche-Orlow and Parker (2005), they reported that the most common demographic features that were reportedly linked to health literacy were education level, age, ethnicity, geographic location, and income level. Overall, education and ethnicity were observed to be significantly associated with health literacy.

The health literacy for the general US population can be divided into four categories. The first is individuals who are proficient in health literacy, and so are able to perform complex and challenging literacy activities. The second tier is individuals with intermediate health literacy with moderate proficiency and are able to perform moderately challenging literacy activities. The third tier is individuals with basic proficiency in health literacy that allows them to perform simple everyday literacy activities. Finally, the fourth tier is individuals who fall below the basic proficiency standard and so are able only to perform simple and concrete health-literacy activities; these individuals may be considered to have low health literacy.

The National Center for Education Statistics (https://nces.ed.gov/pubs93/93275.pdf) estimates that approximately 21% of adult Americans (16 years and older) are health illiterate, i.e., with a lower than basic health-literacy level. This means that their reading standard is equal that of a fifth-grade level or lower, so that they may be unable to read a newspaper or follow written instructions. The National Center for Education Statistics also suggest that about 25% of the US adult population is marginally literate with a reading standard equal to that of the eighth grade (considered the basic literacy level). It is also estimated that one in three older US adults have low health literacy (Nielsen-Bohlman et al. 2004). This is a population whose literacy level is also most likely to decline over time, in relation to, or independent of, conditions that increase in prevalence with age, such as dementia, and the prevalence of low health literacy is particularly high among low-income older adults, such as African Americans (AAs). Older adults in other minority groups, including Hispanics and also people with limited English proficiency or who are non-literate in the English language, have a high prevalence of low health literacy. This statistical data indicates that a large proportion of the US adult population has a basic or below-basic level of literacy and will have difficulty with health literacy as related to printed information and their accuracy of interpreting health-care-related information. In other words, the rate of high-school completion was proportional to the percentage of the health-literacy rate: Individuals in the top quartile of completing high school or higher education (degree level) have the lowest prevalence of low literacy, whereas the prevalence of low literacy is correlated with the bottom quartile by educational standards, predominantly among Hispanic and AA populations in comparison with European-American (EA) populations (Fig. 7.1).

While years of schooling may not be the best proxy for literacy level, there is a strong correlation between general literacy skills (a reflection of the level of education) and health literacy, demonstrating a strong link of limited education with low health literacy. One report indicates that adult patients with limited literacy skills were more likely to report experiencing shame, low self-esteem, and limited social navigational skills, as well as a lack of social support (Wolf et al. 2007). US health literacy is declining with increases in the immigrant, minority, and elderly populations and the increasing demands of health care and society. There are some suggestions that health-literacy skills may be an important mediator of the

7.1 Introduction

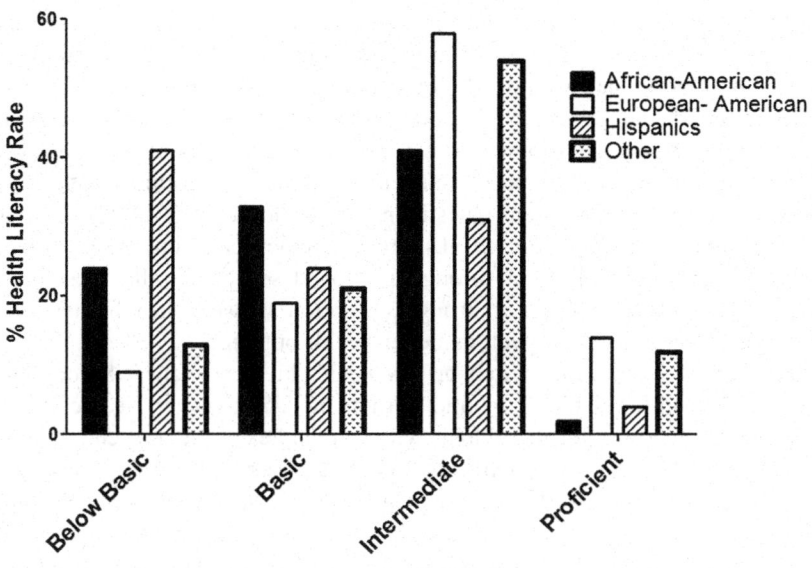

Fig. 7.1 Adult health literacy. Graph demonstrates the % rates of health literacy among US racial and ethnic groups. Data used for making the graph was obtained from the US Department of Education, Institute of Education Sciences, and 2013 National Assessment of Adult Literacy. Data for AA, EA, and Hispanics are shown, and others (refers to Asians, Native Americans, and multi-racial adults)

relationship between socio-environmental and behavioral risk factors and health disparities. Thus, a better understanding of the various components of literacy as it applies to the health-care setting is crucial in order to implement effective health-promoting behaviors or programs for preventative measures, as well as disease treatment. The following sections will consider three factors that may influence health literacy: self-care; the patient-provider relationship; and access to, and utilization of, health care.

Health literacy is different from the ability to understand plain language, whereas plain language is a tool for clear communication that can also be used to improve health literacy. Health literacy, however, means communication skills that are directly related to health issues, including: the ability to fill out a patient form in a hospital or clinical setting; the ability to understand and follow the age-appropriate guidelines for preventative health measures and screening; the ability to articulate a medical issue; and the ability to navigate the health-care system and access information in health insurance plans and so forth.

The definition of health literacy is expanding to encompass listening, speaking, writing, memory span, navigation of the health system, reading, and numeracy, as well as cultural and conceptual knowledge of health. So, health literacy is now considered a multi-dimensional concept involving both the individual and health professionals and takes into consideration the cultural context. An example of a health-literate individual would be someone who can claim and demonstrate knowledge on a health topic (Schulz 2005). Such knowledge is typically measured by a multiple-choice questionnaire that asks questions about the basics and symptoms of a disease, causes, and management, as well as treatment options, such as the Asthma Self-Management Questionnaire (Mancuso et al. 2009) or the diabetes knowledge test (Fitzgerald et al. 1998). Literacy can improve in a general sense (adult basic education) or through improved self-care skills. Results from such knowledge tests indicate a strong correlation between health literacy and effective self-management, as well as better health outcomes.

The cost associated with limited or low health literacy to the US economy is about US$238 billion. This economic burden on US taxpayers is the result of adverse health outcomes for individuals with limited health literacy, culminating in increased use of emergency-room and acute-care services, unnecessary doctor visits, frequent hospitalization, and longer hospital stays, as well as higher rates of re-admissions. Other health costs associated with low health literacy include less likelihood of obtaining flu shots, lower use of screening tools including mammography, and greater likelihood to administer medicines incorrectly (Berkman et al. 2011). In addition, individuals with low health literacy have less knowledge of chronic diseases and have worse self-management for hypertension, diabetes, asthma, and heart failure (Gazmararian et al. 2003). Low health literacy is also associated with a lack of a patient's knowledge of HIV medications and dosing instructions. Thus, low health literacy is associated with the disparities of disease incidence and mortality rates.

7.2 Individual Self-Care

Individuals including the AA population and other minority groups, low-income families, the elderly, and migrants for whom English is a second language disproportionately reside in neighborhoods where they are more likely to be exposed to environmental toxins and hazards, and have limited access to nutritious foods; these are factors that are significantly associated with adverse health. Yet these ethnic and racial minorities are more likely to have poor or limited health literacy and are disproportionately impacted by poor knowledge about the causes of disease and the risk factors associated with diseases, including cardiovascular diseases, cancer, diabetes, HIV/AIDs, infant mortality, mental illness, obesity, and other diseases of major public-health importance. One report indicated that low health literacy was significantly linked to well-established predictors of poor health, including current smoking status, perceived high level of stress, and self-reported general, as well as physical, health (Hoover et al. 2015). Individuals with limited knowledge about the effects of lifestyle factors such as diet, exercise, and smoking may not understand the association between these factors and health outcomes or recognize when they should seek health care. Furthermore, low health-literacy individuals may not understand the significance of health-promoting behaviors including exercise, healthy diets, or taking action after hearing health-related news. In addition, poor literacy has been linked with worse mental-health functioning and worse depression (Lincoln et al. 2006; Wolf et al. 2005); patients with low health literacy are more likely to be passive when it comes to making some health decisions or find it difficult to communicate with their primary care physicians; and this creates a barrier to patient-physician interaction that leads to miscommunication.

In addition to a lack of knowledge about diseases, low health-literacy individuals are more likely to report general poor health than individuals with high health literacy. Poor health-literacy individuals are less likely to use preventative health services and less likely to seek ways to promote general health or self-care activities. They are also more likely to be unwilling to delay gratification (as a coping mechanism), which may adversely affect their health, and are less likely to practice healthy behavior.

In addition, low health-literacy individuals tends to have poor information-processing skills, as well as limited access to communication channels including internet access, and, even when they have access, they are not able to process the information adequately (Freimuth and Mettger 1990). There is also the mistrust by individuals with low health literacy of mainstream institutions and even a deliberate rejection of the establishment position in some instances, due to previous incidents, as discussed in Sect. 7.4. Furthermore, there is a degree of helplessness that impacts their health status, for instance, individuals of low health literacy believe that there is no hope of surviving cancer (Freimuth and Mettger 1990). Thus a concerted effort is needed to reach out to these individuals through outreach programs in which basic and simple language is used to educate them, in the appropriate cultural and language settings, about disease awareness.

7.2.1 *Individual Preventative Measures*

One way to reduce disease incidence and mortality rates, as well as disease disparities, is through prevention and early detection (Marks et al. 2008). However, poor health-literate individuals are less likely to participate in preventive health care or adopt the recommended behavioral measures. Much of the routine prevention is dependent on patients coming into primary health care. However, minorities with low health literacy are typically low income, reside in low-income neighborhoods and therefore face certain unique challenges, such as access to transportation. Lack of adequate transportation is a barrier tor low health-literate individuals to visiting health-care facilities for preventative measures, such as screening for cancer because they often live far away from the health-care-service location. Low health-literacy individuals also lack the knowledge of the resource available to them and how to access these treatment options, and they may also delay seeking care because of the lack of understanding of prevention and/or knowledge about disease symptoms.

It is not surprising that people with low health literacy receive less primary preventative care and interventions (Bennett et al. 1998; Scott et al. 2002), and this is associated with increased disparities in disease incidence and mortality rates. For instance, a role for dietary guidelines, such as the so-called "DASH diet" that consists of a low-fat and low sodium diet and high intake of fruits and vegetables, has been reported to be a safe and powerful tool in the management of hypertension (Feyh et al. 2016). Despite its proven success in controlling hypertension without pharmacological intervention, individuals of low health literacy struggle to adhere to this diet. This suggests that for low health-literate individuals, carefully tailored education intervention by health-care professionals and/or community navigators and patients advocates may be essential in encouraging adherence to this diet.

Several reports demonstrate that behavior-based counseling that emphasizes the harmful effect of nicotine addiction using motivational enhancement tools and social support are effective for smoking cessation (Gritz et al. 2006), in addition to pharmacotherapy intervention. However, there is very little evidence that culturally appropriate interventions have been designed that specifically target the AA and other minority populations with low health literacy for smoking cessation. Specifically tailored interventions are necessary for the poor and health-illiterate population who are particularly sensitive to perceptions of blame for smoking-related illnesses. Such interventions to explain the causal role of nicotine addiction that can be communicated by social workers and family members, as well as by health-care professionals, are necessary for the successful behavior-based intervention in low health-literate individuals with lung cancer (Coughlin et al. 2014; Gritz et al. 2006).

Diabetes specifically Type 2 diabetes (T2D) is a preventable disease through normalization of blood glucose, blood pressure, and lipid levels. There are reports to demonstrate that intensive diabetes self-management, in addition to information technology, can improve glucose control in diabetic patients. However, diabetes self-management is a team effort between health-care providers and patients, raising the challenge for low health-literate individuals, particularly for those for whom English is their second language, such as Latinos, and/or those who do not have health insurance. Such low health-literate individuals would benefit more from one-to-one self-management interventions tailored to their literacy level, as well as circumstances and needs (Gritz et al. 2006; Lopez and Grant 2012).

Advances in therapeutic interventions, such as the combination of antiretroviral treatment, have prolonged the survival rates of individuals living with HIV. Despite these advances, individuals with low health literacy face challenges with HIV-disease management, and one study of AA HIV patients with low health literacy found that these individuals are less likely to keep hospital appointments, do not adhere to their HIV medications, and are most likely to die during hospitalization compared to their high health- literate counterparts (Gakumo et al. 2015). These groups of patients when interviewed responded that information on HIV management should be written in plain English at a lower reading level and preferred the team-based approach for health education. To improve user-friendly health information, printed materials, including test results, medication instructions, insurance and social-service information, and home-care instructions should also be in plain English that can be easily understood. Many of these communication characteristics should also be applied to verbal messages, e.g., use plain language and keep the content simple and actionable. In addition, internet-based information about health should also be easy to navigate.

7.3 Patient Navigation System

A concept that has evolved to help individuals with low health literacy and medically underserved populations to gain increased access to and utilization of health care is the patient navigation system. The patient navigation system is a model service system that encompasses disease prevention, detection, diagnosis, treatment, and survivorship through to the end of life. The concept is meant to include all the skills needed to explore medical care. However, the utilization of the health-care system incorporates plans for multiple non-profit, for-profit advertisement, insurance organizations, and government payers, such as Medicaid. The latter program is one for which millions are eligible but have not enrolled, again, due to a lack of understanding of the benefits and full potential that creates barriers to accessing the health-care system, leading to worse health among individuals with limited literacy. The rules and regulations of how to use health plans vary, as does the degree of understanding what services are covered and how to use various types of programs. For instance, a patient needs to be able to articulate disease symptoms in order to get the right medication from a primary-care physician or know which over-the-counter medication to use. In addition, a patient needs to know how to use medication and understand the side effects and adverse side effects that warrant stopping medication use or seeking alternative medication. Low health-literate patients have difficulty navigating all these health systems. In addition, low health-literate patients have the daunting tasks of using monitoring devices correctly (e.g., glucometer) and also have difficulty interpreting results and even knowing what to do next (e.g., increase the Lasix dose) and, often times, low health-literate patients have to make complex health decisions under time pressure with limited information and clinical uncertainty.

7.4 Mistrust of the Healthcare System

Individuals with low health literacy have been reported to mistrust the health-care system, tend to express pessimism about treatment, and demonstrate lower satisfaction, as well assessing more poorly the quality of health care delivered to them (Kalichman and Rompa 2000). To a large extent, the lack of trust in the medical institution has an historical basis. The AA population in particular recalls the infamous Tuskegee study, which started in the 1930s, where several AA men with syphilis were prevented from receiving penicillin that could have cured the disease, as well as saved their lives. Others recall similar historical events in biomedical research, such as in the human research that included withholding antibiotics from men with rheumatic fever or injecting nursing-home patients with live cancer cells (Jewish chronic disease). Another worrisome incident of human experimentation was the Willowbrook study where mental-health patients were infected with hepatitis to provide medical researchers with a controlled research population for their research into hepatitis. Although, there is now in place institutional review boards to make sure abuses of human rights do not take place anymore, these events are still very raw in the minds of many individuals with low health literacy. When it comes to participation in clinical trials, low health-literate individuals still believe that the health-care provider is experimenting on them or that the mainstream treatment options are not the best for them.

With the completion of the human genome project and a greater understanding of the genetic variation that underlies differences in disease susceptibility and drug metabolism in various ethnic and racial populations, a field largely driven by pharmacogenomics, it is now clear that, when it comes to disease treatment, one size does not fit all. There is therefore a need for diversity in biomedical research, as well as clinical trials. Unfortunately, only a small proportion of patients (e.g., 3–5% of cancer patients) participate in clinical trials, because there is a lack of basic information about the importance of scientific research; how it is designed and reported and the potential benefits versus risks of the research and clinical trials outcomes for health are not well articulated to the general community. The participation rate is even lower in the low health-literacy population and underserved communities (AAs, uninsured, the poor, rural inhabitants) for several reasons, including the mistrust of the health-care system and the lack of knowledge of the potential benefits of clinical research, as mentioned previously. Some reports suggests that up to 32% of US residents would be willing to participate in trials if asked; an additional 38% would be inclined to participate if asked, but had questions/reservations (Comis et al. 2003) indicating that the primary problem with accrual is not the patients attitudes, but the design of clinical trials that potentially disqualify a large sector of the patient population, as well as a lack of information about available trials. The pool of willing patients is further reduced by the reluctance of some physicians to engage in accrual, or even to refer their patients for clinical trials, for fear of losing patients.

7.5 Health Literacy and Professionals

The majority of the health-care providers or professionals are unaware or do not recognize that some of their patients are low health literate and do not understand the health information being provided to them because providers seldom evaluate patients understanding of the disease topic or treatment for that matter. Patients with low health literacy may be less responsive and more reluctant to ask questions, or admit ignorance or even confusion to their physicians. In addition, poor health-literate patients may describe their medical issues quite differently from that normally encountered by health-care professionals, as well as use different descriptions of medical problems than clinicians will use, leading to inaccurate medical information or health histories being given to the health professional, which can often result in misdiagnoses or wrong medication being given to patients (Paasche-Orlow et al. 2006). Some of the strategies that can be used to improve health communication from the health-professional point of view include: employ face-to-face communication with patients to establish a rapport and engage patients in conversations that facilitate understanding of unfamiliar medical terms and makes health information personally relevant and of limited content; limit usage of medical jargon and put oneself in the patient's shoes. In addition, the use of pictures, teaching tools, and repetition of medication information, as well as the provision of information summaries, helps to reinforce the patient's understanding. Another approach is teach back, where patients are asked certain information by their physicians, such as when do you take medication? How many pills and at what time? For how long? And what are the benefits and side effects that might be expected?

7.6 Health Literacy and Culture

In a multicultural society such as the USA, health-care professionals interact with individuals and families of migrants who may come from diverse cultures. For migrants with limited English proficiency or English as their second language, how they communicate and understand the health-care system and how they receive information or even respond to educational information on lifestyle changes, as well as if they understand how treatment options may impact their health. There are many pathways that link health-literacy deficits and adverse health. These include limitations in expressive language (passivity in the medical dialogue), less-detailed medical histories, and lack of involvement in decision making. In addition, patients feel they are not listened to and have difficulty being understood, and also the use of medical jargon may interfere with medical treatment.

Lack of adequate exchanges of information between doctors and patients, as a result of language barriers or different cultural backgrounds (Schouten and Meeuwesen 2006), have been reported to be associated with members of migrant families receiving less-frequent medical care and relatively late diagnoses compared to individuals who speak the native language. One report from a Dutch study demonstrated that ethnic-minority children receive less-frequent medical care for asthma and at relatively later stages of diagnosis compared to the native Dutch children (Urbanus-van Laar et al. 2008). Many of these migrant families also have low incomes, which may also be a confounding factor that may also negatively impact their health status.

Difficulties related to cultural and linguistic factors require that physicians develop tailored care for individuals from such diverse cultures, a concept known as "cultural competence". Cultural competency is the ability of *professionals* to work cross-culturally. It can contribute to health literacy by improving communication and building trust. Plans to develop culturally competent health-literacy programs would require government action or organizational/practitioner action, as well as partnership action. Overall, the evidence indicates that health disparities can be alleviated in part by creating and maintaining a culturally competent health-care system (Anderson et al. 2003).

7.7 What About Cultural Competence and Acculturation?

One of the early definitions of cultural competence is "a set of congruent behaviors, attitudes, and policies that come together in a system, agency, or among professionals that enables effective work in cross-cultural situations". Nowadays, cultural competence encompasses the ability of health-care professionals to provide equal and effective quality care and services that can meet the needs of people with diverse cultural health beliefs and practices. Cultural competence should also take into account the preferred language of communication and health literacy of the patient. Thus, cultural competence is about the needs and the care of the patient. For instance, cultural competence should also consider the beliefs and attitudes of the patients towards disease—some view disease as a punishment from God, whereas some view illness as an issue of fatalism, i.e., disease and death are part of life. Other aspects of cultural competence that a health-care provider must consider are the cultural background of some patients and their attitudes towards authority—some patients may never question authority and that could affect patient-physician communication. Here is the problem: nearly half of all underrepresented minority medical students plan to care for underserved populations, whereas fewer than 20% of other new doctors have such plans (Zambrana and Carter-Pokras 2010), while, by 2050, at least 48% of the US population will be composed of racial and ethnic minorities. Medical students need to be taught to understand the diverse issues and cultural backgrounds, as well as the religious perception of health and disease, of their patients.

Acculturation is the process whereby immigrants incorporate the cultural behavioral patterns of their host country (Satia-Abouta et al. 2002). Acculturation can significantly impact health literacy, particularly for older adult immigrants for whom English is a second language. In addition, other culturally related factors, such as environment and dietary choices, can influence exposure to and understanding of health and preventive information. Studies carried out by Thomson and Hoffmann-Goetz (2011) found that acculturation was an important factor in obtaining information on cancer prevention that influenced cancer-screening participation among Spanish-speaking immigrant women in Canada for whom English is a second language. While low health literacy has been reported in the Latino minority population, studies have shown that the high acculturation of Latinos was significantly associated with increased access to health care, increased physical activity, and decreased breast-feeding behavior, perhaps due to attitudinal changes that accompany acculturation (Ciampa et al. 2013).

7.8 Summary

With demographic shifts in the USA, health-care organizations have the daunting task to address and adapt changes and approaches in the health-care system that will provide information and service to various racial and ethnic groups, including individuals from different cultural backgrounds, language skills and health-literacy levels. Improving the health literacy of individuals with inadequate or marginal literacy skills is one of the Surgeon General's seven public-health priorities, and there is also Healthy People 2010 that has evolved into Healthy People 2020 meant to increase the proportion of persons who report that their health-care providers delivered understandable and satisfactory communication. This requires identifying patients with limited literacy levels and using programs such as discussed above to include the use simple language, short sentences, and simple definitions of technical terms. Dahhan et al. (2012) found that poor adherence to health-care advice may not necessarily be associated with language skills, per se, but rather with low functional health literacy, poor knowledge of disease, and limited comprehension of disease severity. It is important therefore to provide a knowledge-based approach to understanding disease in patients that will promote health literacy and better adherence to health-care advice and practice.

Improving health literacy would also require developing support programs to reduce the negative effects of limited health literacy. This perhaps will require beginning health education very early on in the primary-education curriculum (kindergarten through 12th grade), as well as adult education and community programs. Because of the diverse cultures in the USA, health education has to be tailored to be culturally and linguistically sensitive in order to promote health literacy. Furthermore, interventions are better served by acknowledging the interdependence of the various socio-cultural factors that need to be managed in order to succeed in promoting improved health care for those with limited health literacy (Paasche-Orlow and Wolf 2007). Finally, the development of outreach and community-based programs is important for bringing education and screening services directly to low health-literate individuals, millions of whom are eligible but not enrolled in programs such as Medicaid and other means-tested health programs (Piette et al. 2004) because of the complexity encountered in navigating health-care programs. These measures would help reduce the low health literacy that is associated with health disparities.

References

Anderson, L. M., Scrimshaw, S. C., Fullilove, M. T., Fielding, J. E., & Normand, J. (2003). Culturally competent healthcare systems. A systematic review. *American Journal of Preventive Medicine*, 24(3 Suppl), 68–79. Available from: PM:12668199.

Bennett, C. L., Ferreira, M. R., Davis, T. C., Kaplan, J., Weinberger, M., Kuzel, T., Seday, M. A., & Sartor, O. (1998). Relation between literacy, race, and stage of presentation among low-income patients with prostate cancer. *Journal of Clinical Oncology, 16*(9), 3101–3104 (available from: PM:9738581).

Berkman, N. D., Sheridan, S. L., Donahue, K. E., Halpern, D. J., & Crotty, K. (2011). Low health literacy and health outcomes: An updated systematic review. *Annals of Internal Medicine, 155*(2), 97–107 (available from: PM:21768583).

Ciampa, P. J., White, R. O., Perrin, E. M., Yin, H. S., Sanders, L. M., Gayle, E. A., & Rothman, R. L. (2013). The association of acculturation and health literacy, numeracy and health-related skills in Spanish-speaking caregivers of young children. *Journal of Immigrant and Minority Health, 15*(3), 492–498 (available from: PM:22481307).

Comis, R. L., Miller, J. D., Aldige, C. R., Krebs, L., & Stoval, E. (2003). Public attitudes toward participation in cancer clinical trials. *Journal of Clinical Oncology, 21*(5), 830–835 (available from: PM:12610181).

Coughlin, S. S., Matthews-Juarez, P., Juarez, P. D., Melton, C. E., & King, M. (2014). Opportunities to address lung cancer disparities among African Americans. *Cancer Medicine, 3*(6), 1467–1476 (available from: PM:25220156).

Cutilli, C. C. (2007). Health literacy in geriatric patients: An integrative review of the literature. *Orthopaedic Nursing, 26*(1), 43–48 (available from: PM:17273109).

Dahhan, N., Meijssen, D., Chegary, M., Bosman, D., & Wolf, B. (2012). Ethnic diversity outpatient clinic in paediatrics. *BMC Health Services Research, 12*, 12 (available from: PM:22236336).

Feyh, A., Bracero, L., Lakhani, H. V., Santhanam, P., Shapiro, J. I., Khitan, Z., & Sodhi, K. (2016). Role of dietary components in modulating hypertension. *Journal of Clinical & Experimental Cardiology, 7*(4) (available from: PM:27158555).

Fitzgerald, J. T., Funnell, M. M., Hess, G. E., Barr, P. A., Anderson, R. M., Hiss, R. G., & Davis, W. K. (1998). The reliability and validity of a brief diabetes knowledge test. *Diabetes Care, 21*(5), 706–710 (available from: PM:9589228).

Freimuth, V. S., & Mettger, W. (1990). Is there a hard-to-reach audience? *Public Health Reports, 105*(3), 232–238 (available from: PM:2113680).

Gakumo, C. A., Enah, C. C., Vance, D. E., Sahinoglu, E., & Raper, J. L. (2015). Keep it simple: Older African Americans' preferences for a health literacy intervention in HIV management. *Patient Preference and Adherence, 9*, 217–223 (available from: PM:25678780).

Gazmararian, J. A., Williams, M. V., Peel, J., & Baker, D. W. (2003). Health literacy and knowledge of chronic disease. *Patient Education and Counseling, 51*(3), 267–275 (available from: PM:14630383).

Gritz, E. R., Fingeret, M. C., Vidrine, D. J., Lazev, A. B., Mehta, N. V., & Reece, G. P. (2006). Successes and failures of the teachable moment: Smoking cessation in cancer patients. *Cancer, 106*(1), 17–27 (available from: PM:16311986).

Hoover, D. S., Vidrine, J. I., Shete, S., Spears, C. A., Cano, M. A., Correa-Fernandez, V., Wetter, D. W., & McNeill, L. H. (2015). Health literacy, smoking, and health indicators in African American Adults. *Journal of Health Communication, 20*(Suppl 2), 24–33 (available from: PM:26513028).

Kalichman, S. C., & Rompa, D. (2000). Functional health literacy is associated with health status and health-related knowledge in people living with HIV-AIDS. *Journal of Acquired Immune Deficiency Syndrome, 25*(4), 337–344 (available from: PM:11114834).

Lincoln, A., Paasche-Orlow, M. K., Cheng, D. M., Lloyd-Travaglini, C., Caruso, C., Saitz, R., & Samet, J. H. (2006). Impact of health literacy on depressive symptoms and mental health-related: Quality of life among adults with addiction. *Journal of General Internal Medicine, 21*(8), 818–822 (available from: PM:16881940).

Lopez, L., & Grant, R. W. (2012). Closing the gap: Eliminating health care disparities among Latinos with diabetes using health information technology tools and patient navigators. *Journal of Diabetes Science and Technology, 6*(1), 169–176 (available from: PM:22401336).

References

Mancuso, C. A., Sayles, W., & Allegrante, J. P. (2009). Development and testing of the Asthma self-management questionnaire. *Annals of Allergy Asthma & Immunology, 102*(4), 294–302 (available from: PM:19441600).

Marks, B., Sisirak, J., & Hsieh, K. (2008). Health services, health promotion, and health literacy: Report from the State of the science in aging with developmental disabilities conference. *Disability and Health Journal, 1*(3), 136–142 (available from: PM:21122722).

Nielsen-Bohlman, L., Panzer, A. M., & Kindig, D. A. (2004). *Health literacy: A prescription to end confusion.* USA: National Academies Press.

Paasche-Orlow, M. K., & Parker, R. M. (2005). The prevalence of limited health literacy. *Journal of General Internal Medicine, 20,* 175–184.

Paasche-Orlow, M. K., Schillinger, D., Greene, S. M., & Wagner, E. H. (2006). How health care systems can begin to address the challenge of limited literacy. *Journal of General Internal Medicine, 21*(8), 884–887 (available from: PM:16881952).

Paasche-Orlow, M. K., & Wolf, M. S. (2007). The causal pathways linking health literacy to health outcomes. *American Journal of Health Behaviour, 31*(Suppl 1), S19–S26 (available from: PM:17931132).

Piette, J. D., Wagner, T. H., Potter, M. B., & Schillinger, D. (2004). Health insurance status, cost-related medication underuse, and outcomes among diabetes patients in three systems of care. *Medical Care, 42*(2), 102–109 (available from: PM:14734946).

Satia-Abouta, J., Patterson, R. E., Neuhouser, M. L., & Elder, J. (2002). Dietary acculturation: Applications to nutrition research and dietetics. *Journal of the American Dietetic Association, 102*(8), 1105–1118 (available from: PM:12171455).

Schouten, B. C., & Meeuwesen, L. (2006). Cultural differences in medical communication: A review of the literature. *Patient Education and Counseling, 64*(1–3), 21–34 (available from: PM:16427760).

Schulz, P. J. N. K. (2005). Emerging themes in health literacy. *Studies in Communication Sciences, 5,* 1–10.

Scott, T. L., Gazmararian, J. A., Williams, M. V., & Baker, D. W. (2002). Health literacy and preventive health care use among Medicare enrollees in a managed care organization. *Medical Care, 40*(5), 395–404 (available from: PM:11961474).

Thomson, M. D., & Hoffman-Goetz, L. (2011). Cancer information comprehension by English-as-a-second-language immigrant women. *Journal of Health Communication, 16*(1), 17–33 (available from: PM:21120740).

Urbanus-van Laar, J. J., de Koning, J. S., Klazinga, N. S., & Stronks, K. (2008). Suboptimal asthma care for immigrant children: Results of an audit study. *BMC Health Services Research, 8,* 22 (available from: PM:18218104).

Wolf, M. S., Gazmararian, J. A., & Baker, D. W. (2005). Health literacy and functional health status among older adults. *Archives of Internal Medicine, 165*(17), 1946–1952 (available from: PM:16186463).

Wolf, M. S., Williams, M. V., Parker, R. M., Parikh, N. S., Nowlan, A. W., & Baker, D. W. (2007). Patients' shame and attitudes toward discussing the results of literacy screening. *Journal of Health Communication, 12*(8), 721–732 (available from: PM:18030638).

Zambrana, R. E., & Carter-Pokras, O. (2010). Role of acculturation research in advancing science and practice in reducing health care disparities among Latinos. *American Journal of Public Health, 100*(1), 18–23 (available from: PM:19910358).

Chapter 8
The Impact of Culture on Health Disparities

Abstract Culture denotes the ways of life that are normally transmitted from one generation to another, and these are associated with various ethnic and racial groups. The culture of the African diaspora and other low–socioeconomic (SES) minority populations may influence health behaviors and practices and interactions with the health-care system. Conversely, the cultural assumptions on which the health/care systems, policies, and interventions are based may impact health behaviors and outcomes for minority and low-SES populations. Health disparities can be alleviated in part by creating and maintaining a culturally competent health-care system.

8.1 Introduction

Culture and the significant role it plays in human behavior have been recognized as far back as the time of Hippocrates during the classical Greek era (Dona 1991). Culture encompasses language, learned core values, certain norms and beliefs, and behaviors as well as customs that are shared by a certain group of people and transmitted from one generation to the next. Cultural norms by definition are shared within the various different ethnic groups, along with similar physical traits that distinguish them from other ethnic groups, including primary language, native history, traditions, values, and dietary habits (Griffith et al. 2011).

There is diversity within any particular ethnic group with regards to ties to their country of origin or immigration status and associations with health outcomes. For instance first- and second-generation African migrants to the USA have better health profiles than US-born African Americas (AAs), who are the descendants of slaves and/or whose beliefs and ways of life are historically linked to slavery (Dey and Lucas 2006). Part of the AA population is composed of people whose ancestors have continuously lived away from the African continent for more than 400 years, so they have acclimatized to the Western way of life, and many of their descendants are of mixed race, with at least 20% European ancestry. On the other hand, there is heterogeneity among the African ethnic groups on the native African continent. The African continent is made up of 54 countries with between 1500 and 2000 dialects of languages and diverse arrays of cultural practices. The health advantages reported for recent ethnic migrants could be due to healthier lifestyles in their countries of origin, or fewer experiences of racialized stress and discrimination. However, the longer these migrants remain in the USA, the, they lose their healthy status, perhaps as a result of adopting unhealthy American sedentary or poor dietary lifestyles, as well as the other adversities that minorities face in the USA (Griffith et al. 2011).

The various ethnic groups represented in the USA, according to the US Census Bureau, are quite heterogeneous within themselves. For instance, Asian Americans are a very heterogeneous group. Asia as a continent is made up of more than 20 countries, with over 30 ethnic groups and more than 200 dialects (Chen 1998). In addition, there are distinct cultural, demographic, and levels of SES within the Asian-American population. While this population is often noted as having the highest income among US minority groups, the Hmong Asian-American population have a much lower per capita income ($6000) compared to the USA as a whole ($21,587) (USA Census Bureau website www.census.gov/). Culture may even span various religious organizations, such as Christian and Islamic, or even groups that are not just ethnically or racially distinct but share certain beliefs, ways of life, or disabilities, such as lesbian, gay, bisexual and trans-sexual (LGBT) community, HIV/AIDs patients, and the deaf or other disabled communities.

Cultural factors influence attitudes towards race and ethnicity, beliefs, gender, age, sexual orientation, religion, disability status, SES, geographic location, and other characteristics that influence health and health disparities. The cultural demographics in the USA are diverse in themselves, and this is even reflected in the health-care system, with minorities experiencing persistent healthcare inequalities. According to the 2015 report from the Agency for Healthcare Research and Quality, there are national disparities in both the access and quality of health care in the USA. The AA population and other minority populations have worse health-care indicators (www.ahrq.gov/research/findings/nhqrdr/), and these disparities have persisted for 13 years in a row. Therefore the provision of health care to various ethnic and racial populations must incorporate specific and sensitive aspects of cultural norms that integrate schools, housing, social-services providers, and diet and lifestyle behaviors to meet the needs in each culture.

8.2 Diet and Its Cultural Impact

Poor dietary habits are a major risk factor associated with disparities in the incidence, morbidity, and mortality rates for many chronic diseases, including cardiovascular disease, hypertension, cancer, type II diabetes, and obesity, as chronicled throughout this book. There are differences in the dietary intake, dietary behaviors, and dietary patterns in the various ethnic and racial cultures in the USA.

Minority cultural groups of the AA population, Hispanics, Asian-Americans, American Indians/Alaskan native, in particular (low-SES and poorly-educated) have poor dietary behaviors, such as high intake of diets rich in saturated fats, low intake of fruit, vegetables, and whole-grain foods, and high intake of salt in comparison with the dietary patterns of European Americans (EAs) (Satia 2010).

According to a survey on Behavioral Risk Factor Surveillance, only 21.3% of AAs consumes fruits and vegetables more than five times per day, the lowest of any US racial or ethnic group and non-Hispanic AAs, as well as all Hispanics, were less likely than EAs to meet USDA fruit and vegetable guidelines (Casagrande et al. 2007). There are differences in the dietary habits of recently arrived minority immigrants and US-born ethnic groups. For example, recent African migrants to the USA have a dietary pattern that has a great variety of nutrients, characterized by low-fat, high-protein, complex-carbohydrates, high-fiber intake, in comparison to the US-born AA population who consume more total energy, total and saturated fat, and less fiber and calcium (Lancaster et al. 2006). However, dietary habits and patterns are influenced by so many factors including income level, neighborhood, and availability of fresh fruits and vegetables, conveniences, and knowledge about nutritional choices, as well as adaptation of migrants to the dietary patterns of their host country. Therefore, effective dietary intervention should take into consideration social, economic, and behavioral patterns, as well as cultural norms.

8.3 Religion and Its Cultural Impact

Spirituality is an important factor that has been documented to provide health protection. A nationwide survey of the use of prayer for health concerns reported a significant level. Studies by McCaffrey et al. (2004) found that 35% of respondents used prayer for health reasons, with users reporting high levels of perceived effectiveness. However, most respondents did not discuss prayer with their health-care providers, who may not share in their beliefs in spiritual matters. The role of prayer was highest in the AA population but low among EAs and Hispanics, with prayer prevalence highest among AA women compared with other ethnic or racial groups categorized by gender (Dessio et al. 2004). Millions of AAs have embraced the Christian faith, while some have found faith in other religions, including Islam.

Throughout history, the AA Christian church has been a strong social and religious force of unity for many AAs and continues to occupy a dominant place in the lives of most AA (Chatters et al. 1998). The AA church probably came into existence after emancipation from slavery because at that time AAs were free to establish separate churches, to create their own communities, and to worship in their own culturally distinct ways. Within the churches, AAs were finally able to build strong community organizations and to hold positions of leadership that, until then, had been denied to them in mainstream America. Consequently, the AA church has become the center stage of the AA community, and historically it has provided a wealth of resources and has been deeply entrenched in the daily affairs of AA people (Foluke 1999). Many AAs report a strong feeling of social support when engaged in church-related activities (Carter-Edwards et al. 2004).

Churches offer a variety of resources: human, social, intellectual, capital, and spiritual guidance and can provide an avenue to address areas of health disparity in the AA community. Churches historically have been places where members trust each other, and thus, when education is provided and services are offered, they are more readily accepted. Churches can therefore provide an environment where clinicians can build confidence and competence in their ability to communicate effectively with diverse patient populations. When health-care providers are endorsed by members of the church, participants are much more likely to be interested in beginning a relationship that allows health care to be provided and accepted. The church as an institution provides other services for the community. For example, after slavery ended in the USA, the AA church through various denominations provided the infrastructure for schools (kindergarten through 12th grade) throughout the country and took up the role of social-welfare functions, establishing orphanages and founding colleges and university (Foluke 1999).

Church attendance and religious participation does not only reduce mortality risks, but also improves health statuses and substantially augments the quality of life among many AAs (Hummer et al. 1999; Musgrave et al. 2002), especially for those who attend church on a regular basis and are involved in church activities and functions. One of the primary reasons for increased vulnerability to major illnesses is the limited opportunities to gain health information, even within the AA church. The church can be a valuable asset in the AA and other minority communities, even for those who do not attend church on regular basis. Churches have stepped up their programs of awareness about health conditions, such as HIV/AIDs (Coleman et al. 2006), diabetes (Polzer 2007), and hypertension and heart disease (Laken et al. 2004), smoking cessation, mental illness, and cancer prevention, as well as screening programs. The AA church can offer a wealth of resources for disease prevention and treatment, exercise, and diet, and can play an important role in reducing and eliminating health disparities.

In addition to the AA churches, barbershops and hair salons can serve as locations for providing health-information resources. Community health workers can use their connections in the AA community to promote health services or even recruit candidates for clinical trials from churches, public-housing authorities, places of business such as barbershops, and community-based organizations. In the AA and other minority cultures, health-care professionals need to partner with community and faith-based organizations to create effective groups to eliminate health disparities. This can be accomplished through research, outreach and education, and training to address health disparities. Community health workers are instrumental in providing the information that would facilitate informed decision making among AAs and other minority patients, and improve health outcomes for various health issues, such as cancer, new-born care, and infectious diseases. According to the WHO (World Health Organization 2007), the key attributes of community health workers are that they are members of the communities in which they work, selected by the communities, answerable to the communities for their activities, and supported by the health system, but not necessarily a part of an organization. Through their activities, they can bridge the cultural and health literacy differences between the community and the health-care system, reducing the barriers to achieving health equality.

8.4 Cultural Behavior in Alternative Medicine

The culture of minority groups such as AAs and Hispanics may influence their health behavior towards health care and disease treatment. Minority populations are likely to seek alternative approaches to the Westernized health-care system for disease treatment. Some of these alternative treatments, including the use of chamomile tea to induce sleep and relaxation, are effective, while other alternative treatments, such as breaking an egg on the stomach to treat *susto* (a belief about a form of spiritually induced depression in the Hispanic community) has no effect, and yet other alternative treatments, such as the use of lead-based remedies for treating *empacho* (obstruction of the stomach; indigestion, diarrhea, constipation) among populations of Mexican origins, can be dangerous. Latino populations may use various diets and herbal treatment to treat diseases, instead of taken Western medicines.

It is estimated that about 42% of the US population uses some form of complementary or alternative medicine (CAM), such as herbal medicines, acupuncture, chiropractic, traditional healing, and home remedies, including herbal medicine that is most widely used among the Hispanic population. Various racial and ethnic groups may use various CAM. One study suggests that EAs and minority patients who use CAM do not disclose this information to their health-care providers, whereas only about 2% of minority patients asked their primary physicians questions about the use of alternative medicine (Sleath et al. 2001).

One analysis of the use of alternative-medicine supplements to the 2002 US National Health Interview Survey carried out by Graham et al. (2005) discovered that the use of CAM is prevalent in the EA and Hispanic populations and lowest among the AA population, with EAs using herbal medicine, relaxation techniques, and chiropractic more frequently than in the Hispanic and AA populations. Among the reasons given for the use of CAM is the perceived notion that "CAM with conventional medicine would help". Hispanics, on the other hand, attributed the use of CAM instead of conventional medicine to cost, saying that conventional treatment was too expensive, especially amongst the uninsured. In addition, Hispanics have less access to health professionals than the general population and are therefore more likely to turn to alternative forms of health care, such as folk/home remedies and family or community healers (Pachter 1994). The use of CAM is also most common among women. Interestingly, this cut across all demographics of the female population: Highly educated individuals, high-income individuals without insurance, and persons of fair-to-poor health status have all reported to use CAM. However, there is inconsistency in the reported use of CAM by various racial and ethnic groups. Graham et al. (2005) found high use of CAM by EAs and Hispanics, but low usage among the AA population. Mackenzie et al. (2003) on the other hand, reported higher usage of CAM, with equal prevalence by EAs, AAs, Latinos, Asians, and Native Americans in the USA. This inconsistency could reflect the population cohorts and geographic areas where these surveys were carried out.

Complementary and alternative medicine usage also varies considerably by specific CAM modality. Overall, there is higher use of herbs among Hispanics and AAs than reported in the Graham study. Other smaller studies on the use of CAM in minority populations have been reported, albeit limited by national generalization. One study of Mexican American population in El Paso TX reported 77% of their study population used CAM (Keegan 1996). Yet other reports indicates that Hispanics use more herbal medicine than EAs, suggesting that ethnicity was related to the use of herbal medicines (Dole et al. 2000). Discrepancies in CAM modality, geographic variation of use, biases in language usage, and exclusion of individuals without a telephone may contribute to inconsistencies with CAM usage in various populations (Dole et al. 2000; Mackenzie et al. 2003).

The usage of other alternative medicines known as folk medicine is reported to be at a low rate (0.2%) among Hispanics in a National Health Interview Survey (NHIS). Other previous surveys have estimated the use of folk medicines, such as *curandores* and other traditional medicines, at higher rates of 4–7% (Druss and Rosenheck 1999). The low percentage of folk-medicine usage reported in these surveys is a reflection of the types of herbs surveyed. The type of herbs included in the NHIS survey tended to be commonly used by higher SES populations, such as the EA population, and these are well-processed and manufactured. Whereas the types of herbs used by Hispanics and AAs are mostly non-processed and home-grown herbs, including cat's clay rue, aloe vera, and eucalyptus among the Hispanic population, but these are not named in the NHIS questionnaire (Graham et al. 2005). A popular folk medicine called *curanderismo* is commonly used among the Mexican American and other Latino communities. In addition, community healers in the Latin-Mexican-American community, such as bonesetters, midwifes and *sobadores* (lay healers who use manual-massage techniques to treat diseases such as conventionally recognized ailments, as well as culture-specific folk illnesses) are visited more often than traditional health-care centers. Other folk medicines such as Esperitismo, in which mental and spiritual healing is carried out by healers using energy and/or trance, are used in Latino populations (Harwood 1981).

A better understanding of CAM used among minority populations will enable clinicians to provide a more culturally sensitive care to the diverse minority patient populations for successful delivery of health services to minorities.

8.4 Cultural Behavior in Alternative Medicine

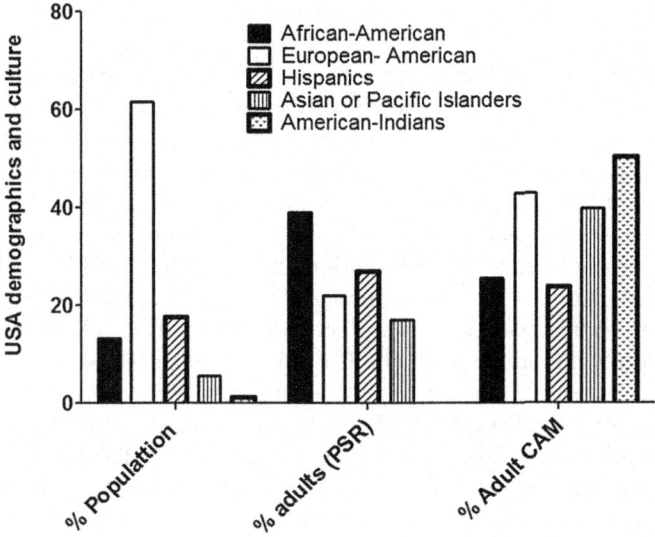

Fig. 8.1 A graph of US demographics and culture. This graph demonstrates the proportion of various US racial and ethnic groups, the % of adult USA population that are religious (PSR; pray, read scriptures, and attend religious studies) and use CAM (complementary alternative medicine). Data from the 2014 US Department of health and health services, US Census Bureau and Pew research

Overall, while minority populations including AAs, Hispanics and American-Indians account for less than 40% of the US population, they account for a significant fraction of the US population who are religious and/or users CAM. For instance, AA adults accounts for the highest US population who are religious (defined as individuals who pray, read bible scriptures, or attend religious education), whereas American Indians, perhaps the least populous of the US ethnic and minority groups, are make up the highest fraction of the US population to use CAM (Fig. 8.1).

8.5 Cultural Competence and Linguistics

Cultural and linguistic competence can help reduce disparity. Acculturation, such as positive assimilation into the American culture, enables immigrants to better navigate the health-care system, and this can have positive health outcomes. On the other hand, negative assimilation, such as cumulative exposure to toxic physical environments and social stresses and the length of stay in the USA, can negatively impact health outcomes. Healthy-immigrant effects have been reported for several minority-immigrant groups to the USA with various outcomes. Hispanics migrants to the USA have a long-standing advantage of low mortality and better health compared to US-born Hispanics, and this advantage probably comes from favorable health behaviors and other sociocultural protective factors that enable these migrants to cope better with stress. However, this health disadvantage has not been observed for some important chronic conditions, such as diabetes and the debilities of old age (Riosmena et al. 2013).

Other reports suggest that the healthy-immigrant effect may not be applicable among twenty-first century African immigrants. Studies carried out by O'Connor et al. (2014), wherein they assessed glucose-tolerance, beta-cell function, greater visceral adiposity, blood pressure, and BMI, among other biometric parameters, in healthy African migrants, as well as AAs, found that, while African migrants were less obese compared to the AA population in their study, they were at a higher risk for diabetes and heart disease (i.e., had poorer cardiometabolic health) than the AA population. Historically, African migrants acquired obesity and T2DM and CVD, only after living in the US, however the recent global epidemic of cardiometabolic diseases suggests the possibility that immigrant health may be changing for not only Africans but other minority populations. Furthermore, the healthy-migrant paradox could also be skewed by the potential for undiagnosed disease that can lead to inaccurate health assessment of immigrants' population. The healthy-migrant or protective effect is not sustained over time, within and across generations in the USA. Recent reports by Koku et al. (2016) indicate the increased prevalence of HIV/AIDs among sub-Saharan African immigrants in the USA, and this raises the suggestion of disaggregation of the sub-Saharan African population from the AA-black demographic population in order to identify disease incidence and mortality rates in this population, so that resources for prevention and treatment can be appropriately targeted.

Cultural competence (discussed in Chap. 7) and linguistic competence, i.e., the ability to communicate information in a suitable manner (cultural context) that makes it easy to understand, is very important in the health-care setting for minority populations. For instance, minority patients who believe they have not received the best care because of a healthcare professional mannerism or attitude because of their race or ethnic group tend to ignore doctors' advice and put off care that is medically needed. There is also the perception that physicians give less attention and less information to AAs and individuals of lower SES. There is a need for more culturally comprehensive diagnostic and treatment models that incorporate spiritual belief, the use of complementary alternative medicine, and appropriate language to match the level of health literacy (discussed in Chap. 7). Evidence has shown that culturally sensitive care models are effective in reducing depressive symptoms among ethnically and culturally diverse communities (Beauboeuf-Lafontant 2007).

8.6 Culturally Sensitive Medical Care

Racism and racial segregation in the US health-care system, including medicine, nursing, and dentistry, up to the 1970 is well documented, and many will argue that it still goes on. Up until the implementation of the Medicare program in the summer of 1966, nearly all hospitals segregated minority patients in separate wards. Typically, minority patients, including AAs, Hispanics, and Native Americans, were kept in the basement or otherwise cold or hot areas or, simply put, did not have access to hospitals. In addition to the disparity in access to hospital beds, there was disparity in utilization, treatment, intervention and other services.

The culture of minority and low-SES populations may influence health behavior and practices and interactions with the health-care system based on Anglo-American culture. On the other hand, the culture of health professionals may influence their health-care practices and interaction with culturally diverse patients. The health-care professionals who understand their patients' culture may influence their interactions with culturally diverse patients, the treatment they provide, and continuity of care. The cultural assumptions on which the health-care systems, policies, and interventions are based may impact health behaviors, and outcomes for minority and low-SES populations and all these interactive factors once successfully integrated with each other will provide better health-are for minorities and bridge health disparities.

In the USA, most medical schools did not open their doors to minority students until well after World War II. Howard University College of Medicine and Meharry Medical College were established specifically to educate black medical students, and they also admitted Jews and women. Thus minority institutions such as Howard University have a unique mission to not only educate minority health-care professionals but to also provide minority patients with culturally sensitive health care.

8.7 Summary

The effect of cultural systems on health outcomes is huge, therefore to neglect the role of culture in health and health care is a major barrier to the advancement of high standards of healthcare, as well as the elimination of health disparities (Napier et al. 2014). Culture is related to health promotion, disease prevention, early detection, access to health care, and the trust and compliance needed to establish comprehensive models to deliver quality and effective health care, including behavioral health and primary care within the context of demonstrating respect for the cultural orientation of the patient.

In order to better understand the role of culture in health disparities, investigators should, first of all, adopt a definition of "culture" that clearly distinguishes it from related concepts such as ethnicity, race, and SES. Secondly, there should be models designed to effectively guide research and intervention with culturally diverse populations. Such models must specify the way in which culture relates to health behavior and outcomes, as well as to the sources of cultural variation, such as ethnicity and SES. Thirdly, there must be the implementation of culturally appropriate methodological approaches and statistical techniques for testing theory-based hypotheses concerning the structure of relations among the multiple factors influencing heath disparities. Finally, research is needed to identify, measure, and scientifically demonstrate aspects of culture that drive disparities in health outcome. This should empirically test propositions concerning how population characteristics of patients and healthcare professionals relate to culture, psychological functioning, and behaviors relevant to health disparities.

References

Beauboeuf-Lafontant, T. (2007). You have to show strength: An exploration of gender, race, and depression. *Gender and Society, 21*, 28–51.
Carter-Edwards, L., Skelly, A. H., Cagle, C. S., & Appel, S. J. (2004). "They care but don't understand": Family support of African American women with type 2 diabetes. *The Diabetes Educator, 30*(3), 493–501. Available from: PM:15208847.
Casagrande, S. S., Wang, Y., Anderson, C., & Gary, T. L. (2007). Have Americans increased their fruit and vegetable intake? The trends between 1988 and 2002. *American Journal of Preventive Medicine, 32*(4), 257–263. Available from: PM:17383556.
Chatters, L. M., Levin, J. S., & Ellison, C. G. (1998). Public health and health education in faith communities. *Health Education & Behavior, 25*(6), 689–699.
Chen, M. S., Jr. (1998). Cancer prevention and control among Asian and Pacific Islander Americans: Findings and recommendations. *Cancer, 831*, 856–864.
Coleman, C. L., Holzemer, W. L., Eller, L. S., Corless, I., Reynolds, N., Nokes, K. M., et al. (2006). Gender differences in use of prayer as a self-care strategy for managing symptoms in African Americans living with HIV/AIDS. *Journal of the Association of Nurses in AIDS Care, 17*(4), 16–23. Available from: PM:16849085.
Dessio, W., Wade, C., Chao, M., Kronenberg, F., Cushman, L. E., & Kalmuss, D. (2004). Religion, spirituality, and healthcare choices of African-American women: Results of a national survey. *Ethnicity and Disease, 14*(2), 189–197. Available from: PM:15132203.
Dey, A. N., & Lucas, J. W. (2006). Physical and mental health characteristics of U.S.- and foreign-born adults: United States, 1998–2003. *Adv. Data, 369*, 1–19. Available from: PM:16541709.
Dole, E. J., Rhyne, R. L., Zeilmann, C. A., Skipper, B. J., McCabe, M. L., & Low, D. T. (2000). The influence of ethnicity on use of herbal remedies in elderly Hispanics and non-Hispanic whites. *Journal of the American Pharmaceutical Association (Washington), 40*(3), 359–365. Available from: PM:10853536.
Dona, G. (1991). Cross-cultural psychology as presaged by Hippocrates. *Cross-Cultural Psychology Bulleting, 25*, 2.
Druss, B. G., & Rosenheck, R. A. (1999). Association between use of unconventional therapies and conventional medical services. *JAMA, 282*(7), 651–656. Available from: PM:10517718.
Foluke, G. (1999). *The old-time religion: A holistic challenge to the Black church*. New York: Winston-Derek.
Graham, R. E., Ahn, A. C., Davis, R. B., O'Connor, B. B., Eisenberg, D. M., & Phillips, R. S. (2005). Use of complementary and alternative medical therapies among racial and ethnic minority adults: Results from the 2002 national health interview survey. *Journal of the National Medical Association, 97*(4), 535–545. Available from: PM:15868773.

References

Griffith, D. M., Johnson, J. L., Zhang, R., Neighbors, H. W., & Jackson, J. S. (2011). Ethnicity, nativity, and the health of American Blacks. *Journal of Health Care for the Poor and Underserved, 22*(1), 142–156. Available from: PM:21317512.

Harwood, A. (1981). In A. Harwood (Ed.), *Ethnicity and medical care Mainland Puerto Ricans* (pp. 397–481). Cambridge, MA: Harvard University Press. Ref Type: Journal (Full).

Hummer, R. A., Rogers, R. G., Nam, C. B., & Ellison, C. G. (1999). Religious involvement and U. S. adult mortality. *Demography, 36*(2), 273–285. Available from: PM:10332617.

Keegan, L. (1996). Use of alternative therapies among Mexican Americans in the Texas Rio Grande Valley. *Journal of Holistic Nursing, 14*(4), 277–294. Available from: PM:9146186.

Koku, E. F., et al. (2016). *Journal of Health Care for the Poor and Underserved, 27*(3), 1316–1329. doi:10.1353/hpu.2016.0128

Laken, M. A., O'Rourke, K., Duffy, N. G., Swinton, R., & Jordan, J. (2004). Use of the internet for health information by African-Americans with modifiable risk factors for cardiovascular disease. *Telemedicine and E-Health, 10*(3), 304–310. Available from: PM:15650525.

Lancaster, K. J., Watts, S. O., & Dixon, L. B. (2006). Dietary intake and risk of coronary heart disease differ among ethnic subgroups of black Americans. *Journal of Nutrition, 136*(2), 446–451. Available from: PM:16424126.

Mackenzie, E. R., Taylor, L., Bloom, B. S., Hufford, D. J., & Johnson, J. C. (2003). Ethnic minority use of complementary and alternative medicine (CAM): A national probability survey of CAM utilizers. *Alternative Therapies in Health and Medicine, 9*(4), 50–56. Available from: PM:12868252.

McCaffrey, A. M., Eisenberg, D. M., Legedza, A. T., Davis, R. B., & Phillips, R. S. (2004). Prayer for health concerns: Results of a national survey on prevalence and patterns of use. *Archives of Internal Medicine, 164*(8), 858–862. Available from: PM:15111371.

Musgrave, C. F., Allen, C. E., & Allen, G. J. (2002). Spirituality and health for women of color. *American Journal of Public Health, 92*(4), 557–560. Available from: PM:11919051.

Napier, A. D., Ancarno, C., Butler, B., Calabrese, J., Chater, A., Chatterjee, H., et al. (2014). Culture and health. *Lancet, 384*(9954), 1607–1639. Available from: PM:25443490.

O'Connor, M. Y., Thoreson, C. K., Ricks, M., Courville, A. B., Thomas, F., Yao, J., et al. (2014). Worse cardiometabolic health in African immigrant men than African American men: Reconsideration of the healthy immigrant effect. *Metabolic Syndrome and Related Disorders, 12*(6), 347–353. Available from: PM:24814168.

Pachter, L. M. (1994). Culture and clinical care. Folk illness beliefs and behaviors and their implications for health care delivery. *JAMA, 271*(9), 690–694. Available from: PM:8309032.

Polzer, R. L. (2007). African Americans and diabetes: spiritual role of the health care provider in self-management. *Research in Nursing & Health, 30*(2), 164–174. Available from: PM:17380517.

Riosmena, F., Wong, R., & Palloni, A. (2013). Migration selection, protection, and acculturation in health: A binational perspective on older adults. *Demography, 50*(3), 1039–1064. Available from: PM:23192395.

Satia, J. A. (2010). Diet-related disparities: Understanding the problem and accelerating solutions. *Journal of the American Dietetic Association, 109*, 610–615.

Sleath, B., Rubin, R. H., Campbell, W., Gwyther, L., & Clark, T. (2001). Ethnicity and physician-older patient communication about alternative therapies. *Journal of Alternative and Complementary Medicine, 7*(4), 329–335. Available from: PM:11558775.

World health Organization. (2007). Community health workers: What do we know about them? The state of the evidence on programmes, activities, costs and impact on health outcomes of using community health workers. Evidence and information for policy. Department of Human Resources for Health. Geneva, Switzerland.

Chapter 9
Psychological Factors and Health Disparities

Abstract Stress and psychological distress caused by perceived racial discrimination or other social factors may elicit negative emotional responses. These, in turn, can trigger adverse biological responses and negative health behaviors, and eventually lead to adverse health outcomes. The concept of "allostatic load" is used to demonstrate how environmental stresses including psychosocial ones can culminate in health disparities.

9.1 Introduction

Health and wellness or disease outcomes are determined by dynamic interactions between biological, psychological, behavioral, and social factors. These interactions occur during early development and throughout an individual's lifetime. Psychological factors influence health directly through biological mechanisms and indirectly through a plethora of behavioral and environmental factors, as discussed throughout this book. Environmental factors that can impact an individual's psychological well-being include low socioeconomic status (SES), depression, poor work conditions, social inequalities, racism, hostility, and income level, whereas behavior and lifestyle factors such as tobacco smoking, excessive alcohol consumption, or risky sexual behaviors can also have psychological effects.

Social scientists have discovered that living in environmental conditions of economic and social deprivation can be psychologically harmful. The constant exposure to distressing environments, such as racial segregation and poverty, can reinforce the restrictions on an individual's welfare causing frustrations that can lead to higher levels of anger, anxiety, depression, and/or stress. However, the mechanisms whereby distressing environmental exposures are mediated through psychological factors to effect adverse health are not well known. However, higher levels of acute and chronic stress that are some of the manifestations of psychological disorders are found among low-SES families who live in low-income segregated neighborhoods where there in increased neighborhood stressors, including the lack of safety and exposure to violence in comparison with high-SES families who live in safe neighborhoods and do not experience such neighborhood stressors.

Chronic diseases have replaced infectious diseases as the leading cause of mortality and morbidity in the USA, and the increased incidence and mortality rates from chronic diseases are huge public-health concerns. As discussed in the introductory chapter (Chap. 1), African Americans (AAs) and other racial and ethnic minority populations are disproportionally affected by increased incidences of chronic diseases, including CVDs, cancer, diabetes, hypertension, and HIV/AIDs in comparison with their European-American (EA) counterparts. Furthermore, AA and other minority populations experience higher infant-mortality rates, shorter life expectancies, and higher rates of homicide deaths. Individual behavior contributes a significant proportion of the increased incidence of chronic diseases, as well as mortality rates (discussed in Chap. 6). Therefore, the study of human behavior or psychology will provide more insights into understanding the disparities associated with AA and other minorities' health.

Our emotions and behavior affects our moods, bodies, and ultimately health. For instance, having a positive emotional attitude in life is correlated with longevity and good health, whereas fear and anger, which tend to increase stress levels and the associated psychological responses, may increase an individual's susceptibility to various diseases. One study found that patients who suffer from psychological distress, such as anxiety or depression, often also have physical manifestations of symptoms such as headaches, back pain, gastric distress or heartburn, dizziness, and bowel or bladder irregularities. In some instances, patients may need medical care for both psychological and physical complaints. However, in many instances, relief of psychological distress such as depression is able to eliminate the need for medical care, suggesting that various physical symptoms such as chronic pain are the manifestation of underlying depressive disorders (Turk and Salovey 1984). Therefore, the ability to elucidate the biological pathways that link psychological issues and physical symptoms would be a major medical breakthrough; unfortunately, this remains an unachieved major challenge for health professionals.

Several investigations have looked at the effect of mood on physical health. In one study by Croyle and Uretsky (1987) which involved transient mood experimentation, they observed that subjects who experienced negative moods were more likely to judge their health status negatively and were likely to experience more physical symptoms as well as be more pessimistic about potential improvements in their health. On the other hand, subjects who experienced positive moods were more likely to judge their health favorably, indicating that moods clearly affect health judgment and have favorable health outcome. Other reports indicate that moods influence risk-reducing behaviors, such as seeking medical treatment when sick, attitudes towards smoking, and exercise, all of which have health ramifications.

One potential mechanism that links mood and physical health outcomes is that mood alters physiological processes that affect immune signaling. For instance, one study reported that psychiatric in-patients who were hospitalized with major depressive disorder were observed to have abnormal immune responses, including the inability of lymphocytes to repair DNA damaged by irradiation, in comparison with non-psychiatric low-distress controls (Kiecolt-Glaser et al. 1985). This observation provides evidence for the direct pathway through which distress can suppress immune signaling, giving rise to increased susceptibility to diseases.

Moods and emotions can affect an individual's behavior. Studies have shown that behavior can be changed through behavioral interventions to successfully teach new behaviors and reduce risky behaviors. However, maintaining behavioral changes over a long period of time is not a small feat, because the root cause of an individual behavior (e.g., emotions and moods) has biological underpinnings and consequences that are influenced by SES, family interactions, community and workplace relationships, and other sources. In addition, policies at the local, state, and national levels can indirectly influence behavior and behavioral changes. For instance, racial desegregation at the national level can remove some of the distress faced in minority communities who feel socially marginalized. Therefore, changing unhealthy behavior is not simply a matter of "will power" but requires coordinated efforts at the individual, community, and even government levels to be successful. This chapter looks at the various psychological factors that are associated with health disparities.

9.2 Environmental Stressors

Stress is recognized as a state of mental or emotional condition whereby the result of adverse environmental factors exceeds individuals' physiological adaptive capacity to the extent that their psychological responses may place them at risk of adverse health outcomes (Cohen et al. 1995). Individuals of low SES, such as AA and other minority populations, typically report lower levels of resilient resources (ability to thrive and survive adversity), such as being in control of themselves and their surroundings, having social support, or feeling socially integrated, according to the Gallo and Matthew reserve capacity model (Gallo and Matthews 2003). This suggests that such variables may indeed serve as one link in the chain connecting low SES with poor physical health. Other reports suggest that one of the reasons why low-SES individuals have fewer resilience resources needed to deal with stressful events compared to individuals with higher SES (Matthews et al. 2008; Prescott et al. 2007) is that constant exposure to stress depletes their few resilient resources, leaving individuals more vulnerable to future strains and unable to replenish resources for future needs.

Social-science and social-epidemiologic research indicates that psychological stresses due to environmental hazards and other societal factors can lead to acute and chronic changes in the immune functioning of the human body and give rise to a dysfunctional immune system, which is needed to fight diseases in the first place. For instance, the AA population and other minority groups residing in poor neighborhoods are more susceptible to violence and pollutants, which leads to differential experience of environmental stresses compared to the EA population who live in safe, clean, and good neighborhoods with access to excellent community resources. Some reports indicate that individuals living in low-SES environments have a high incidence of depressive symptoms or disorders, hostile cognition, and angry emotions because of the constant exposure to environmental stressors, as well as psychological distress (Gallo and Matthews 2003). In addition, a low level of educational attainment is linked to individuals who are more vulnerable to stress. One report indicates that, for any given stressful experience, the poorly educated individuals reported greater distress and physical symptoms in comparison with their better-educated counterparts (Grzywacz et al. 2004). The psychosocial stresses experienced by the AA population, if not ameliorated by other resources, can directly contribute to health disparity.

9.3 Psychological Stress and Socioeconomic Status

There is a popular belief that psychosocial processes might play a role in the association of SES and health disparity. Indirect research has connected SES to various types of stresses and connected stress with health and disease processes on the other hand. However, the various studies that have investigated the direct association of SES and stress have reported inconsistent findings and limited data in direct support for the association of stress and SES. Most of these studies have investigated life events or perceived stressful events linked with SES, including social status, education, income, occupational status, and health outcomes, such as CVDs, hypertension, blood pressure, and diabetes.

One study investigated whether psychosocial stress (using metabolic syndrome as a predictor of health outcomes) may mediate SES and health outcomes. In this large Copenhagen City Heart study of a total of 6038 subjects including 3462 women and 2576 men aged 20–97 years, they measured seven components of metabolic syndrome (waist-to-hip ratio, high-density lipoprotein (HDL) cholesterol, triglycerides, systolic blood pressure (SBP), blood glucose, C-reactive protein (CRP) and fibrinogen), and their association with aspects of SES, such as educational status and predictive indicators such as psychosocial and behavior factors (Prescott et al. 2007). They observed a high inverse association between SES and metabolic syndrome, such that individuals who had attained more than a high-school education had better metabolic syndrome outcomes. On the other hand, psychosocial factors such as depression and fatigue were not consistently associated with high metabolic-syndrome scores. Also, behavioral factors such as increased physical activity showed variable associations with metabolic syndrome, whereas heavy smoking was associated with increased metabolic syndrome. Thus, this report did not support a direct role for psychosocial nor behavioral factors in mediating the association between SES and metabolic syndrome, and other groups have reported similar null findings for a role of psychosocial processes in explaining the association of SES and health outcomes (Avendano et al. 2006).

Another study examined if low SES was associated with increased metabolic syndrome (an important predictor of coronary heart disease and diabetes) as a result of stressful experiences in over 400 healthy women who were studied for a period of over twelve years. Results found low SES was positively linked to increase metabolic syndrome. A potential mechanism for this association fits the reserve capacity model mentioned in Sect. 9.2, as several measures of adverse life experiences based on the reserve capacity model demonstrated that these low SES individuals have depleted available capacity reserves which could partially account for the association of stress and increase metabolic syndrome (Matthews et al. 2008). This data suggests that reserve capacity and emotions serve as potential psychosocial pathways through which SES may relate to metabolic syndrome. Another report suggests that chronic stress on the job such as risk of injury and disability and lack of health-care insurance contributes to the association of low SES and health outcomes, including coronary heart disease (Marmot et al. 1997; Wamala et al. 2000). One job-related Scottish study of psychological stress and health outcomes of individuals at risk of cardiovascular disease reported that foremen (with higher SES) reported higher stress than lower-level employees (Macleod et al. 2005), indicating a positive association of higher SES and stress.

While education, income, and occupation are factors that capture both resources and significant components of SES, there are various limitations in using these factors to investigate associations with psychosocial factors and health. This is because the quality and meaning of education, as well as the potential implications for generating wealth, vary across demographic groups, such as age/gender, racial or ethnic groups, or even the country of origin. Income does not provide comprehensive information about purchasing power or standards of living that vary across demographic group and community levels. Occupational measures cannot be used for individuals that are not employed. The effect of SES on health begins early in life and extends into adulthood. All these mediating factors make it difficult to link psychosocial stresses with SES and health outcomes (Matthews and Gallo 2011), as shown in the relatively few studies. There are also gender differences in SES, and this may cause additional challenges to the psychological context of SES and health outcomes. One study suggests that men may have higher incomes with higher educational attainment or occupational standards in comparison with women. On the other hand, low-SES women may experience cumulative stress as a result of heading single-parent households, domestic violence, or gender discrimination on the job (Thurston et al. 2005).

A critical review by Matthews et al. (2010) of all studies addressing the role of psychosocial factors in SES and health disparities at that time concluded that psychosocial factors may play a critical role in the origins of an association of SES and health outcomes, particularly at critical developmental stages of childhood. There are several factors that account for the absence or partial association of psychosocial stress with SES and health outcomes (already mentioned). This is because stress is a multifaceted and complex construct, and there are a number of factors that can influence its association with SES, including the duration of exposure and severity of the stressful experience being assessed. Many large surveillance studies rely on brief, personal accounts that are not validated by these constructs (Khang et al. 2009; Prescott et al. 2007). Thus, such studies often fail to adequately capture the contributions these variables make to SES–physical health associations. In addition, studies that rely on self-reporting can also create biases that can lead to under- (or over-) estimates of association. Nonetheless, the dispute over whether stress is an important mediator for SES and health outcomes requires additional empirical evidence. Thus, while stress may be an important determinant for the association of SES and health outcome, it may not be the primary determinant of SES and health association. Additional studies are needed to clarify the inconsistent observation of SES, psychological stress, and health disparities.

9.4 Biological Mechanism of Psychological Stress

Stress is a condition of the mind and body's interaction resulting from experiences such as anxiety and frustration because they push individuals beyond their abilities to successfully handle a situation, such as meeting a work-schedule deadline, constant daily hassle, insecurity, poor health, and other interpersonal social issues, and the molecular mechanisms underlying psychological stress provide an example of gene-environment interaction (discussed in Chap. 10).

The body's response to environmental stress is cascade activation and the expression of several hormones, which is initiated in the central nervous system in response to external stimulus such as violence and culminates in a physiological response. However, the molecular pathway whereby the brain translates environmental stress into the final biological response is not clearly understood. Nonetheless, there is evidence that dysregulation of these physiological responses to stress can have biological consequences that are associated with adverse health and health disparities. The well characterized biological pathway, whereby signals from the brain are transmitted through the body to execute physiological responses, is the so-called hypothalamic-pituitary-adrenal (HPA) axis system.

Signals from the central nervous system in the form of chemical messengers or electrical potential are conveyed to the HPA axis which then triggers a cascade synthesis and release of hormones including corticotrophin releasing hormone (CRH), adrenocorticotrophic hormone, and glucocorticoids (cortisol) (Weinberg et al. 2001). The amount of cortisol released then stimulates the synthesis and release of adrenaline and noradrenaline which leads to various "flight and fight" physiological responses (Fig. 9.1). The prolonged and chronic activation of the stress-response system, such as perpetual exposure to economic deprivation and poor and violent low-income neighborhoods, is believed to lead to "wear and tear" on the human organ system, resulting in stress-associated diseases, a phenomenon known as allostatic load (discussed in Sect. 9.6).

9.4 Biological Mechanism of Psychological Stress

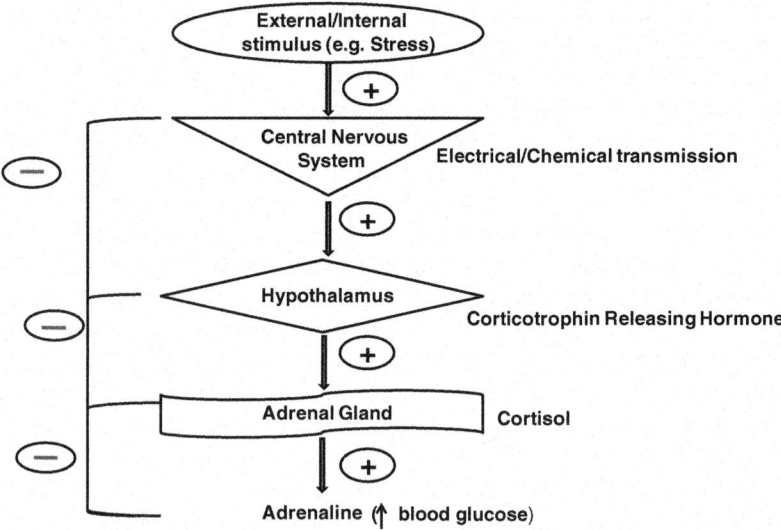

Fig. 9.1 A schematic diagram demonstrating the cascade activation of hormonal signal in response to an environmental stimulus such as stress. An example of typical hormonal cascade activation is initiated by signals sent to the central nervous system, which in turn leads to activation (+) and expression of corticotrophin releasing hormone (CRH) from the hypothalamus. THE CRH in turn activates the release of cortisol from the adrenal gland, and one of the effects of increased cortisol level is to stimulate the synthesis of adrenal to provide the energy needed to deal with the stressful situation. Once threshold activation is achieved, there are negative/inhibitory signals (−) that are initiated to stop additional release of these hormones

Several investigations have demonstrated that environmental exposures, such as early life stressors in animal and human studies, can alter gene expression via epigenetic mechanisms and consequently alter physiologic responses. This provides a classic example of gene-environment interaction, i.e., how the environment can impinge upon the genome using epigenetic mechanisms (discussed in Chap. 11). One such study was carried out using a stress-induced mouse model designed to exhibit stress-induced social-avoidance behavior in response to chronic stress (Elliott et al. 2010). When these mice were exposed to chronic stress to assess the effect of epigenetic changes and expression of the corticotrophin releasing factor (CRF), stress-induced aberrant DNA methylation of the CRF-gene promoter region was observed, and this event was associated with the silenced expression of CRF that consequently led to avoidance behavior. On the other hand, when the mice were treated with the DNA methyltransferase inhibitor 5′azacytisdine, this drug was able to reverse the methylation and induce gene expression of CRF. In addition, treatment of mice with the anti-depressant imipramine was also able to induce CRF mRNA expression and reverse the social-avoidance behavior, providing additional evidence that chronic stress induced aberrant DNA methylation in this mouse model. Other studies have reported that stress regulated DNA methylation and other epigenetic changes, such as histone modifications, in adult mice, suggesting that regulation of DNA methylation may be a primary mechanism underlying stress-induced behavioral changes in adult mice.

Another study carried out in a rat model demonstrated that differences in maternal care of newborn pups can give rise to epigenetic profiles of the hippocampal neurons in the pups that help regulate reactivity to stress and behavior in the adult rats. In this study, individual pups that were less nurtured as newborns were more reactive and anxiety-prone as adults (Meaney et al. 2007). Recent research provides preliminary evidence that similar epigenetic pathways may be operative in humans. For instance, it has been found that, in a number of teenage suicide victims with a history of childhood abuse, there was an association with methylation differences at the GR locus in the hippocampus (McGowan et al. 2009). Other studies found that child abuse was significantly associated with DNA methylation at the serotonin transporter protein (SLC6A4) locus, a gene whose dysregulation is associated with a wide range of disorders, including migraine, major depression, autism, and alcoholism (Beach et al. 2010). One limitation to this study is that the methylation analysis was carried out in the blood lymphoblasts from subjects, and this does not provide direct evidence of DNA methylation changes in the central nervous system. Nevertheless, these observations suggest that both early postnatal (or even prenatal), as well as childhood environmental exposures, can shape the epigenome of offspring with enduring effects on stress physiology and related behavioral outcomes.

Several epidemiological studies indicate that behavioral alterations in response to traumatic psychological events can be transmitted to offsprings, even if the offsprings themselves did not experience the traumatic events. One study that investigated the transgenerational impact of early-life stress analyzed the behavioral pattern of mice that were separated from their mothers from day one until day 14. They observed that these mice demonstrated depressive-like behavior, as well as altered response to new and aversive environment (Franklin et al. 2010). They also observed that this behavioral pattern of depressive-like behavior was transmitted to male offspring despite the fact that these males were reared normally. A potential mechanism for the altered behavioral characteristics indicated changes in DNA methylation patterns of gene promoter regions in the germline, as well as in the brain of these mice. This study highlights the negative impact of early-life stressors and behavioral changes that can affect several generations. Psychological stressors can use aberrant epigenetic phenomenon to exert trans-generational effects on health outcomes. This provide evidence in support of adverse psychological impacts on the next generation, and even grand offspring, suggesting that the full health costs of psychological stressors may not be realized for several generations. The importance of intergenerational and/or intragenerational social disorders has already been identified for several illness, including schizophrenia (Goldberg and Morrison 1963), chronic bronchitis (Meadows 1961) and epilepsy (Harrison and Taylor 1976), and is likely to include other mental illnesses and severely disabling diseases (West 1991).

9.5 Different Categories of Stress

There are three different categories of stress, which are described next.

9.5.1 Positive Stress

Positive stress is associated with a brief increase in heart rate and mild elevations of stress-hormone (cortisol and adrenaline) levels based on the "fright and fight" model to handle an immediate situation. Acute stressors (lasting minutes) are associated with adaptive and increased expression of some level of natural immunity, as well as an alteration of some functions of immune response in response to environmental exposure. For instance, receiving an immunization injection for flu or other normal experience can initiate a signal transduction for the release of a stress hormone. In this case, a positive stress response can ensue in a satisfactory way, creating a sense of accomplishment and mastery and control.

9.5.2 Tolerable Stress

This is a physiological state of stress which occurs within a limited time period but much longer than a positive stress. This type of stress can induce some form of damage to the neural circuitry of the central nervous system (e.g., prolonged exposure to cortisol can cause neural death in the hypothalamus). This type of stress can be caused by the death of a loved one, a long illness, or some natural disaster. Coping mechanisms in the form of protective relationships can help bring the body's response to such stressful experience back to baseline.

9.5.3 Prolonged Stress

Chronic and prolonged elevations of stress hormones can be caused by several factors, including low SES and the associated neighborhood violence, child maltreatment, family chaos, and food insufficiency that are typically seen in low-SES AA and minority populations. Other causes of chronic stresses include recurrent physical and/or emotional abuse and family violence, and these can have damaging adverse effects on physical and mental health. The timing of exposure to chronic stress is also important. Exposures can occur during the prenatal stage, infancy, childhood, adolescence, adulthood, or aging with early-life stress exposures being the most impactful on the overall health outcome of the individual.

Chronic stress underlies the etiology, as well as the progression, of many diseases, such as CVDs, diabetes, infections, immune dysfunction, and associated conditions that can impair growth and cognitive functioning, cancer, and mental problems, including depression and anxiety. In addition, chronic stress can lead to increase in visceral fat mass, obesity, and increased risk of type 2 diabetes. Overall, chronic stress is associated with physical and mental illness, such as producing wear and tear (measured by allostatic load and discussed in Sect. 9.6) on the CVS, which can lead to disorders such as strokes and heart attacks. Such chronic stressors are associated with suppression of both cellular and humoral immunity (Segerstrom and Miller 2004) and inflammatory responses (Miller et al. 2008) that ultimately deregulate the immune response. While chronic stress can be associated with psychological disorders and increased risk of adverse health, the effects of chronic stress and adverse health can be further compounded by individuals attempting to cope with these experiences through health-damaging behaviors such as tobacco smoking and excessive alcohol consumption. On the other hand, stress-, reduction programs such as cognitive-behavioral interventions have been demonstrated to reduce cortisol level and increased cardiovascular survival, during a standardized psychosocial challenge.

Based on observation of the body's physiological responses to stressors in order to regain homeostasis, McEwen (1998) conceptualized a health-model known as allostasis or allostatic load as the mediator of neuroendocrine, autonomic metabolic and immune system responses to stressors. Several markers associated with allostatic load can be measured in response to stress that can be directly correlated with health outcomes as discussed in Sect. 9.6.

9.6 Measurement of a Stress Indicator (Allostatic Load)

Allostatic load partially explains increased mortality rate in AAs independent of SES and health behaviors. Allostatic load reflects cumulative physiological imbalance as a result of repeated chronic stressors in daily life that may accumulate from early childhood throughout the lifespan of an individual. Allostatic load is determined using measurements that include levels of hormones that are secreted in response to stress (cortisol and primary or direct mediators) and/or biomarkers that reflect the effects of these hormones on the body (secondary indirect mediators). Duru et al. (2012) carried out longitudinal studies using the National Health and Nutrition Examination Survey (NHANES III) between 1988 and 1994 involving 40,000 people to investigate the role of allostatic load and mortality rates in various racial and ethnic groups. In this study, allostatic-load measurements included metabolic markers (e.g., waist-to-hip ratio, glycated hemoglobin), cardiovascular markers (e.g., systolic blood pressure, diastolic blood pressure, total cholesterol, triglycerides, homocysteine), and inflammatory markers [e.g., albumin, C-reactive protein (a measure of inflammation)]. The results demonstrated higher allostatic load scores to be significantly associated with higher mortality rates of CVDs and diabetes in AAs in comparison with EAs after adjusting for education, poverty, and health-insurance status.

Early-life adversity as determined by childhood SES disadvantages [e.g., marked by welfare payments, perceived as low-income and with less-educated parents] and other stressors, such as the death or divorce of parents, as well as parental physical abuse, can be measured by the outcome of cumulative allostatic load. One report found that the association of childhood physical abuse with allostatic load remained after adjusting for adult educational attainment, social relationships, and health behaviors with the association stronger for secondary stressor indicators, including inflammation, cardiovascular function, and lipid metabolism (Friedman et al. 2015).

Other reports suggests an inverse association between allostatic-load score and SES, such as increased allostatic load in direct association with low SES (Karlamangla et al. 2005; Seeman et al. 2004). One multi-ethnic study of atherosclerosis by Merkin et al. (2014) used sub-clinical data from 6814 men and women aged 45–84 years including EA, AA, Chinese, and Hispanic populations from various US communities. The study examined the effect of childhood and adult SES on changes in allostatic load over a period of time. The allostatic-load measures in this study including metabolic indicators (e.g., waist-hip ratio, triglycerides, low density lipoprotein, cholesterol, HD LDL, glucose) and cardiovascular measures (systolic blood pressure, resting heart rate and pulse). Overall Merkin et al. (Merkin et al. 2014) observed higher education (reflection of higher SES) was associated with slower increase in allostatic load over time, indicating that the link between SES and health outcomes may vary over time as a result of the accumulation of biological risk.

The direct association of allostatic load and SES may reflect some of the adverse low SES-related exposures, which contribute to adverse health outcomes, including accelerated aging process and the increased dysregulation of bodily functions (Seeman et al. 2004). On the other hand, a more favorable SES may slow or even reverse the aging process. Overall, changes in allostatic-load measurement can be used as an indicator of a disease-risk score, which can be followed up to improve assessment of mortality risk.

9.7 Prenatal Stress

Maternal stress during pregnancy has been described as a risk factor for the health of the developing fetus and is also a predictor of the future health consequences for the individual that persist throughout lifespan. Several human and animal studies demonstrate that maternal stress during pregnancy may also have consequences for cognition and learning, stress reactivity, other emotional and behavioral responses, and future health outcome. As mentioned above and throughout this book, low SES is significantly associated poor health outcome. One of the direct mechanistic pathways whereby maternal low-SES and its associated chronic-stress levels affects the developing fetus is that chronic stress can modulate the level of placental corticotrophin-releasing hormone (CRH) and glucocorticoids via the HPA axis as discussed in Sect. 9.4. Excessive CRH release may have important adverse effects, such as disrupting fetal nervous-system programming and causing growth impairment, and is also associated with the likelihood of premature birth. Thus, excessive CRH release during pregnancy as a result of chronic stress may be linked to increased risk of childhood mental illness, poor school performance, and other adverse outcomes in adulthood.

Work carried out by Erickson et al. (2001) found that pregnant women with excessive secretions of placental CRH are at significantly increased risk of preterm birth, and preterm birth in turn is associated with a shorter gestation period and risk of a wide variety of developmental problems and later adverse health outcomes in adulthood. Other reports have implicated a role for CRH and childhood temperament. In one study that assessed infant temperament at two months of age and maternal CRH concentration at 19, 25 and 31 weeks of gestation (Davis et al. 2005), they found that maternal stress related to high CRH concentration may also influence infant temperament. The study demonstrated that infants of mothers with low concentrations of CRH in maternal blood at 25 weeks of gestation scored lower in fear and distress at two months of age, whereas the CRH concentration levels at 19 and 32 weeks of gestation did not show significant association with infant temperature, suggesting the possibility that there is a critical period during which exposure to excess CRH impacts childhood temperament. These data indicate that the prenatal exposure to CRH at critical periods during development may exert effects that persist into the postnatal period. It is possible that CRH acts directly on regions of the brain that regulates the characteristics of temperament.

Other pathways, including postpartum maternal psychological state, may independently influence infant temperament, as well as maternal perception of infant temperament. Neuroscience research on brain development suggests that in utero exposures to toxins, such as high levels of lead, a neurotoxin that affects IQ and school achievement in low-SES children, in the blood. Environmental stresses such as poor nutritional sufficiency can also influence neural mechanisms and cognition and emotion. In addition, alcohol, cocaine, and tobacco use during pregnancy can all affect child development and are associated with significant behavioral changes later in life, such as increased rates of illicit substance use in adolescence (Hackman et al. 2010).

Other studies have investigated maternal stress and the immune response to allergies in their offsprings. For instance, one investigation examined maternal-childhood SES, cord blood immunoglobulin E (IgE) levels (indicator for early atopic risk), and repeated wheezing using data from Hispanic, AA and other foreign born mothers involved in the urban pregnancy cohort known as the Asthma Coalition on Community Environment and Social Stress (ACCESS) project. The study found that mothers with low SES and more susceptible to environmental stresses were significantly more likely to have newborns with increased IgE levels and repeated wheezing in comparison with mothers of higher SES (Sternthal et al. 2011). However, the study found that prenatal stress, household allergens such as cockroach allergens and mouse urinary protein, or traffic-related pollution did not significantly associate with cord blood IgE levels. The result from this study supports the transgenerational effects (discussed in Sect. 9.4) of early-life exposures based on the observation that early-life environmental stresses, both psychological and physical, were related to the mother's own childhood experience, which can be transmitted into adulthood, pregnancy, and consequently influence her child's development. While other studies have shown indirect associations between wheezing and psychological, as well as behavioral, factors, one report actually suggests a direct mechanism between early postnatal stress and repeated wheezing independent of smoking and breast-feeding behaviors, as well as allergen exposure, birth weight, or lower respiratory infections (Wright et al. 2002).

9.8 Parental Care and Stress

There are abundant reports in the literature to demonstrate that early-life experiences shape an individual's general physical and mental well-being for the entire lifespan, such that adversity during early life can have detrimental effects on health in later life. Several indirect observations indicate that maternal-childhood adverse psychosocial experiences, such as low-SES related violence, sexual abuse, and neglect were significantly associated with adolescent, early adulthood, and mid-life health outcomes, including increased risk of CVD, respiratory illness, and obesity, and most associations are long lasting, so they did not attenuate with age (Clark et al. 2010). Researchers have identified that negative and hostile family environments characterized by recurrent episodes of anger, conflict, or neglect and such psychosocial factors can be one intermediary pathway linking low childhood SES and adult metabolic functioning, inflammatory markers, and blood pressure (Lehman et al. 2005, 2009). Other studies have shown that postnatal parental stress and depression that reduces parental care and involvement during childhood also has adverse health effects on the child. There is a link between childhood maltreatment and adult mental, as well as the increased susceptibility to adverse physical, health such as depression, heart diseases, and diabetes as indicated my allostatic markers such as high C-reactive protein expression and inflammatory markers.

One model proposes that early-life adversity and its associated psychosocial stresses can disrupt biological responses in the HPA axis (Fig. 9.1), causing life-long reprogramming of the neuroendocrine and immune function that increases susceptibility to asthma and related diseases (Wright and Enlow 2008). Variations in parental care mediate intellectual and emotional well-being of a child as demonstrated in animal studies that have shown that licking and grooming of pups can have positive effects on cognition and emotional development by modulating the HPA axis. Positive psychosocial behavior, such as tactile stimulation by mothers, stimulates the release of increased growth hormones and decreased CRH release in offspring (Schanberg et al. 1984). On the other hand, pups who suffer prolonged separation from mothers demonstrate increased levels of glucocorticoids and decreased expression of growth factors; the cross-talk between glucocorticoids and certain growth factors at the optimal level is essential for normal physiological regulation, such as growth and development. However, the aberrant glucocorticoids and growth-factor expression can be reversed by tactile stimulation from mother, such as licking and grooming, suggesting that maternal stimulation can promote an endocrine-paracrine signaling system to promote growth and development. In addition, pups with high licking and grooming mothers demonstrate enhanced spatial learning and memory ability (Liu et al. 2000), as well as reduced physiological responses to acute stress as adults, in comparison with pups that received low licking and grooming (Liu et al. 1997).

There are also observations from human studies to suggest that the HPA-axis can be modulated by trauma and disrupted as evidenced by neglect and abuse of foster children who appear to have abnormal adrenal-cortisol release, suggesting that maltreated children who lack maternal warmth may display related characteristics, such as being less likely to respond well to stressful situations or less likely to regulate their emotions (Fisher et al. 2000). Other supporting studies come from middle-school children exposed to cumulative psychosocial (family violence and low SES) and physical (crowding, substandard housing) risk factors who demonstrated significantly higher levels of allostatic load, which could be alleviated by maternal warmth and care (Evans and Kim 2007). Thus, maternal warmth and care can buffer the adverse effects of early-life exposures such as low SES on adult metabolic symptoms (Miller et al. 2011). Interestingly, parental care in the form of parent-child verbal communication and discipline, as well as displays of sensitivity to the emotional needs of a child, have positive outcomes for the emotional and intellectual well-being of a child, regardless of SES status. High-quality parent–child interactions are associated with resilience among children who live in stressful, impoverished low SES environments.

9.9 Cognitive Stimulation in the Home Environment

One psychological factor that influences health outcome is cognitive stimulation in the home environment. The quality of the home environment includes availability of books, access to computers, educational programs on television, and other media source, trips, and parental communication that can stimulate cognition in the growing child. These resources vary depending on the SES of the home and can explain the association of SES on cognitive ability in children (for example, reading and mathematics skills), even when maternal IQ has been controlled for. One longitudinal study found that the level of cognitive stimulation in early childhood predicted quite well the language-related skills in low-SES adolescents independently of the quality of parental care and maternal intelligence. On the other hand, differences in parental interactions, such as time spent talking and giving attention to children, is associated with language skills in children. Low-SES children are exposed to a narrower range of vocabulary through less parental interaction and may often be prohibited from talking. Thus, children of low SES may build vocabularies at a slower pace when compared to higher-SES children and who received positive social influences (Walker et al. 1994). It is estimated that the size of vocabulary for US three-year-olds with supervised study from higher SES, such as professional families, is twice as large as for children from low-SES families, such as those on welfare (Hart and Risley 1995).

Thus, among low-SES families, such as AA and other minority families, lack of resources and parent-child interactions can adversely affect health outcomes. On the other hand, one longitudinal study demonstrated that among low-SES (but not high-SES) families, positive social relationships (such as high emotional support) were associated with reduced risk of cardiovascular disease and inflammation over an 18-month period (Vitaliano et al. 2001).

There is a cumulative effect of the adverse childhood experiences of children of low SES, which is directly correlated with intelligence and academic achievement from early childhood through to adolescence. Studies that analyzed brain activity using neuroimaging to assess language task in five-year-old children (Raizada et al. 2008) demonstrated that children from higher SES families and who are exposed to a richer language environment have greater volume in Broca's area, a part of the brain whose activity is an indicator of child's linguistic environment, in comparison with low-SES children who have limited language vocabulary, suggesting that weaker language skills of low-SES children are related to reduced underlying neural specialization connected to speech and other language skills.

One study of eastern Finnish men found that respondents, who experienced low SES in childhood and limited upward mobility in terms of economic opportunity, exhibited poorer cognitive profiles in comparison with those who started life in low SES but then attained a higher education and income (Turrell et al. 2002). This finding would suggests that SES across all stages of life can influence cognitive abilities in the later stages of life, however with regards to cognition, beginnings do not necessarily equate with destiny, as low-SES circumstances in childhood may be overcome to some extent by later higher economic opportunities.

9.10 Community Stressors and Health

Several environmental factors in low-SES communities have important psychological effects and poor health outcomes in AA and other minority populations. For instance, constant exposure to noise pollution, violence, radiation, extreme temperatures, unsafe water supply, and neighborhood filth can all contribute to chronic stresses and induce physiological changes that make the body more susceptible to illness. Other environmental toxic exposures, e.g., mold, heavy metals, fluorocarbons, unsafe housing, and limited play and green spaces also have psychological impacts on individual health. Furthermore, psychosocial conditions, including crowded living conditions in low-SES communities, social disorganization, fear, higher neighborhood crime rates or the perception of crime, and economic deprivation are linked to adverse psychological outcomes including anxiety depression, posttraumatic stress disorder, and substance abuse. Studies have reported that stress due to racial discrimination is associated with high blood pressure, mental health, and excessive alcohol consumption. Social psychology provides direct evidence of key mediating mechanisms or pathways, by which environmental pressures linked to a group's position in the social structure translate into psychological perceptions and experiences, psychophysiological responses, and ultimately into health.

9.11 Psychosocial Relationships in Community and Health

Some reports have assessed psychosocial benefits to communities, such as the presence of social support, a community with integrated social groups or a communities with high SES (social capital), have found these factors to have a positive psychosocial effect (Rasmussen et al. 2009; Uchino 2006). These observations indicate that a sense of mastery or control over various aspects of life, such as self-esteem or optimism, can have favorable effects on health outcomes.

The importance of social relationships and support and health outcomes is underscored by other studies that indicate that lack of social relationships such as family and friends can adversely affect the health outcome of individuals. One study showed increased mortality rates in patients who have sparse social networks and low social support, in comparison with those who have a positive social network or family support (House et al. 1988), suggesting that social isolation may be a major risk factor for increased mortality rate. Other supporting observations of social isolation and poor health outcomes indicate that individuals with limited social networks including family and friends or live alone have higher CVDs incidence, as well as mortality rates when compared to individuals who are well-connected socially (Kaplan et al. 1988). The link between social isolation and high CVD risk and death was highly significant among the Finish men analyzed in this study, whereas there was no strong or consistent association between social isolation and high CVD risk and death in the Finish women in this study.

Studies in the 1970s that looked at social environments, including neighborhoods, organizations to which we belong, and workplaces, also support a positive role for social relationship in buffering against stressful events and poor health (Yen and Syme 1999). Other studies confirm an inverse relationship between positive social relationships and mortality risk (Schoenbach et al. 1986). Schoenbach et al. observed that lack of a social network, such as marital status, church activities, and other social networks among older subjects, was significantly associated with increased mortality rates.

Yet other studies, such as work carried out by Chen et al. (2011) have shown that there are some individuals from low-SES backgrounds who live in adverse environmental conditions. Yet, despite the persistent and severe adversity, they do not get sick so frequently, which defies the trend of low SES association with poor health, including asthma. Chen et al. (2011) proposed the so-called "shift-and-persist" approach to explain how such individuals stay well despite their circumstances. The "shift-and-persist" approach suggests that such individuals are able to adjust themselves through finding positive outcomes in whatever the situation may be, while staying optimistic about the future and pursuing future-oriented goals. Such individuals are less likely to display negative responses to psychological factors, which in turn reduces their stress hormone levels, as well as inflammatory responses, and ultimately reduces their risk of adverse health outcomes.

Other observations indicates that, among a study sample of adults who were all from low-SES families, but experienced high childhood maternal warmth, the adults demonstrated reduced expressions of pro-inflammatory gene networks and decreased inflammatory (IL-6) responses in vitro microbial stimulation tests, in comparison with adults whose childhood experience was low in maternal warmth and care. Supporting data suggests that positive family relationships during childhood are associated with faster recovery of heart rate and blood pressure to normal levels after an acute stressor, whereas adults who experienced childhood adversity, such as the loss of a parent, required a prolonged recovery of heart rate and blood pressure to normal levels (Luecken et al. 2005).

9.12 Resilience and Psychological Impact on Health

Numerous daily adversities and challenges are faced by low-SES populations including AA and other minorities. AA and other minority populations of low SES typically report lower resilient resources, such as lack of social support, or not feeling in control of circumstances and environment (Gallo and Matthews 2003). These parameters may serve as one link in the chain of events connecting low SES with poor physical health. Four studies found evidence of a mediating role for these variables (Matthews et al. 2010) and health outcomes. Moreover, strong support was identified in a study of men performed by Bosma and colleagues (Bosma et al. 1999), who found that about a one-third to two-third excess incidence of coronary heart problems in low SES groups which could be attributed to generalized control beliefs (Bosma et al. 2005). Control beliefs could contribute to health outcomes through a variety of pathways, such as problem solving (e.g., active attempts to cope) or depression, because of a low sense of control can be equated with helplessness (a known correlate of depression).

On the other hand, naturally occurring coping mechanisms, such as optimism and other successful adaptation to challenges such as low SES and environmental stresses, appear to mitigate some of the adverse health outcomes for low-SES populations. One model proposed to explain developing resilience in the face of adversity is "shift strategies". Shift strategies enable an individual to adjust to the environmental factors in such a way that they are cognizant of their environmental stressors but adapt various strategies to modulate the effects of the stresses, such as not easily getting upset, while at the same time keeping focus on their goals. The ability to adjust to a stressful situation is a coping style that is referred to in the literature as "secondary control coping" (Heckhausen and Schulz 1995). Observations indicate that shift strategies have the potential benefit of mitigating adverse physical health. For instance, better emotion-regulation abilities are linked to lower allostatic load, a measure of adverse health (Kinnunen et al. 2005). Shifting strategies can also alter clinical disease outcomes (Affleck et al. 1987) as demonstrated in patients who survived heart attack and attributed their chances of survival to appreciating evaluating the benefits derived from misfortune. Furthermore, the ability to manage one's emotions is a general indicator of better self-reported health and less sickness (Schutte et al. 2007).

Another model that provides resilience in the face of adversity is persistence. Persistence deals with the ability to find meaning in difficult circumstances faced in low-SES or other adverse situations by staying optimistic, hopeful, and maintaining the pursuit of goal pursuits, while enduring such adversity with strength and optimism about the future (Updegraff et al. 2008). One report that investigated low-SES adults who managed to maintain good physical health in comparison with high-SES adults reported self-development, such as setting goals, following through, not giving up despite adversity, and striving to achieve the things they wanted in life (Markus et al. 2004). In addition, having an optimistic outlook on life makes it easier for individuals to find appropriate emotional responses to unsolvable problems (Aspinwall and Richter 1999) and makes individuals more likely to reinterpret or change the trajectory of their emotional response to stressful events (Carver et al. 1993).

Individuals who are optimistic and lead a purposeful life have better immune responses to infections and overall better health outcomes. For instance, optimism is associated with lower levels of inflammatory markers such as IL-6 (Roy et al. 2010) and lower expression levels of IL-6 receptor, a marker that increases proinflammatory signals from IL-6 (Friedman et al. 2007) and which are implicated in cardiovascular disease. Other reports suggest that persistence is also associated with good clinical outcomes. Notably, optimistic and hopeful individuals with high self-esteem live longer and are less likely to suffer CVDs in comparison with individuals who are less optimistic or hopeful about life (Everson et al. 1996). Overall, "shift and persist" may have physiological benefits for dealing with stress and could lead to better health outcomes regardless of SES.

Numerous published studies have identified key factors in mediating resilience on the child, family, and neighborhood levels that buffers individuals against SES adversities (Masten and Coatsworth 1998). For instance, good schools promote better academic outcomes, and a warm, family nurturing environment provides children with the temperament, cognitive ability, and self-confidence which buffers against adversities, such as behavioral problems and academic difficulty in children.

9.13 Psychosocial Factors and Adverse Health Outcomes in African Americans

Very limited studies have investigated psychological distress among AAs despite this population being socially disadvantaged at several levels. One study used data from the 2001–2003 National Survey of American Life to investigate several social and economic predictors of psychological distress in the AA population comprising 18-year-olds and older. This study identified several factors including young age, lower income, lower education attainment, and lower self-reported health status and childhood health that were strongly associated with psychological distress. In addition, material hardship and a history of previous incarceration of a family member, as well as homelessness, were significantly associated with increased psychological distress (Mouzon et al. 2016). Another study found that AA women, in particular, are more susceptible to stressful events through factors such as network stress, motherhood, and childbirth, employment and financial hardship, and personal illness and injury, as well as victimization and single parenthood (Stevens-Watkins et al. 2014). This study further reported that the combination of employment and parenting increased stress and consequently increased incidence and mortality rates for diabetes and hypertension in AA women in comparison with EA women. The unique role of AA women in society, with regards to their gender and racial position, may increase susceptibility to adverse life events and chronic stressors that can often result in psychological distress.

9.14 Psychosocial Factors and Psychological Implications of Health Disparities

Besides SES, there are many other psychosocial factors including racial prejudice, discrimination of various forms, a lack of social network, stigmatization, and environmental hazards that can have psychological impact on individual and population health. The effects of these psychosocial factors for low-SES AA and other minority populations can significantly affect their health as described next.

9.14.1 Anxiety and Depression

Individuals of low SES without community or family support often report not being in control of their circumstances or being able predict events in order to obtain desired outcomes. Cynicism, suspicion, and/or resentment may build up in these individuals and manifest themselves in anger and hostility, as well as anxiety. AA and other minority populations experience external stresses due to victimization and violence or internal stresses such as rejection. Both types of stresses are linked to adverse health outcomes in individuals belonging to minority populations (Clark et al. 1999). The feeling of anxiety is associated with increased risks for coronary heart disease and sudden cardiac death (Everson-Rose and Lewis 2005a). Individuals who experience high levels of hostility are at an increased risk of strokes, myocardial infarctions, and coronary heart diseases, as well as premature mortality (Everson-Rose and Lewis 2005b; Krantz and McCeney 2002).

In addition to depression and anxiety, there is abundant literature documents that low SES is also associated with psychological characteristics, including loss of interest or pleasure in activities or social interactions, and this could often be accompanied by weight loss or weight gain (Gallo and Matthews 2003). Studies documented depression about future cardiovascular morbidity and mortality outcomes (Rozanski et al. 1999). Individuals of low SES also experience insomnia, fatigue, and feelings of guilt or worthlessness that can manifest themselves in mental disorders, such as suicidal thoughts and other chronic illnesses including kidney disease, hypertension, and diabetes. Recurrent episodes of depression and anger in low-SES families can manifest in family conflict that can result in neglecting of nurturing children and results in children lacking the experiences needed to develop effective social-emotional skills, as well as being vulnerable to a wide range of emotional and physical disorders. In essence, family and community environments in low SES that is fraught with violence and hostility culminate in shaping individual psychological characteristics and behaviors that results in adverse health (Matthews et al. 2010).

9.14.2 Psychological, Emotional, and Social Well-Being

Mental health is the psychological, emotional, and social well-being of an individual. Several factors influences mental health, such as the individual genetic factors or brain chemistry, life experiences including abuse or traumatic experiences, and a family history of mental problems. Other psychosocial factors, such as racism, discrimination, low SES, mistrust, fear, and cultural and social influences can influence mental health. Several of these adverse psychosocial factors are over-represented in AA and other minority populations, including immigrants and refugees, victims of violence, and homeless people, as well as individuals with chronic disease and disability. When there is violence in a neighborhood, both adults and children experience more mental health problems (Stockdale et al. 2007; Xue et al. 2005). In addition, individuals of low-SES can develop personalities characterized by high hostility and pessimism because of mistrust and cynicisms about others (Heinonen et al. 2006; Kawachi et al. 1997).

9.14.2.1 Psychosocial Factors and Mental Health Disparity in Children and Adolescents

Attention-deficit/hyperactivity disorder (ADHD) is primarily a genetic disorder with a strong familial predisposition. The ADHD condition is a common childhood mental disorder diagnosed in about 7% of children and youths (Pliszka 2007). When parents and teachers were given specific criteria for the characteristics of ADHD, AA children were more likely to be rated higher on these criteria. Despite the high prevalence of ADHD in AA children in comparison with EA children, children of EAs are one-and-a-half times more likely to be treated for ADHD (Miller et al. 2009). The disparity in the treatment of ADHD persisted even after confounding factors such as SES were controlled for in one study (Olfson et al. 2003). Some of the reasons for this disparity is that EA parents who are affluent and well educated are knowledgeable about this condition and also have strong emphasis on academic success, so would pursue treatment for their affected children. AA parents, on the other hand, are less knowledgeable about this condition and may worry that drug treatment for ADHD is simply the schools trying to make their children conform to their standards, and there are also issues with lack of access for health care in the AA community. Youths with an ADHD diagnosis often have other comorbid psychiatric disorders, including oppositional defiant disorder (ODD), anxiety disorders, depressive disorders, and increased rates of smoking (Pliszka 2007).

Few studies have documented the prevalence of mental illness in US children or the prevalence of mental illness in various racial and ethnic groups. Generally, depression, anxiety disorders, attention-deficit/hyperactivity disorder (ADHD), and substance-abuse disorders are the most commonly reported mental health problems of youth in the USA (Anon 2000). However, various estimates indicate that 10–21% of US children have a diagnosable mental illness resulting in functional impairment (Costello et al. 2003; Roberts et al. 1998). Two reports have suggested similar frequencies of mental health disorders in youths from various racial and ethnic groups such as AAs and EA populations in the general community (Zimmerman 2005; Zwaanswijk et al. 2003). A more comprehensive national report of mental health among US youths by the Youth Risk Behavior Surveillance System (YRBSS) found that Hispanic youths had higher behavioral and emotional issues commonly associated with mental-health disorders as evidenced by higher rates of suicide attempts in the Hispanic youths in comparison with other racial and ethnic groups (Eaton et al. 2010).

Several mechanisms have been proposed to explain the higher prevalence of mental health in ethnic minorities, in particular the Hispanic youth population, demonstrating that ethnicity or race is a risk factor for youths' mental health (Kodjo and Auinger 2004; Muroff et al. 2008; Slade 2004). Several indicators suggest that the underlying cause of higher mental health in one population versus the other is low SES, which in turn leads to poorer mental health status and outcomes for minority youths. Minority youths of low SES disproportionally live in chronic states of poverty or severe poverty, which has cumulative effects on mental health. Poverty can also influence family dynamics, causing household stresses and conflicts that can result in poor parent–youth interactions, and this too is linked to the likelihood for increased risk of mental disorders as observed for AA youths (Natsuaki et al. 2007). The accumulating evidence has shown that exposure to family and community poverty is linked to increased mental disorders such as depression and associated behavioral disorders such as substance abuse and criminal activity (Kodjo and Auinger 2004; Leslie et al. 2007; Natsuaki et al. 2007). Mental health issues in minority youths are also compounded by the lack of health-care access, particularly the lack of health insurance and other access to mental-care services.

9.14.2.2 Psychosocial Factors and Mental Health Disparity in Adults

Mental-health disorders are common illnesses among US adults. The National Institute of Mental Health data for 2014 estimates that about 18.1% of all Americans struggle with a mental illness regardless of their race (https://www.nimh.nih.gov/health/statistics/prevalence/any-mental-illness-ami-among-us-adults.shtml). When the prevalence of mental health is stratified by race and ethnic groups, Native Hawaiians/Other Pacific Islanders have the highest incidence of any other US racial and ethnic group. Then prevalence of mental disorders in the AA population is less than the EA population, however the AA population is 1.2-times more likely to have serious psychological distress and associated mental disorders in comparison with their EA counterparts.

Mental health is a topic that many individuals within the AA community consider a taboo and often do not discuss. Depression is one of the most common mental illnesses, but it is under-recognized and often under-treated among the AA population, in particular among AA men. Depression is a serious problem for AA men. Ignoring those problems or pretending that they don't exist won't make them go away. Depression is treatable by counseling, psychotherapy, and medication.

Mental-health disorders are one of the risk factor for increased incidence of suicides in the USA. Suicide is the third leading cause of death among AAs aged 15–24 years. Less than half of all Americans with a mental disorder get the treatment that is needed, and only about 50% of AA patients get treatment for their mental disorder in comparison with the EA population. As a result of the under-diagnosis and under-treatment of mental disorders in AA men, they are more than four times as likely to commit suicide as AA women, even though the prevalence of mental disorders is higher in AA women. Other reasons why so few AAs receive mental-health care include the stigma associated with the condition. People with mental disorders are referred to as psychos, weirdos, crazies, basket cases, and wackos. Such a stigma keeps many people away from seeking help for issues like depression. Also there is lack of access to care, and a lack of health insurance, as well as a lack of health-literate professionals who understand the AA culture and that of other minority populations. The Surgeon General's Report on Mental Health notes striking disparities in mental health care for AAs and other US minority populations, indicating that ethnic minorities are less likely to receive services, and/or receive poorer quality of mental-health care. Since minority populations are also under-represented in mental-health research, overall, such disparities impose a great burden from these disabilities on minority people.

9.14.3 Racism and Health

Stress and psychological distress caused by perceived racial discrimination or other factors may elicit negative emotional responses. These, in turn, can connect to adverse biological processes and negative health behaviors, and eventually to disease. The concept of "allostatic load" discussed in Sect. 9.6 is used to indicate how psychosocial factors can culminate in health disparities. There is data to indicate that low-SES populations, in particular AAs and other minorities who self-reported experiences of racial discrimination, exhibited increased risks of psychological distress (Krieger et al. 2011). Perceived discrimination may contribute to poorer self-reported health among AAs through heightened levels of stress and depression. Thus, in addition to inequity in material resources and access to healthcare, the high prevalence of adverse health seen in minority population could also be caused by social marginalization with the underlying causes being the concentration of poverty in low-SES populations and neighborhoods (Smith et al. 2008).

9.14.4 Psychological Stressors and Stigma

From a sociological perspective, stigma is defined as "the co-occurrence of labeling, stereotyping, separation, status loss, and discrimination in a context in which power is exercised" (Link and Phelan 2001). Stigmatization can occur at various levels: stigmatization that occurs at the global level such as genocide, disruption of certain cultures, and oppression or slavery are traumatic assaults of historical proportion that have generational consequences with regards to health. At the individual level, stigma can be manifested as stereotypes, prejudice, and discrimination. The concept of stigma encompasses broader status and characteristics beyond racism to include sexual orientation, disability, mental illness, incarceration, HIV status, and obesity.

According to US medical data (National Center for HIV/AIDs 2010), although AA comprised about 12% of the US population, they accounted for 45% of all newly diagnosed HIV cases in the period 2007–2010. Moreover, black men who have sex with men bear the greatest burden of all races/ethnicities and transmission groups. Stigmatization affects screening and diagnosis. For instance, 77% of the AA population are more likely to report having been tested for HIV in comparison with 49% of the EA population, and yet AAs are often diagnosed with a later stage of the HIV disease (Kaiser Family Foundation 2017). Reports indicate that once a person is diagnosed with HIV, he/she is marked forever with the HIV stigma, and this may discourage people from getting tested in the first place. There is also a stigma when it comes to treatment, as AAs and other minorities are less likely to receive antiretroviral treatment compared to the EA population with HIV. When receiving HIV care, people living with HIV perceive an explicit stigma based on their race and SES, as well as HIV status. AAs may also perceive a stigma and prejudice at the level of the care provider, as AAs report receiving poorer care, limited access to care, and have less confidence in the care providers (Kinsler et al. 2007). Low-SES AAs living in poor neighborhoods have higher mortality rates from HIV/AIDs than other racial and ethnic groups and are less likely to remain alive nine years after diagnosis, as a result of stigmatization and other factors that disproportionally affect health outcomes in low-SES minorities.

A variety of stigmatized circumstances leads to many forms of resource-reducing events, such as employment, wages, mortgage and other loans, housing, the quality and quantity of education, and access to good healthcare. Several reports indicate that a stigma can also lead to social isolation. For instance, the fear of rejection and negative evaluation can cause stigmatized individuals to conceal their identities by avoiding close relationship for fear of others discovering the stigma. Thereby, this forces stigmatized individuals to relate only to other individuals who are also stigmatized (Pachankis 2007). Other reports indicate that the experience of stigmatization can lead to inappropriate coping behaviors, such as smoking and drinking that are associated with increased risk of several diseases (Paradies 2006).

Hatzenbuehler et al. (2013) review of the literature on stigma indicates that psychological stress plays an important role in the stigma process, whereby stigmatized individuals, as a result of discrimination and unfair treatment, are exposed to excess stress causing adverse physiological response (indicated by higher allostatic load), including diastolic blood pressure and increased cortisol output, contributing to adverse health outcomes. Hatzenbuehler et al. (2013) suggest that stigmatization of AAs and other minority populations in the USA can contribute to disparities that are associated with adversity in mental and physical health. Stigmatization can lead to inability to access multiple resources, such as legislative policies and interpersonal and psychological factors that could otherwise be useful in minimizing the adverse health outcome in low-SES populations. However, stigma may be one factor in a myriad of external factors that might contribute to differences in health outcomes. Overall, stigma influences several physical and mental conditions that affect millions of the US population through multiple mechanisms.

9.14.5 Prejudice and Discrimination

Social prejudice and discrimination, based on race or ethnic group or certain features, has widespread and negative effects on health. Prejudice, based on irrational assumptions about particular population or communities, creates ignorance and denies opportunities to the victims of prejudice, while by the same token limiting the experiences and perspectives of those showing prejudice. For instance, assuming that all AAs are lazy may affect the chances on any AA person getting a job, irrespective of educational status or experience. On the other hand, assuming that all Asian-Americans are smart may give an Asian-American an advantage in the job market compared to other ethnic and racial groups that may be more or equally qualified, or even more educated and skilled. Preconceived prejudice of high-SES members (predominantly EA) against those of low SES (AAs and other ethnical minorities) leads to low SES-groups being discriminated against in job promotions, which affects their financial resources. In addition, discrimination can also limit access of low-SES people to several resources important for good health that high SES can easily obtain. Such insidious prejudice that is felt on a daily basis can lead to violence and crime, and adversely affect the health of AA and other minority populations (Macdonald and Leary 2005). Individuals in the health professions may hold implicit prejudices against low-SES patients that can influence the quality and access to healthcare received by AA patients. For instance, AA patients often perceive EA physicians as cold or unfriendly, even though the physicians themselves did not recognize the impact of their implicit bias on their behavior (Penner et al. 2010).

9.14.6 Psychological Stress and Blood Pressure

Persistent or long-term exposure to stress is associated with numerous poor health conditions, including high blood pressure, increase buildup of fat in blood vessels and around the abdomen, type 2 diabetes, increased susceptibility to infection, and atrophy of brain cells (Brunner et al. 2007; Epel et al. 2004; Ferrie et al. 2002; Gianaros et al. 2007). One study reported gender differences in blood pressure in response to psychosocial stress. In an article by Bindon et al. (1997) that investigated the differences in blood pressure of 134 Samoa men and women who lived on the American Samoa island, they observed that men had higher blood pressure than women in response to psychosocial stress due to lifestyle incongruity, and similarly men also demonstrated increased blood pressure in comparison with their female spouse for the same household tasks. This study suggests that men and women may respond differently to psychosocial stress, however other factors, such as cultural and societal norms, may come into play. Additional studies are necessary to confirm this observation.

9.14.7 Psychological Stress and Stroke

Some reports indicate an association of negative emotions, such as chronic stress, depression, and anxiety, with low SES and poor health outcomes such as stroke (Avendano et al. 2006).

9.15 Summary

Psychological studies that examine individual behaviors and lifestyle choices have demonstrated that several factors, including low SES, poor education, racism, discrimination, and so many other factors, are over-represented in AA and other minority populations and can result in adverse health outcomes and potentially contribute to disparities in mental and physical health based on psychological mechanisms. Health psychology applies psychological principles to physical-health areas such as: lowering high blood pressure, controlling cholesterol, managing stress, alleviating pain, ending smoking, moderating risky behaviors, encouraging regular exercise, encouraging regular medical/dental exams, and encouraging safer behaviors. Psychosocial and environmental factors can affect individual health at any stage of life with the in utero environment of the growing fetus and early childhood being most impactful for long-term health outcomes. Thus, chronic psychological stress that can impair neurocognitive abilities can lead to various affective and behavioral disorders in both language and educational development that can result in compromised academic performance and increased risk of mental illness or future absences of economic success. Nowadays, there are various psychological intervention tools for changing the behaviors implicated in chronic diseases, and for relieving pain, reducing stress, improving adherence, and helping those living with chronic illness. In addition, the science of psychology helps identify risk factors associated with adverse health, contributes to the enhancement of health through prevention and treatment of disease through behavioral modifications and psychological rehabilitation and overall improvement of the health-care system, and also can improve the shaping of public opinion with regard to health.

References

Affleck, G., Tennen, H., Croog, S., & Levine, S. (1987). Causal attribution, perceived benefits, and morbidity after a heart attack: An 8-year study. *Journal of Consulting and Clinical Psychology, 55*(1), 29–35. Available from: PM:3571655.

Anon. (2000). *Report of the Surgeon general's conference on children's mental health*: A national action agenda. Department of health and human services. US Public Health Service.

References

Aspinwall, L. G., & Richter, L. (1999). Optimism and self-mastery predict more rapid disengagement from unsolvable tasks in the presence of alternatives. *Motivation and Emotion, 23*, 221–245.

Avendano, M., Kawachi, I., Van, L. F., Boshuizen, H. C., Mackenbach, J. P., Van den Bos, G. A., et al. (2006). Socioeconomic status and stroke incidence in the US elderly: The role of risk factors in the EPESE study. *Stroke, 37*(6), 1368–1373. Available from: PM:16690902.

Beach, S. R., Brody, G. H., Todorov, A. A., Gunter, T. D., & Philibert, R. A. (2010). Methylation at SLC6A4 is linked to family history of child abuse: An examination of the Iowa adoptee sample. *American Journal of Medical Genetics Part B: Neuropsychiatric Genetics, 153B*(2), 710–713. Available from: PM:19739105.

Bindon, J. R., Knight, A., Dressler, W. W., & Crews, D. E. (1997). Social context and psychosocial influences on blood pressure among American Samoans. *American Journal of Physical Anthropology, 103*(1), 7–18. Available from: PM:9185949.

Bosma, H., Schrijvers, C., & Mackenbach, J. P. (1999). Socioeconomic inequalities in mortality and importance of perceived control: Cohort study. *BMJ, 319*(7223), 1469–1470. Available from: PM:10582929.

Bosma, H., Van Jaarsveld, C. H., Tuinstra, J., Sanderman, R., Ranchor, A. V., van Eijk, J. T., et al. (2005). Low control beliefs, classical coronary risk factors, and socio-economic differences in heart disease in older persons. *Social Science and Medicine, 60*(4), 737–745. Available from: PM:15571892.

Brunner, E. J., Chandola, T., & Marmot, M. G. (2007). Prospective effect of job strain on general and central obesity in the Whitehall II study. *American Journal of Epidemiology, 165*(7), 828–837. Available from: PM:17244635.

Carver, C. S., Pozo, C., Harris, S. D., Noriega, V., Scheier, M. F., Robinson, D. S., et al. (1993). How coping mediates the effect of optimism on distress: A study of women with early stage breast cancer. *Journal of Personality and Social Psychology, 65*(2), 375–390. Available from: PM:8366426.

Chen, E., Miller, G. E., Kobor, M. S., & Cole, S. W. (2011). Maternal warmth buffers the effects of low early-life socioeconomic status on pro-inflammatory signaling in adulthood. *Molecular Psychiatry, 16*(7), 729–737. Available from: PM:20479762.

Clark, R., Anderson, N. B., Clark, V. R., & Williams, D. R. (1999). Racism as a stressor for African Americans. A biopsychosocial model. *The American Psychologist, 54*(10), 805–816. Available from: PM:10540593.

Clark, C., Caldwell, T., Power, C., & Stansfeld, S. A. (2010). Does the influence of childhood adversity on psychopathology persist across the lifecourse? A 45-year prospective epidemiologic study. *Annals of Epidemiology, 20*(5), 385–394. Available from: PM:20382340.

Cohen, S., Kessler, R. C., & Gordon, L. (1995). Personality characteristics as moderators of the relationship between stress and disorder. In Cohen, S., Kessler, R. C., Gordon, L. U. (Eds.), *Measuring stress* (pp. 3–26). Oxford University Press.

Costello, E. J., Mustillo, S., Erkanli, A., Keeler, G., & Angold, A. (2003). Prevalence and development of psychiatric disorders in childhood and adolescence. *Archives of General Psychiatry, 60*(8), 837–844. Available from: PM:12912767.

Croyle, R. T., & Uretsky, M. B. (1987). Effects of mood on self-appraisal of health status. *Health Psychology, 6*(3), 239–253. Available from: PM:3595548.

Davis, E. P., Glynn, L. M., Dunkel, S. C., Hobel, C., Chicz-Demet, A., & Sandman, C. A. (2005). Corticotropin-releasing hormone during pregnancy is associated with infant temperament. *Developmental Neuroscience, 27*(5), 299–305. Available from: PM:16137987.

Duru, O. K., Harawa, N. T., Kermah, D., & Norris, K. C. (2012). Allostatic load burden and racial disparities in mortality. *Journal of the National Medical Association, 104*(1–2), 89–95. Available from: PM:22708252.

Eaton, D. K., Kann, L., Kinchen, S., Shanklin, S., Ross, J., Hawkins, J., et al. (2010). Youth risk behavior surveillance—United States, 2009. *MMWR Surveillance Summaries, 59*(5), 1–142. Available from: PM:20520591.

Elliott, E., Ezra-Nevo, G., Regev, L., Neufeld-Cohen, A., & Chen, A. (2010). Resilience to social stress coincides with functional DNA methylation of the Crf gene in adult mice. *Nature Neuroscience, 13*(11), 1351–1353. Available from: PM:20890295.

Epel, E. S., Blackburn, E. H., Lin, J., Dhabhar, F. S., Adler, N. E., Morrow, J. D., et al. (2004). Accelerated telomere shortening in response to life stress. *Proceedings of the National Academy of Sciences of the United States of America, 101*(49), 17312–17315. Available from: PM:15574496.

Erickson, K., Thorsen, P., Chrousos, G., Grigoriadis, D. E., Khongsaly, O., McGregor, J., et al. (2001). Preterm birth: Associated neuroendocrine, medical, and behavioral risk factors. *Journal of Clinical Endocrinology and Metabolism, 86*(6), 2544–2552. Available from: PM:11397853.

Evans, G. W., & Kim, P. (2007). Childhood poverty and health: Cumulative risk exposure and stress dysregulation. *Psychological Science, 18*(11), 953–957. Available from: PM:17958708.

Everson, S. A., Goldberg, D. E., Kaplan, G. A., Cohen, R. D., Pukkala, E., Tuomilehto, J., et al. (1996). Hopelessness and risk of mortality and incidence of myocardial infarction and cancer. *Psychosomatic Medicine, 58*(2), 113–121. Available from: PM:8849626.

Everson-Rose, S. A., & Lewis, T. T. (2005a). Psychosocial factors and cardiovascular diseases. *Annual Review of Public Health, 26,* 469–500. Available from: PM:15760298.

Everson-Rose, S. A., & Lewis, T. T. (2005b). Psychosocial factors and cardiovascular diseases. *Annual Review of Public Health, 26,* 469–500. Available from: PM:15760298.

Ferrie, J. E., Shipley, M. J., Stansfeld, S. A., & Marmot, M. G. (2002). Effects of chronic job insecurity and change in job security on self reported health, minor psychiatric morbidity, physiological measures, and health related behaviours in British civil servants: The Whitehall II study. *Journal of Epidemiology and Community Health, 56*(6), 450–454. Available from: PM:12011203.

Fisher, P. A., Gunnar, M. R., Chamberlain, P., & Reid, J. B. (2000). Preventive intervention for maltreated preschool children: Impact on children's behavior, neuroendocrine activity, and foster parent functioning. *Journal of the American Academy of Child and Adolescent Psychiatry, 39*(11), 1356–1364. Available from: PM:11068890.

Franklin, T. B., Russig, H., Weiss, I. C., Graff, J., Linder, N., Michalon, A., et al. (2010). Epigenetic transmission of the impact of early stress across generations. *Biological Psychiatry, 68*(5), 408–415. Available from: PM:20673872.

Friedman, E. M., Hayney, M., Love, G. D., Singer, B. H., & Ryff, C. D. (2007). Plasma interleukin-6 and soluble IL-6 receptors are associated with psychological well-being in aging women. *Health Psychology, 26*(3), 305–313. Available from: PM:17500617.

Friedman, E. M., Karlamangla, A. S., Gruenewald, T. L., Koretz, B., & Seeman, T. E. (2015). Early life adversity and adult biological risk profiles. *Psychosomatic Medicine, 77*(2), 176–185. Available from: PM:25650548.

Gallo, L. C., & Matthews, K. A. (2003). Understanding the association between socioeconomic status and physical health: Do negative emotions play a role? *Psychological Bulletin, 129*(1), 10–51. Available from: PM:12555793.

Gianaros, P. J., Jennings, J. R., Sheu, L. K., Greer, P. J., Kuller, L. H., & Matthews, K. A. (2007). Prospective reports of chronic life stress predict decreased grey matter volume in the hippocampus. *Neuroimage, 35*(2), 795–803. Available from: PM:17275340.

Goldberg, E. M., & Morrison, S. L. (1963). Schizophrenia and social class. *The British Journal of Psychiatry, 109,* 785–802. Available from: PM:14080574.

Grzywacz, J. G., Almeida, D. M., Neupert, S. D., & Ettner, S. L. (2004). Socioeconomic status and health: A micro-level analysis of exposure and vulnerability to daily stressors. *Journal of Health and Social Behavior, 45*(1), 1–16. Available from: PM:15179904.

Hackman, D. A., Farah, M. J., & Meaney, M. J. (2010). Socioeconomic status and the brain: Mechanistic insights from human and animal research. *Nature Reviews Neuroscience, 11*(9), 651–659. Available from: PM:20725096.

Harrison, R. M., & Taylor, D. C. (1976). Childhood seizures: A 25-year follow up. Social and medical prognosis. *Lancet, 1*(7966), 948–951. Available from: PM:57348.

Hart, B., & Risley, T. R. (1995). *Meaningful differences in the everyday experience of young American children*. Baltimore, Maryland: Brookes Publishing.

Hatzenbuehler, M. L., Phelan, J. C., & Link, B. G. (2013). Stigma as a fundamental cause of population health inequalities. *American Journal of Public Health, 103*(5), 813–821. Available from: PM:23488505.

Heckhausen, J., & Schulz, R. (1995). A life-span theory of control. *Psychological Review, 102*(2), 284–304. Available from: PM:7740091.

Heinonen, K., Raikkonen, K., Matthews, K. A., Scheier, M. F., Raitakari, O. T., Pulkki, L., et al. (2006). Socioeconomic status in childhood and adulthood: Associations with dispositional optimism and pessimism over a 21-year follow-up. *Journal of Personality, 74*(4), 1111–1126. Available from: PM:16787430.

House, J. S., Landis, K. R., & Umberson, D. (1988). Social relationships and health. *Science, 241* (4865), 540–545. Available from: PM:3399889.

Kaplan, G. A., Salonen, J. T., Cohen, R. D., Brand, R. J., Syme, S. L., & Puska, P. (1988). Social connections and mortality from all causes and from cardiovascular disease: Prospective evidence from eastern Finland. *American Journal of Epidemiology, 128*(2), 370–380. Available from: PM:3394703.

Karlamangla, A. S., Singer, B. H., Williams, D. R., Schwartz, J. E., Matthews, K. A., Kiefe, C. I., et al. (2005). Impact of socioeconomic status on longitudinal accumulation of cardiovascular risk in young adults: The CARDIA study (USA). *Social Science and Medicine, 60*(5), 999–1015. Available from: PM:15589670.

Kawachi, I., Kennedy, B. P., Lochner, K., & Prothrow-Stith, D. (1997). Social capital, income inequality, and mortality. *American Journal of Public Health, 87*(9), 1491–1498. Available from: PM:9314802.

Khang, Y. H., Lynch, J. W., Yang, S., Harper, S., Yun, S. C., Jung-Choi, K., et al. (2009). The contribution of material, psychosocial, and behavioral factors in explaining educational and occupational mortality inequalities in a nationally representative sample of South Koreans: Relative and absolute perspectives. *Social Science and Medicine, 68*(5), 858–866. Available from: PM:19121885.

Kiecolt-Glaser, J. K., Stephens, R. E., Lipetz, P. D., Speicher, C. E., & Glaser, R. (1985). Distress and DNA repair in human lymphocytes. *Journal of Behavioral Medicine, 8*(4), 311–320. Available from: PM:2936891.

Kinnunen, M. L., Kokkonen, M., Kaprio, J., & Pulkkinen, L. (2005). The associations of emotion regulation and dysregulation with the metabolic syndrome factor. *Journal of Psychosomatic Research, 58*(6), 513–521. Available from: PM:16125518.

Kinsler, J. J., Wong, M. D., Sayles, J. N., Davis, C., & Cunningham, W. E. (2007). The effect of perceived stigma from a health care provider on access to care among a low-income HIV-positive population. *AIDS Patient Care and STDs, 21*(8), 584–592. Available from: PM:17711383.

Kodjo, C. M., & Auinger, P. (2004). Predictors for emotionally distressed adolescents to receive mental health care. *Journal of Adolescent Health, 35*(5), 368–373. Available from: PM:15488430.

Krantz, D. S., & McCeney, M. K. (2002). Effects of psychological and social factors on organic disease: A critical assessment of research on coronary heart disease. *Annual Review of Psychology, 53*, 341–369. Available from: PM:11752489.

Krieger, N., Kosheleva, A., Waterman, P. D., Chen, J. T., & Koenen, K. (2011). Racial discrimination, psychological distress, and self-rated health among US-born and foreign-born Black Americans. *American Journal of Public Health, 101*(9), 1704–1713. Available from: PM:21778504.

Lehman, B. J., Taylor, S. E., Kiefe, C. I., & Seeman, T. E. (2005). Relation of childhood socioeconomic status and family environment to adult metabolic functioning in the CARDIA study. *Psychosomatic Medicine, 67*(6), 846–854. Available from: PM:16314588.

Lehman, B. J., Taylor, S. E., Kiefe, C. I., & Seeman, T. E. (2009). Relationship of early life stress and psychological functioning to blood pressure in the CARDIA study. *Health Psychology, 28* (3), 338–346. Available from: PM:19450040.

Leslie, L. K., Plemmons, D., Monn, A. R., & Palinkas, L. A. (2007). Investigating ADHD treatment trajectories: Listening to families' stories about medication use. *Journal of Developmental and Behavioral Pediatrics, 28*(3), 179–188. Available from: PM:17565284.

Link, B. G., & Phelan, J. C. (2001). Conceptualizing stigma. *Annual Review of Sociology, 27*, 363–385.

Liu, D., Caldji, C., Sharma, S., Plotsky, P. M., & Meaney, M. J. (2000). Influence of neonatal rearing conditions on stress-induced adrenocorticotropin responses and norepinepherine release in the hypothalamic paraventricular nucleus. *Journal of Neuroendocrinology, 12*(1), 5–12. Available from: PM:10692138.

Liu, D., Diorio, J., Tannenbaum, B., Caldji, C., Francis, D., Freedman, A., et al. (1997). Maternal care, hippocampal glucocorticoid receptors, and hypothalamic-pituitary-adrenal responses to stress. *Science, 277*(5332), 1659–1662. Available from: PM:9287218.

Luecken, L. J., Rodriguez, A. P., & Appelhans, B. M. (2005). Cardiovascular stress responses in young adulthood associated with family-of-origin relationship experiences. *Psychosomatic Medicine, 67*(4), 514–521. Available from: PM:16046362.

Macdonald, G., & Leary, M. R. (2005). Why does social exclusion hurt? The relationship between social and physical pain. *Psychological Bulletin, 131*(2), 202–223. Available from: PM:15740417.

Macleod, J., Davey, S. G., Metcalfe, C., & Hart, C. (2005). Is subjective social status a more important determinant of health than objective social status? Evidence from a prospective observational study of Scottish men. *Social Science and Medicine, 61*(9), 1916–1929. Available from: PM:15916842.

Markus, H. R., Ryff, C. D., Curhan, K. B., & Palmersheim, K. A. (2004). In their own words: Well-being ai midlife among high school and college educated adults. In O. G. Brim, C. D. Ryff, & R. C. Kessler (Eds.), *How healthy are we? A national study of well-being at midlife* (pp. 273–319). Chicago IL: University of Chicago Press.

Marmot, M. G., Bosma, H., Hemingway, H., Brunner, E., & Stansfeld, S. (1997). Contribution of job control and other risk factors to social variations in coronary heart disease incidence. *Lancet, 350*(9073), 235–239. Available from: PM:9242799.

Masten, A. S., & Coatsworth, J. D. (1998). The development of competence in favorable and unfavorable environments. Lessons from research on successful children. *American Psychologist, 53*(2), 205–220. Available from: PM:9491748.

Matthews, K. A., & Gallo, L. C. (2011). Psychological perspectives on pathways linking socioeconomic status and physical health. *Annual Review of Psychology, 62*, 501–530. Available from: PM:20636127.

Matthews, K. A., Gallo, L. C., & Taylor, S. E. (2010). Are psychosocial factors mediators of socioeconomic status and health connections? A progress report and blueprint for the future. *Annals of the New York Academy of Sciences, 1186*, 146–173. Available from: PM:20201872.

Matthews, K. A., Raikkonen, K., Gallo, L., & Kuller, L. H. (2008). Association between socioeconomic status and metabolic syndrome in women: Testing the reserve capacity model. *Health Psychology, 27*(5), 576–583. Available from: PM:18823184.

McEwen, B. S. (1998). Protective and damaging effects of stress mediators. *The New England Journal of Medicine, 338*(3), 171–179. Available from: PM:9428819.

McGowan, P. O., Sasaki, A., D'Alessio, A. C., Dymov, S., Labonte, B., Szyf, M., et al. (2009). Epigenetic regulation of the glucocorticoid receptor in human brain associates with childhood abuse. *Nature Neuroscience, 12*(3), 342–348. Available from: PM:19234457.

Meadows, S. H. (1961). Social class migration and chronic bronchitis. A study of male hospital patients in the London area. *British Journal of Preventive and Social Medicine, 15*, 171–176. Available from: PM:14471917.

Meaney, M. J., Szyf, M., & Seckl, J. R. (2007). Epigenetic mechanisms of perinatal programming of hypothalamic-pituitary-adrenal function and health. *Trends in Molecular Medicine, 13*(7), 269–277. Available from: PM:17544850.

Merkin, S. S., Karlamangla, A., Roux, A. V., Shrager, S., & Seeman, T. E. (2014). Life course socioeconomic status and longitudinal accumulation of allostatic load in adulthood: Multi-ethnic study of atherosclerosis. *American Journal of Public Health, 104*(4), e48–e55. Available from: PM:24524526.

Miller, G. E., Chen, E., Sze, J., Marin, T., Arevalo, J. M., Doll, R., et al. (2008). A functional genomic fingerprint of chronic stress in humans: Blunted glucocorticoid and increased NF-kappaB signaling. *Biological Psychiatry, 64*(4), 266–272. Available from: PM:18440494.

Miller, G. E., Lachman, M. E., Chen, E., Gruenewald, T. L., Karlamangla, A. S., & Seeman, T. E. (2011). Pathways to resilience: Maternal nurturance as a buffer against the effects of childhood poverty on metabolic syndrome at midlife. *Psychological Science, 22*(12), 1591–1599. Available from: PM:22123777.

Miller, T. W., Nigg, J. T., & Miller, R. L. (2009). Attention deficit hyperactivity disorder in African American children: What can be concluded from the past ten years? *Clinical Psychology Review, 29*(1), 77–86. Available from: PM:19008029.

Mouzon, D. M., Taylor, R. J., Keith, V. M., Nicklett, E. J., & Chatters, L. M. (2016). Discrimination and psychiatric disorders among older African Americans. *International Journal of Geriatric Psychiatry*. Available from: PM:26924389.

Muroff, J., Edelsohn, G. A., Joe, S., & Ford, B. C. (2008). The role of race in diagnostic and disposition decision making in a pediatric psychiatric emergency service. *General Hospital Psychiatry, 30*(3), 269–276. Available from: PM:18433660.

National Center for HIV/AIDs, (2010). https://www.hivlawandpolicy.org/resources/new-hiv-infections-united-states-2010-centers-disease-control-and-prevention-national

Natsuaki, M. N., Ge, X., Brody, G. H., Simons, R. L., Gibbons, F. X., & Cutrona, C. E. (2007). African American children's depressive symptoms: The prospective effects of neighborhood disorder, stressful life events, and parenting. *American Journal of Community Psychology, 39*(1–2), 163–176. Available from: PM:17294122.

Olfson, M., Gameroff, M. J., Marcus, S. C., & Jensen, P. S. (2003). National trends in the treatment of attention deficit hyperactivity disorder. *American Journal of Psychiatry, 160*(6), 1071–1077. Available from: PM:12777264.

Pachankis, J. E. (2007). The psychological implications of concealing a stigma: A cognitive-affective-behavioral model. *Psychological Bulletin, 133*(2), 328–345. Available from: PM:17338603.

Paradies, Y. (2006). A systematic review of empirical research on self-reported racism and health. *International Journal of Epidemiology, 35*(4), 888–901. Available from: PM:16585055.

Penner, L. A., Dovidio, J. F., West, T. V., Gaertner, S. L., Albrecht, T. L., Dailey, R. K., et al. (2010). Aversive racism and medical interactions with black patients: A field study. *Journal of Experimental Social Psychology, 46*(2), 436–440. Available from: PM:20228874.

Pliszka, S. (2007). Practice parameter for the assessment and treatment of children and adolescents with attention-deficit/hyperactivity disorder. *Journal of the American Academy of Child and Adolescent Psychiatry, 46*(7), 894–921. Available from: PM:17581453.

Prescott, E., Godtfredsen, N., Osler, M., Schnohr, P., & Barefoot, J. (2007). Social gradient in the metabolic syndrome not explained by psychosocial and behavioural factors: Evidence from the Copenhagen city heart study. *European Journal of Preventive Cardiology, 14*(3), 405–412. Available from: PM:17568240.

Raizada, R. D., Richards, T. L., Meltzoff, A., & Kuhl, P. K. (2008). Socioeconomic status predicts hemispheric specialisation of the left inferior frontal gyrus in young children. *Neuroimage, 40*(3), 1392–1401. Available from: PM:18308588.

Rasmussen, H. N., Scheier, M. F., & Greenhouse, J. B. (2009). Optimism and physical health: A meta-analytic review. *Annals of Behavioral Medicine, 37*(3), 239–256. Available from: PM:19711142.

Roberts, R. E., Attkisson, C. C., & Rosenblatt, A. (1998). Prevalence of psychopathology among children and adolescents. *American Journal of Psychiatry, 155*(6), 715–725. Available from: PM:9619142.

Roy, B., Diez-Roux, A. V., Seeman, T., Ranjit, N., Shea, S., & Cushman, M. (2010). Association of optimism and pessimism with inflammation and hemostasis in the multi-ethnic study of atherosclerosis (MESA). *Psychosomatic Medicine, 72*(2), 134–140. Available from: PM:20100888.

Rozanski, A., Blumenthal, J. A., & Kaplan, J. (1999). Impact of psychological factors on the pathogenesis of cardiovascular disease and implications for therapy. *Circulation, 99*(16), 2192–2217. Available from: PM:10217662.

Schanberg, S. M., Evoniuk, G., & Kuhn, C. M. (1984). Tactile and nutritional aspects of maternal care: Specific regulators of neuroendocrine function and cellular development. *Proceedings of the Society for Experimental Biology and Medicine, 175*(2), 135–146. Available from: PM:6364149.

Schoenbach, V. J., Kaplan, B. H., Fredman, L., & Kleinbaum, D. G. (1986). Social ties and mortality in Evans County, Georgia. *American Journal of Epidemiology, 123*(4), 577–591. Available from: PM:3953538.

Schutte, N. S., Malouff, J. M., Thorsteinsson, E. B., Bhullar, N., & Rooke, S. E. (2007). A meta-analytic investigation of the relationship between emotional intelligence and health. *Personality and Individual Differences, 42*, 921–933.

Seeman, T. E., Crimmins, E., Huang, M. H., Singer, B., Bucur, A., Gruenewald, T., et al. (2004). Cumulative biological risk and socio-economic differences in mortality: MacArthur studies of successful aging. *Social Science and Medicine, 58*(10), 1985–1997. Available from: PM:15020014.

Segerstrom, S. C., & Miller, G. E. (2004). Psychological stress and the human immune system: A meta-analytic study of 30 years of inquiry. *Psychological Bulletin, 130*(4), 601–630. Available from: PM:15250815.

Slade, E. P. (2004). Racial/ethnic disparities in parent perception of child need for mental health care following school disciplinary events. *Mental Health Services Research, 6*(2), 75–92. Available from: PM:15224452.

Smith, L. A., Bokhour, B., Hohman, K. H., Miroshnik, I., Kleinman, K. P., Cohn, E., et al. (2008). Modifiable risk factors for suboptimal control and controller medication underuse among children with asthma. *Pediatrics, 122*(4), 760–769. Available from: PM:18829799.

Sternthal, M. J., Coull, B. A., Chiu, Y. H., Cohen, S., & Wright, R. J. (2011). Associations among maternal childhood socioeconomic status, cord blood IgE levels, and repeated wheeze in urban children. *Journal of Allergy and Clinical Immunology, 128*(2), 337–345. Available from: PM:21704362.

Stevens-Watkins, D., Perry, B., Pullen, E., Jewell, J., & Oser, C. B. (2014). Examining the associations of racism, sexism, and stressful life events on psychological distress among African-American women. *Cultural Diversity and Ethnic Minority Psychology, 20*(4), 561–569. Available from: PM:25313434.

Stockdale, S. E., Wells, K. B., Tang, L., Belin, T. R., Zhang, L., & Sherbourne, C. D. (2007). The importance of social context: Neighborhood stressors, stress-buffering mechanisms, and alcohol, drug, and mental health disorders. *Social Science and Medicine, 65*(9), 1867–1881. Available from: PM:17614176.

Thurston, R. C., Kubzansky, L. D., Kawachi, I., & Berkman, L. F. (2005). Is the association between socioeconomic position and coronary heart disease stronger in women than in men? *American Journal of Epidemiology, 162*(1), 57–65. Available from: PM:15961587.

Turk, D. C., & Salovey, P. (1984). "Chronic pain as a variant of depressive disease". A critical reappraisal. *The Journal of Nervous and Mental Disease, 172*(7), 398–404. Available from: PM:6726210.

Turrell, G., Lynch, J. W., Kaplan, G. A., Everson, S. A., Helkala, E. L., Kauhanen, J., et al. (2002). Socioeconomic position across the lifecourse and cognitive function in late middle age. *The*

Journals of Gerontology. Series B, Psychological Sciences and Social Sciences, 57(1), S43–S51. Available from: PM:11773232.

Uchino, B. N. (2006). Social support and health: A review of physiological processes potentially underlying links to disease outcomes. *Journal of Behavioral Medicine, 29*(4), 377–387. Available from: PM:16758315.

Updegraff, J. A., Silver, R. C., & Holman, E. A. (2008). Searching for and finding meaning in collective trauma: Results from a national longitudinal study of the 9/11 terrorist attacks. *Journal of Personality and Social Psychology, 95*(3), 709–722. Available from: PM:18729704.

Vitaliano, P. P., Scanlan, J. M., Zhang, J., Savage, M. V., Brummett, B., Barefoot, J., et al. (2001). Are the salutogenic effects of social supports modified by income? A test of an "added value hypothesis". *Health Psychology, 20*(3), 155–165. Available from: PM:11403213.

Walker, D., Greenwood, C., Hart, B., & Carta, J. (1994). Prediction of school outcomes based on early language production and socioeconomic factors. *Child Development, 65*(2 Spec No), 606–621. Available from: PM:8013242.

Wamala, S. P., Mittleman, M. A., Horsten, M., Schenck-Gustafsson, K., & Orth-Gomer, K. (2000). Job stress and the occupational gradient in coronary heart disease risk in women. The Stockholm female coronary risk study. *Social Science and Medicine, 51*(4), 481–489. Available from: PM:10868664.

Welberg, L. A., Seckl, J. R., & Holmes, M. C. (2001). Prenatal glucocorticoid programming of brain corticosteroid receptors and corticotrophin-releasing hormone: Possible implications for behaviour. *Neuroscience, 104*(1), 71–79. Available from: PM:11311532.

West, P. (1991). Rethinking the health selection explanation for health inequalities. *Social Science and Medicine, 32*(4), 373–384. Available from: PM:2024152.

Wright, R. J., Cohen, S., Carey, V., Weiss, S. T., & Gold, D. R. (2002). Parental stress as a predictor of wheezing in infancy: A prospective birth-cohort study. *American Journal of Respiratory and Critical Care, 165*(3), 358–365. Available from: PM:11818321.

Wright, R. J., & Enlow, M. B. (2008). Maternal stress and perinatal programming in the expression of atopy. *Expert Review of Clinical Immunology, 4*(5), 535–538. Available from: PM:19838310.

Xue, Y., Leventhal, T., Brooks-Gunn, J., & Earls, F. J. (2005). Neighborhood residence and mental health problems of 5- to 11-year-olds. *Archives of General Psychiatry, 62*(5), 554–563. Available from: PM:15867109.

Yen, I. H., & Syme, S. L. (1999). The social environment and health: A discussion of the epidemiologic literature. *Annual Review of Public Health, 20,* 287–308.

Zimmerman, F. J. (2005). Social and economic determinants of disparities in professional help-seeking for child mental health problems: Evidence from a national sample. *Health Services Research, 40*(5 Pt 1), 1514–1533. Available from: PM:16174145.

Zwaanswijk, M., Van der Ende, J., Verhaak, P. F., Bensing, J. M., & Verhulst, F. C. (2003). Factors associated with adolescent mental health service need and utilization. *Journal of the American Academy of Child and Adolescent Psychiatry, 42*(6), 692–700. Available from: PM:12921477.

Part III
Gene-Environment Interactions

Chapter 10
Gene-Environment Interactions in Health Disparities

Abstract The risks of many common and complex diseases in individuals belonging to one population or diverse populations consist of complicated interactions of genes and the environment. Studies are unraveling the genetic, epigenetic, and environmental components of socioeconomic factors down to dependent behaviors, ranging from alcohol dependence and drug addiction to smoking behavior, and disease susceptibility, suggesting a multifactorial basis for diseases. The emerging understanding of epigenetics is complementing traditional social and environmental models of disease causation, and it is helping to explain "nature-nurture" interaction that can be mapped onto categories such as race or ethnicity to explain health disparities.

10.1 Introduction

The current scientific evidence to explain the differences in disease susceptibility of individuals belonging to one population or in diverse populations demonstrates that genetic factors or environmental factors are independently associated with a few diseases, whereas the majority of diseases are caused by the complex interaction between genetic and environmental factors in health disparities.

Epidemiological evidence in support for the role of genes in disease causation comes from the following observations. First, there is greater disease prevalence in first-degree relatives in comparison with spouses. Second, monozygotic twins share higher disease concordance in comparison with dizygotic twins, as well as an earlier age of disease onset among familial, in comparison with non-familial, cases. Third, there is strong disease-phenotype correlation between parents and biological children in comparison with parents and fosters or non-biological children. This evidence provides strong support that disease clusters in families who share genes and, in addition, may share some common family environment. In this case, a role for gene and the environment interaction may contribute to disease causation, as well as progression.

Epidemiological evidence in support for the role of environment and disease risk comes from studies of migrants populations from geographic areas of low rates of disease incidence to areas to higher rates of incidence. For instance, one study reports dramatic increase in the incidence of colorectal cancer of Japanese migrants from their native rural Japan to Hawaii for the years 1886–1924, as a result of adopting a diet that is rich in red meat (Marchand 1999). Other evidence is reported of Chinese men, who in their native country have the lowest incidence of prostate cancer in the world. However, second- and third-generation male descendants of Chinese migrants to the USA and who have adopted a Western diet have a significantly higher risk for prostate cancer, comparable to European Americans (EAs) and significantly more than men in their native China, clearly suggesting an environmental component (diet) to the increased disease risk (Brawley et al. 1998). Yet, other reports from Europe support a potential role for gene-environmental interaction for the high prevalence of obesity and type 2 diabetes among African migrants to Europe, in comparison to the native African population (Agyemang et al. 2014). The higher prevalence of obesity and diabetes among the African immigrants has been attributed to a change in life style, including smoking and lack of physical activity, as well as psychological stress.

Environmental risk factors mean different things to different health professionals: A nutritionist will consider food pyramids when talking about the environment, a toxicologist will be looking at pollution and toxic waste when considering environmental impact, whereas a psychologist will be looking at the nurturing environment of family or community. But all of these different environmental components can alter gene expression and physiological responses via epigenetic mechanisms.

A potential role for the epigenome in disease risk is demonstrated by monozygotic twins who share identical genomic DNA, yet demonstrate differences in disease susceptibility when exposed to different environments, indicating that their epigenome may be altered by the environmental exposures. Thus, modification of the epigenome in response to environmental exposure also contributes to differential susceptibilities to disease incidence and/or progression. Studies have shown that the epigenome of the developing fetus is particularly sensitive to dysregulation by environmental factors during embryogenesis through neonatal development into adolescence and old age (Weidman et al. 2007). The importance of prenatal exposures and health outcomes in adulthood is highlighted by epidemiological studies that have shown that individuals who were exposed to high levels on diethylstilbestrol (DES) in utero, during the first trimester of pregnancy, have increased incidence of cancer and other reproductive disorders in later years (Newbold et al. 2006), with increased disease incidence passed on to subsequent generations.

10.1 Introduction

The classical view of the genetic basis of disease is that it results from changes in the genes, such as mutation, deletion, or chromosomal amplification, which are closely associated with dynamics in gene expression (discussed in Chap. 2). However, gene expression is not only determined by the DNA sequence but also by epigenetic programs, such as chromatin/histone modification, DNA methylation, and noncoding RNA (discussed in Chap. 3). These epigenetic processes, while stable, are not static but rather dynamic and reversible with differential outcomes for gene expression. Given its dynamic nature, the "epigenome is referred to as an interface between the environment and the genome". In principal, aberrant epigenetic alteration during embryogenesis will have a profound effect of the epigenetic program of the organism because this can be transmitted over consecutive mitotic divisions and in adult stem cells and/or somatic cells during postnatal development with potential transgenerational consequences.

Research that is focused solely on the genetic determinants of health disparities might lead investigators to ignore the important contribution of social and environmental determinants to health disparities, while promoting reliance on medical intervention at the expense of social, behavior, and political factors (Sankar et al. 2004). On the other hand, pointing to the multiple social determinants of health, such as SES, residential segregation, lack of access to healthy foods, poor nutritional choices, toxic environmental exposures, and racial discrimination does not completely resolve health disparities. This is because social determinant factors can impact genetic traits to trigger differences in disease risk and susceptibility, even for different racial and ethnic populations subjected to the same social determinant factors. Therefore studies undertaken to understand the causes of underlying health disparities should take into consideration the interaction between genetic and environmental factors.

Overall, there is a complex and multifactorial inter-connected process including the genome (in terms of genetic variation), epigenome alterations, socioeconomic factors, behavioral and psychological factors, and other environmental interactions that culminate in alteration of gene expression, physiological responses, and consequently impact health outcomes. In the past, few studies have incorporated some of these risk factors when attempting to identify predictors of future patterns of disease. With the completion of the human-genome sequencing and technological advances in genomic studies, we now have powerful genetic tools to dissect the contributory role of genomics in the disease process. Future advances in genomic studies with new methods for assessing the impact of environmental factors on individual genetic profiles (genetic variants) and perhaps epigenome profile will help in understanding the role of gene-environment interaction in health disparities.

10.2 Fetal Origin of Health Disparities

10.2.1 The Role of Diet

There is accumulating data to reference fetal origins to CVDs, allergies, asthma, hypertension, diabetes, obesity, and cancer, as well as mental illness and even conditions that are typically associated with old age, such as arthritis, osteoporosis, and neurodegenerative diseases. This demonstrates that, the in utero environment, the arrays of nutrition, pollutants, drugs, infection, and hormones that a growing fetus gets exposed to during gestation, particularly during the first trimester, as well as a pregnant mother's health, stress level, and psychological state of mind influence not only the health of a new-born child, but also this can have long-term effects on the health of an individual from the prenatal stage through teenage years and into adulthood. Thus the nine months of gestation have a powerful influence on the permanent wiring of the brain and the functioning of different organs in the body, including the heart, liver, and the pancreas.

The molecular mechanism whereby the in utero environment influences the genome of the growing fetus is via epigenome programming, which comprises DNA methylation, histone modification, and microRNA. Szyf et al. (2007) proposed that the epigenome programming of the developing fetus is particularly sensitive to maternal nutrition and exposures to other environmental toxins, as well as psychological stress. In addition, exposure to various environmental toxins might affect long-term established epigenetic programs of the brain. The consequence of epigenetic changes is modulation in gene expression similar to genetic alterations. There is evidence to suggest that some of the effects of early environmental exposure on the biological effects and disease phenotype may be passed down from one generation to the next through epigenetic pathways (as discussed in Sect. 9.4).

Work carried out by David Barker and his collaborators correlated the health outcomes of some 15,000 adults and their birth weights and discovered an unexpected link between pre-natal nutrition and other early-life exposures and association with disease risks in adulthood (Paneth et al. 1996). Barker et al. discovered a link between low birth weight (an indication of poor prenatal nutrition) and increased risk of heart disease in the individual's middle age and proposed that, when a developing fetus is faced with inadequate food supply, it will divert nutrients to the most important organ, which is the brain, and starve the other organs, such as the heart, which can result in weakened heart and related problems later on in life. This observation led Barker to make his "fetal origin of adult diseases" hypothesis. This hypothesis, although was initially received with skepticism, has now been supported by observations that smaller birth size is a predictor for high blood pressure (Adair and Dahly 2005), insulin resistance, and diabetes (Yajnik 2004), as well as an elevated risk of suffering or dying from CVDs (Huxley et al. 2007).

One of the best described examples of how the in utero environment can influence future health outcomes is described by Dutch famine studies (Painter et al. 2005). Towards the end of the Second World War (November 1944 to May 1945), a cohort of the Dutch population who resided in German-occupied western Holland had only very limited food supplies; rations were as low as 400–800 calories per day (less than a quarter of the recommended adult caloric intake) for several months. Observations indicated that children who were conceived during this period were small for their small gestational age (SGA) (Painter et al. 2008). Furthermore, compared to their siblings who were conceived during periods of normal food supply, these SGA individuals displayed different DNA methylation patterns, where the methylation of imprinted insulin-like growth factor II (*IGF2*) gene was shown to be lower.

Later on in life, people who were conceived during the nutritional deprivation (SGA) were observed to have a higher prevalence to many diseases in comparison with unexposed people that were conceived at the same time. These individuals were observed to have an increased risk of adult-onset obesity, diabetes, higher HDL/LDL (high-density lipoprotein/low-density lipoprotein) cholesterol ratio, cardiovascular disease, and renal dysfunction. In addition, these individuals were also observed to have higher blood pressure under stress, and females exposed to famine during gestation were more likely to develop breast cancer. The people conceived during the famine period generally rated their health as poorer compared to unexposed people. Interestingly, the second-generation children born to members of this utero-deprived cohort were also SGA, suggesting a generational transmission of this phenomenon (Painter et al. 2008). Overall, adults of SGA, when compared to other adults born before or conceived after this period of starvation, had higher incidences of obesity and coronary heart disease.

African-American (AA) mothers have higher rates of low-birth-weight infants in comparison with EA mothers in the USA. This racial disparity in birth outcomes is linked to environmental factors, in particular, socioeconomic status (SES) and diet or other psychosocial factors, and there is evidence that these patterns can have multi-generational consequences. For instance, low-birth-weight children are often born to pregnant women exposed to malnutrition or food shortage in low SES-families across diverse geographical, social, and political contexts (Brinkman et al. 2010). Studies suggest that low-birth weight is a predictor of high blood pressure, elevated cortisol reactivity, and early signs of diabetes in older African-American (AA) children and adolescents (Oberg et al. 2007), as well as other related cardiovascular conditions, such as end-stage renal disease in adults (Fan et al. 2000).

A potential biological mechanism linking exposure to the in utero environment, such as dietary factors and disease phenotype, is via epigenetic DNA methylation process (Godfrey and Barker 2000). As discussed in Chap. 3, DNA methylation is the process whereby a dietary methyl group from S-adenosylmethionine (SAM) is added to the cytosine (C) nucleotide that precedes a guanine (G) nucleotide in a C-phosphate-G (CpG) context to form 5-methylcytosine. Dietary methyl groups are abundant in folate, a group of water-soluble B vitamins found in high concentration in green leafy vegetables and fruits and regulate DNA methylation and the one-carbon metabolism pathway for DNA synthesis (Duthie 2011). The importance of the DNA-methylation process and diet has been demonstrated in animal studies. Rat offspring that were exposed to maternal diet of suboptimal nutrition during critical period of gestation were found to have hypermethylation of Hnf4 alpha gene, a gene which encodes for a transcription factor with a known biological role in type 2 diabetes. The DNA hypermethylation leads to silencing of Hnf4 alpha expression, suggesting that abnormal DNA-methylation event in poor nutritional environment may play a role in type 2 diabetes (Sandovici et al. 2011). Interestingly, it was also found that the methylation level increased in association with age, and this was more pronounced in rats exposed to poor nutritional diets.

As previously mentioned, epigenetic modification can be passed on to offspring and even grandchildren via germline inheritance of the epigenetic pattern, including evidence for direct transmission through both matrilineal and patrilineal germlines. This finding builds on animal studies of transgenerational transmission of certain diseases. In one study, F_1-generation pregnant rats fed on protein-restricted diets during pregnancy showed lower methylation and increased expression of the tissue-specific peroxisome proliferator-activator receptor gamma (PPAR-gamma) and glucocorticoid receptor (GR) gene-promoter regions in comparison to F_0-generation controls that were fed normal amounts of protein. Interestingly, the F_2 generation that was fed normal amounts of protein showed similar methylation pattern as F_1 offspring (Burdge et al. 2007), suggesting intergenerational transmission of the epigenetic program to the second generation.

Other supporting evidence of intergenerational transmission comes from a study carried out by Torrens et al. (2008) in female Wistar rats fed protein-restricted diets during pregnancy in comparison with the control group fed with normal amounts of protein. The study observed that restricted diets led to increased blood pressure and endothelial dysfunction not only in the F_1 progeny of female rats, but the phenotype was transmitted even to the second-generation progeny through the maternal line. This observation of environmental challenges during pregnancy in the F_0 generation that can be transmitted to the second and third generation supports the occurrence of intergenerational consequences due to environmental exposure. These observations are revolutionary as it reveals how environmental exposure can shape the biology and health across the life cycle and even within a lineage.

Although similar studies have not been carried out in humans, one piece of epidemiological evidence suggests that increased risk and high mortality rates of cardiovascular disease in 3rd-generation grandchildren can be linked to a paternal grandfather who was exposed to food shortage during his childhood (Pembrey 2010). The accumulating evidence indicates that availability of essential dietary nutrients during critical periods of gestation can use epigenetic processes, including DNA methylation, to modulate gene expression with physiological consequences that persist throughout the life course of an individual, with health outcomes that may persist for several generations (Harrison and Langley-Evans 2009; Li et al. 2010).

The accumulating body of evidence indicates that maternal diet has an effect on the offspring's body composition. One study in humans to ascertain the role for DNA methylation changes in neonates and future risk to adiposity carried out methylation analysis of several candidate genes in genomic DNA extracted from umbilical cord tissues from healthy neonates and correlated analysis of maternal pregnancy diets to risks of child's adiposity at nine years of age (Godfrey et al. 2011). The analysis led to the observation that a low-carbohydrate diet during early pregnancy was associated with increased methylation of retinoid X receptor alpha (RXRA) gene, whose biological action may include developmental influences on later metabolic risk, indicating that epigenetic changes at birth could be associated with a child's later risk of adiposity.

Extensive epidemiological data from both human and animal studies demonstrates that nutritional exposures during crucial periods in embryonic development have consequential physiological effects on health such that nutritional deficiencies are associated with diseases, including CVD, T2D, obesity, and cancer. The accumulating data clearly shows that lifetime nutrition exposure is now recognized as an important influence for overall health from infancy to adulthood and is also important in disease risk because diet can influence epigenetic processes such as DNA methylation by regulating the availability of substrates for the enzymatic function of DNA methyltransferases. Thus, dietary differences between populations can help explain some of the disparities associated with health using epigenetic mechanisms.

With regards to dietary factors, AA serum concentration of vitamin C, vitamin E, and carotenoids (e.g., alpha-carotene, beta-carotene, and lutein and zeaxanthin, - essential nutrients and antioxidant which are protective against cancer and other diseases) are statistically and significantly lower than in EAs as evidenced by one cross-sectional study of 164 generally healthy non-smoking AAs and EAs 20–45 years of age (Watters et al. 2007). In addition, AA individuals report diets less rich in fruits and vegetables when compared to EA individuals. The lower intake of vitamin E may influence differential methylation pattern of genes involved in vitamin E biosynthetic pathway in the two populations. There are differences in the dietary patterns in the AA and EA population, in particular, when comparing high-SES EAs with low-SES AAs, as well as the variance in metabolic rates between the two groups, and this may contribute to changes in epigenetic patterns that result in differential susceptibilities to cancer.

10.2.1.1 Genetic Mutation in Enzymes in Dietary Pathways

Findings from animal studies and in vitro experiments, which indicates that epigenetic changes can alter effects of dietary exposure and metabolism into heritable gene expression patterns, offer profound insight into understanding human-disease risk. Many enzymes, including DNA methyltransferases, histone methyltransferases, histone acetyltransferase, and histone deacetylases that play important roles in epigenetic gene regulation, utilize co-substrates generated by cellular metabolism (Kaelin and McKnight 2013).

As mentioned above, one of the most-studied examples of how diet can affect epigenetic DNA methylation is via folate consumption. Folic acid (vitamin B9) is an essential substrate in the metabolic pathway for synthesis of S-adenosyl methionine, which provides the methyl donor group for histone and DNA methylation reactions. Deficiency in dietary folate during early embryogenesis results in numerous health risks, particularly metabolic dysfunction at all stages of life (McKay and Mathers 2016). On the other hand, a protective effect of high dietary intake of folate has been reported for colorectal cancer and lymphatic leukemia, whereas increased risk of esophageal, prostate, and stomach cancers has been linked to high levels of folate, and results are mixed for breast cancer (Van Guelpen et al. 2006). Thus a role for folate metabolism in cancer is important.

There are two pathways whereby folate is either utilized for DNA methylation or DNA synthesis, a process catalyzed by the enzyme methylenetetrahydrofolate reductase (MTHFR). The substrate 5,10-methylenetatrahydrofolate for this reaction promotes DNA synthesis, whereas the product of the MTHFR reaction 5-methyltetrahydrofolate promotes DNA methylation. Thus the availability of the donors for DNA methylation is regulated by the enzymatic activity of MTHFR. Some reports have observed genetic variants (SNPs) in the enzyme MTHFR. One report suggests that specific heterozygotes in SNP alleles can reduce the enzymatic activity by about 35%, whereas homozygote SNP alleles can reduce activity by as much as 70% (Van Guelpen et al. 2006). Thus, these SNPs in MTHFR can mimic a life-long reduced exposure to folate; such polymorphism might increase availability of folate for DNA synthesis and hence cell proliferation and increasing cancer risk. On the other hand, high levels of available methyl donors for increased DNA methylation can result in gene silencing of tumor suppressor genes such as glutathione-s-transferase (GSTPπ) and increase carcinogenesis. Other reports indicate that the amount of methyl substrates can inhibit the enzymatic action of DNA methyltransferase and DNA methylation (Choi and Friso 2010). Several SNPs with various allelic frequencies have been reported in other populations and are correlated with differential methylation patterns and differences in cancer susceptibility. For instance, SNPs in various enzymes that play roles in folate-metabolism have been associated with differential susceptibility to breast cancer in AA women when compared with EA women (Gong et al. 2015a). Other studies have reported polymorphisms in DNA methyltransferases, which influence the activity of these enzymes (Singal et al. 2005). However, there are no studies that have reported polymorphisms in the DNA methyltransferases that are associated with dietary patterns in various racial and ethnic groups.

10.2.2 The Role of Hormonal Exposure

In additional to dietary exposure, other reports suggest that in utero exposures to hormones such as estrogen and testosterone may be linked to future disparities in prostate cancer risk. One report found that AA women have higher levels of testosterone and estrogen in the circulating maternal blood in comparison with EA women, suggesting that high levels of circulating estrogen and testosterone during early gestation may be associated with increased prostate cancer incidence in AA men (Henderson et al. 1988). Experimental studies whereby mice and rats exposed to estrogens resulted in chronic prostatic inflammation and prostate cancer led the renowned prostate cancer researcher Donald S. Coffey to propose that estrogen exposures might be at the root of the prostate-cancer epidemic in the USA, noting that prostate cancers are common in geographic regions where breast cancer is also common (Coffey 2001).

Additional evidence for a role of hormonal exposure and cancer risk comes from studies carried out by Ho et al. (2006), who demonstrated that active environmental estrogens, such as bisphenol A or estradiol, increase disease incidence, including prostate cancer. In their analysis, they established a carcinogenesis rat model for brief perinatal exposure to synthetic estrogens and observed that this permanently altered growth and differentiation of the prostate gland, increasing susceptibility to adult-onset precancerous lesion and prostate tumors in the aged-rat model (Ho et al. 2006). This study also demonstrated that disruption of endocrine signaling as a result of increased exposure to estradiol was associated with permanent changes in the DNA-methylation patterns of multiple cell-signaling genes, including PDE4D4 (phosphodiesterase type 4), an enzyme responsible for cyclic AMP breakdown, suggesting that PDE4D4 could serve as a potential biomarker for prostate-cancer risk assessment as a result of abnormalities in hormonal signals. Their analysis provides a direct link between developmental high doses of bisphenol A or estradiol exposure and carcinogenesis of the prostate gland. Bisphenol A leaches from food and beverage containers, as well as dental sealants, and is found in the serum of humans with higher concentration in placental and fetal tissues; thus, public health approaches that limit the exposure to environmental bisphenol A could contribute to diseases prevention.

Another report on the importance of hormonal exposure during fetal development indicated that inadequate exposure to ultraviolet B (UVB) radiation that can be blocked by heavy skin pigmentation in AA women during pregnancy can prevent the conversion of the pre-hormone to the hormonal form of vitamin D (Fuller 2000). Low levels of serum vitamin D in the in utero environment can disrupt calcium homeostasis, leading to premature and low-birth-weight infants, and this is associated with increased risk to various diseases.

10.2.3 The Role of Air Pollution

In addition to environmental nutritional deficiency and hormonal exposures, there is mounting epidemiological evidence to indicate that maternal exposure to air pollution is linked to increased risk of delivering low-birth-weight babies who have increased susceptibility to various diseases, such as hypertension, coronary heart disease, type 2 diabetes, and abnormal lipid metabolism, and overall increased mortality and morbidity in childhood and adulthood. Many of these air pollutants, such as carbon monoxide, nitrogen dioxide, and sulfur dioxide, are typically from traffic and industrial emissions in low-SES residential areas that are often inhabited by AA and other minority populations.

One study investigated the association between exposure to particulate matter (similar to maternal smoking) in Allegheny County, PA (USA), an industrial area with factories, chemical plants, coking facilities, a cement kiln, and steel and other heavy industrialization, as well as the contribution from traffic emissions. Their results indicated increased risk of mothers giving birth to low-birth-weight babies, particularly for pregnant mothers that were exposed to the particular pollutant during the first trimester of pregnancy. These environmental exposures may cause abnormalities in the placenta and DNA damage and disrupt endocrine signaling, similar to exposure to bisphenol A (Xu et al. 2011) as already discussed.

Other neighborhood or workplace pollutants found in the atmosphere or the water system, include asbestos or chemicals pollutants such as lead, mercury, cadmium, nickel, and chromium, as well as metal ions. These pollutants have been reported to alter global as well as gene-specific promoters of epigenetic DNA-methylation levels, leading to alteration in the expression of key regulatory genes, and this can contribute to higher disease risk (Aguilera et al. 2010). For instance, chromium, cadmium, and nickel have been demonstrated to inhibit the expression of DNA methyltransferases, thereby reducing global histone H4 acetylation and increase histone H3 lysine 9 demethylation, silencing the expression levels of important regulatory genes (Aguilera et al. 2010) and may contribute to increased incidence of cancer. In addition, some of these compounds are found in the food we consume and in countless household items, such as cosmetics, cleaning products, and plastics. Thus, public efforts to limit exposures to these compounds would contribute to reducing adverse health disparities.

10.2.4 The Role of Parental Substance Abuse

Substance abuse, including tobacco smoking, alcohol binge drinking, and cocaine and opioid usage during pregnancy, is a major public-health concern because it has adverse health effects for both the mother and the growing fetus. Several epidemiological reports indicate that prenatal exposure to abused substances can result in neurological defects (cognition delays and disorders, such as Attention Deficit

Hyperactivity Disorder ADHD) and endocrine disruption in the growing fetus that can persist into adulthood, contributing to chronic diseases such as asthma, diabetes, and certain types of cancer.

Although human studies of the long-term effects of in utero exposures to abused substances and, in particular tobacco smoke, are lacking, there are numerous scientific reports based on animal studies to indicate that maternal smoking and, in particular nicotine exposure alone during pregnancy, is associated with a wide array of adverse health outcomes for the offspring throughout life. A recent review by Bruin et al. (2010) suggests that in utero nicotine exposure has damaging effect (neuroteratogen) on central-nervous-system development, including the disruption of critical neural pathways in the developing brain, and this can result in numerous adverse postnatal neurobehavioral outcomes, such as attention-deficit hyperactivity disorders, learning disabilities, and other disorderly behavioral problems. In addition, in utero exposure to nicotine has been shown to cause growth restriction and low birth weight. Other adverse health outcomes, as a result of exposure to intrauterine tobacco smoke, include abnormalities in pulmonary function, reduced fertility in both men and women, and increased risk of childhood cancers such as brain tumors and leukemia/lymphoma.

All psychoactive drugs enter the growing fetus blood circulation by the process of passive diffusion, and the exposure of the fetus to various drugs has been associated with various disorders. For instance, exposure to alcohol is associated with fetal-alcohol-spectrum disorder (FASD describes the full range of abnormal neuroanatomical, and neurodevelopmental, as well as organ abnormalities, associated with prenatal alcohol exposure); exposure to opioids leads to neonatal abstinence syndrome (NAS), whereas tobacco smoke has long-term developmental and behavioral teratogenic effects. These effects can span toxic-induced structural abnormalities, metabolic or functional deficits, growth retardation, and psychological/behavioral abnormalities. The effects to other drugs such as cocaine is less clear, though some reports suggests adverse effects on cognitive development (Konijnenberg 2015). Results of prenatal exposure to these drugs can be manifest in physical dependence of the child to NAS that is evidenced by tremors, irritability, and excessive crying. However, some effects do manifest later on in life. Fisher et al. (2011) found that, in over 1073 youths who were identified at birth to have been exposed to prenatal drugs including cocaine, there were significant individual differences in behavioral dysregulation and associated functional difficulties. The functional difficulties were higher in the youths that were exposed to higher levels of the substances.

The role of genetics with regards to alcohol exposure is the process whereby alcohol is eliminated by the liver's oxidative enzymes. Alcohol dehydrogenase (ADH) metabolizes 90–95% of alcohol to acetaldehyde which is, in turn, oxidized by aldehyde dehydrogenase (ALDH) to acetate, which then is degraded into carbon dioxide and water. The fetus has low hepatic ADH activity, so it is the maternal pattern of ethanol elimination that determines fetal exposure and also the rate-limiting step for metabolizing to carbon dioxide and water. Several reports of genetic variants (also described in Chap. 2) in enzymatic activity, involved in the alcohol metabolic pathway, in particular polymorphisms in the ADH genes that increase ethanol oxidation can increase elimination, whereas the genetic variants that decrease ADH activity lead to decreased catabolism and can result in increased risk of FASH (Pollard 2007). In the AA population, a genetic variant, ADH1B*3 seems to be associated with reduced risk of FASD.

In addition, differences in genetic polymorphisms of metabolic activation and detoxification pathways in various maternal population can be associated with the differential susceptibility to tobacco and other drugs of substance abuse on fetal growth. The low birth weight of infants born to smoking mothers has been linked to genetic variants in the aryl hydrocarbon receptor gene whose protein product functions in detoxification of xenobiotic chemicals such as the highly carcinogenic polycyclic mine hydrocarbons and nitrosamines found in tobacco and cigarette smoke (Pollard 2007). Fathers can also compromise the developmental outcomes and subsequent well-being of their children and grandchildren. For instances, abnormalities in their sperm are prevalent in men who use recreational drugs or smoke and these contribute to DNA damage and other birth defects independent of, or in association with, maternal-induced damages to the growing fetus.

In addition to a role for genetic polymorphism in contributing to tobacco-related birth abnormalities, prenatal exposure to tobacco also alters both global and gene-specific epigenetic DNA methylation and silencing of several genes such as PECAM1, ARHGAP24, and AMOTL2, which play roles in angiogenesis in cardiovascular development, and this could lead to the increased risk of cardiovascular diseases in later years of development and adulthood. Genes whose expression are altered by DNA methylation include the DNA-repetitive elements AluYb8 and LINE1, as well as the carcinogenic detoxification enzyme glutathione S-transferase P (GSTPI), thus variants in detoxification genes in addition to epigenetic alterations may modulate the effects of in utero exposure to tobacco smoke and other recreational drugs to the growing fetus (Breton et al. 2009). Other reports indicate that prenatal exposure to cocaine in pregnant rats induce methylation changes and the silencing in gene expression of protein kinase C (PKC) epsilon type, and this led to increased susceptibility of adults to ischemia and reperfusion injury, suggesting a role for epigenetic process in utero programming of PKC-epsilon gene expression in the pattern of heart development (Zhang et al. 2007).

10.2.5 The Role of Maternal Stress

Several reports from human and animal studies demonstrates that, in addition to the adverse effects of poor nutrition and environmental toxins, exposure of the growing fetus to maternal stress, anxiety, and depression can also have profound effects on the developing fetus, with consequences of life-time risks to psychological and neurological issues. Studies from the Dutch hunger during the winter of 1944, where pregnant women were subjected to deficient nutrition (described previously) and associated secondary stress, indicated a link between increased neurological

10.2 Fetal Origin of Health Disparities

disorders in adults that were born to women under these stressful circumstance in comparison to children born to women during the same period who had enough food and did not undergo such stressful experiences. The risk of schizophrenia in adults who were conceived at the peak of the famine period was significantly higher than for any other period during the famine (Susser et al. 1998).

Similar neurological disorders have been reported for individuals born during the Chinese famine. Between 1959 and 1961, the Chinese leader Mao Zedong, with the support of the Chinese Communist Party, pressed for heavy industrialization in the country as a way to economic revolution by forcing peasant farmers from farm work to mining for steel production. As a result, grain production plummeted, causing one of the world's largest famines, in which some 30 million died. Studies found that individuals born to women who suffered from the famine were twice as likely to develop schizophrenia as those gestated at other times (Xu et al. 2009). These studies suggest that the exposure of the developing fetus to in utero stressful environment, such as historical periods of stress or famine, are more likely to lead to increased risk of schizophrenia in adulthood. Maternal malnutrition, such as deficiencies in certain micro and macronutrients, as well as maternal stress, may have disrupted neural development, contributing to the illness. Prenatal exposure to distress, anxiety, and depression is also linked to autism, as well as other psychiatric disorders (Werner et al. 2007), indicating that prenatal environment influences childhood temperament. Other reports indicate that maternal depression during pregnancy was linked to increased risk of adolescent depression, and one report suggests that the risk of depression in adolescent who were exposed to antenatal depression was 4.7-times greater than in offspring who were not exposed (Pawlby et al. 2009).

The process whereby the maternal stress level in utero environment can be felt by the developing fetus is mediated by placental function. The placenta is highly sensitive to maternal stress and distress, and maternal stress, anxiety, and depression are measured by cortisol level. Studies have shown that at birth infants exposed to higher maternal plasma cortisol also have an increased cortisol level (Davis et al. 2011). Other neurobiological observations indicate that prenatal exposure to maternal distress was linked to reduced gray matter volumes in the prefrontal cortex, medial temporal lobe, and other areas involved in learning and memory, and this may render the developing individual more vulnerable to neurodevelopmental and psychiatric disorders, as well as cognitive and intellectual impairment (Buss et al. 2010).

Scientific evidence demonstrates a potential role of epigenetic mechanism in the regulation of neurobiological behavior. For instance, there is widespread differential methylation of several genes with biological roles in growth and development including the imprinted insulin growth factor (IGF2) gene and INSIGF, IL10, ABCA1, GNAS3AT and MEG3 genes in adult cohort that were prenatally exposed to nutritional deficiencies during the Dutch famine. This observation provides support that adverse early life exposure can induce aberrant epigenetic changes in humans that persist throughout life (Heijmans et al. 2008).

Other reports suggest that prenatal exposure to maternal depression and stresses can induce DNA-methylation changes. One study that analyzed cord blood samples from infants born to mothers with elevated rates of depression in the third trimester and who also had increased cortisol levels (a stress indicator) reported increased DNA methylation of the NR3C1 gene. The NR3C1 gene encodes for the glucocorticoid receptor, which plays an important biological function in regulating HPA axis, thus increased DNA methylation of NR3C1 would disrupt the normal HPA signaling (discussed in more detail in Sect. 10.3). This abnormal epigenetic effect was observed in the infant blood sample and reflects in-utero environmental conditions of the developing fetus. However, other studies have established that these epigenetic marks established during in utero exposure are maintained beyond infancy, noting that children and adolescent (ages 10–19 years) born to women who have experienced spousal stress in the form of intimate-partner violence during pregnancy demonstrated increased NR3C1 DNA methylation levels in whole blood samples (Radtke et al. 2011).

Other supporting data has come from animal studies under controlled laboratory conditions, whereby the exposure of animals to prenatal stress can induce epigenetic variation within the brain regions involved in the behavioral characteristics associated with prenatal stressors. In mice, chronic variable-stress exposure during the first trimester increased corticosterone response to stress and increased depressive-like behavior. In addition, these animal studies also demonstrated that protein restriction and prenatal stress during pregnancy resulted in adult male offspring with decreased DNA methylation of the CRH gene and increased methylation of NR3C1 gene in the hypothalamic tissue of adult male offspring, supporting important epigenetic alterations during early-life exposures that is persistent throughout life and can be transmitted to subsequent generations.

10.2.6 Prenatal Predisposition to Kidney Diseases

If early environmental exposures have life-time influence on adult health, where in the body are the "memories" of these early experiences stored and maintained? A plausible explanation involves a change in growth of a tissue or organ. According to the Barker's hypothesis mentioned above, when resources are restricted, such as from maternal nutritional deficiencies, it can cause a shift in nutritional supplies away from other organs, including the kidney, pancreas, and the heart towards the most important organs in the developing fetus, such as brain (Koleganova et al. 2009), and this potentially affects the growth and development of organs such as the kidney, the pancreas, and the heart. For instance, individuals that were prenatally undernourished have characteristically smaller kidneys with fewer nephrons that can contribute to increase risk of hypertension and renal failure later in life (Luyckx and Brenner 2005). Thus, a limited supply of essential nutrients during the critical period of fetal development affects the developing kidneys and results production of a diminished number of nephrons, increasing an individual's susceptibility to albuminuria and the risk to chronic kidney disease, as well as hypertension. The mechanism involves epigenetic DNA methylation and histone modification that alter gene expression in kidney development. Alterations in the number and composition of muscle cells in individuals born with low birth weight could contribute to insulin resistance in adulthood (Jensen et al. 2007). In addition, the composition and number of body-fat cells present in various adipose tissues could be altered under fetal-malnourishment conditions (Zhang et al. 2007).

10.3 Mechanisms of Epigenetic Programming and Maternal Care

Research on the effects of maternal care, as evidenced by studies in animal models, suggests that, in addition to diet and exposure to environmental toxins, early-life experiences can also have long-term impact on behavior and the response to stress, as well as susceptibility to disease. Studies carried out in rats demonstrate that the adult offspring of mothers that demonstrated pup licking/grooming and arched-backing nursing in the first week of life resulted in reduced fear and more modest response to stress in comparison to pups who were neglected by their mothers (Francis et al. 1999; Weaver et al. 2006). These highly groomed pups exhibited regular feedback-inhibition of the stress response and consequently less HPA-axis activity in comparison with the less-groomed pups, and this stress response persisted into adulthood (Hyman 2009). The highly groomed pups that received licking/grooming on a regular basis demonstrated a high expression of the glucocorticoid receptor (GR or NR3C1 gene mentioned previously) at the RNA and protein levels. The function of glucocorticoids in part is mediated by signaling through glucocorticoid receptors (GR) in the hypothalamus. Circulating glucocorticoids act on GR in the hypothalamus to regulate HPA activity, and this includes a feedback inhibition of the stress response mechanism, which targets the corticotrophin releasing hormone (CRH). The CRH synthesis and its downstream signals culminate in a stress response, such that glucocorticoids are released, and this is involved in the negative-feedback inhibition of CRH synthesis and minimizing HPA response to stress (Francis et al. 1999).

On the other hand, rat pups who have not received frequent licking/grooming by their mothers in infancy demonstrated increased activation of the hypothalamic-pituitary-adrenal axis (HPA) under mild stress conditions (Meaney 2001). The molecular mechanism whereby there is increased HPA activity is mediated by epigenetic alterations, including the role of DNA-methylation changes in the gene promoter region of GR. Because methylation impedes access of transcription factors to the gene's promoter region, the increased methylation triggered by lack of maternal care silenced the expression of the GR gene, thus reducing the level of GR expressed in the hypothalamus. The DNA methylation of GR can inhibit this mechanism of negative-feedback inhibition of glucocorticoids signals that target the CRHs and disrupt homeostasis in hormonal signaling.

Similar epigenetic alterations including DNA-methylation changes in response to childhood abuses has been reported in human beings (McGowan et al. 2009). Studies by McGowan et al. demonstrated that children abused in early childhood exhibited higher DNA methylation in the promoter region of the glucocorticoid receptor. The DNA-methylation pattern was found to be stable into adulthood (Weaver et al. 2004). Social and environmental adversity experienced in low-SES children similar to that of low-grooming pups can result in abnormal epigenetic programming and changes in the gene expression of important regulatory proteins that can stably impact behavior and health outcomes later in life.

One other study observed increased expression of glucocorticoids to be associated with decreased methylation of the nerve growth factor-inducible protein A (NGFI-A) (Meaney and Szyf 2005) in response to maternal care. The protein product of NGFI-A may function in regulating growth, maintenance, and proliferation of neurons and may also regulate the HPA axis. This suggests that maternal care may trigger changes in gene expression via epigenetic mechanisms including DNA methylation and histone modification to mediate changes in the pups' growth and neuronal activity. Thus, social behavior in one subject can affect epigenetic programing in another subject. However, the DNA-methylation process is reversible, such that the increased availability of L-methionine (diet), a precursor for DNA methylation, leads to hypermethylation of NGF1-A, reduced GR expression, and altered HPA response to stress. This suggests that, in theory, dietary interventions or reversing epigenetic processes, including the use of histone deacetylase inhibitor (Trichostatin A; TSA) or DNA methyltransferase inhibitor (5″ Aza-cyticidine), can reverse the maternal effect and behavioral response to stress.

10.4 Epigenetic Programming in Early Life

There is scientific interest in epigenetic programming during early childhood and its impact on human behavior and long-term health outcomes. A fundamental question is whether the epigenetic programming, as described in the animal studies such as differences in response of rat pups to maternal care, could also account for the behavioral differences observed in individuals in response to environmental stress, or whether such epigenetic programing is stable throughout the life span of the individual or this can be reversible.

Animal experimentation has provided insight into the nature of epigenetic programming in response to maternal care. In one study, the drug HDAC inhibitor (TSA) was injected into rat brains to assess their epigenetic effects. The injection of TSA into the brains of adult offspring of low-grooming rats demonstrated increased acetylation and reduced DNA methylation, with the concomitant induction in gene expression of GR to levels that are remarkably similar to adult offspring of highly groomed adult rats (Weaver et al. 2004). Thus, even though the epigenetic mechanism is highly stable resulting in long term-changes in gene expression, it is not so static that it cannot be reversed at a later stage (Szyf 2001), particularly with availability of substrate for the methylation process providing a link between dietary intake and alterations in epigenetic programming in the brain. Other supporting evidence indicates that epigenetic programming of several genes (such as cytokines), which regulate human immune signaling, can be altered or reversed later in life in response to environmental exposure (Bruniquel and Schwartz 2003; Falek et al. 2000; Fitzpatrick et al. 1999; Northrop et al. 2006).

The maternal care of rat pups model demonstrates that significant epigenetic programming arises after embryogenesis is completed and that it could be triggered by social cues. However, several questions remain: first, whether environmental exposures after birth affects epigenetic programming throughout life or if epigenetic programming is restricted to fetal development; second, whether environmental exposures at different time points in life alter the epigenetic program that causes physiologically changes and consequently late-onset of diseases. Finally, can environmentally induced epigenetic changes contribute to shaping societal change and promote positive social behavior or culture? These questions remain to be answered and would have broad-ranging implications on our understanding of social, physiological, and pathological processes and their relationships.

10.5 Infant and Child Gene-Environmental Conditions

Early infancy is characterized by intense brain development, which is highly sensitive to interactions with caregiving adults (Shore 1999). Infants and children who experience chronic stress or adverse social factors such as low SES or family conflict show distinct patterns of neurotransmitter expression and structural changes in brain activity and development that can impact memory, educational attainment, and the ability to cope with subsequent stressors (Gunnar et al. 1997; Shore 1999). Several of these adverse factors are over-represented in AA and other minority populations and contribute to health disparities.

Scientific evidence indicates that both prenatal and postnatal environmental exposures can synergistically affect the health outcomes of an individual. As with the case of the Dutch famine study, individuals who are born small and later experienced rapid weight gain in infancy and childhood, as a result of a change in appetite regulation and later nutritional abundance, are associated with increased adult diseases (Adair and Cole 2003). Conditions under which infants and children are raised, such as SES of the family, education, housing and neighborhood, employment insecurity, and health-related behaviors such as smoking and diet, can have long-term effects on health. Just like low birth weight, small size in infancy is also linked to adverse health outcomes in adulthood, including higher risk for CVD, obesity, and diabetes. On the other hand, several studies have demonstrated that breast-fed infants had lower risk of hypertension, obesity, and diabetes in adulthood. One systematic review of published epidemiological studies involving more than 69,000 participants demonstrated that breast feeding protects against obesity

(Arenz et al. 2004). There are hormones in breast milk, such as growth factors, e.g., insulin growth factor, which inhibit adipocytes differentiation in vitro, and leptin, which plays a role in metabolic regulation in infants and could play a role in lowering childhood obesity.

10.6 The Role of Gene-Environment Interactions in Disease Disparities

Some of the most common chronic diseases of youths and adults in the USA are asthma, diabetes mellitus, obesity, hypertension, dental disease, attention-deficit/hyperactivity disorder (ADHD), mental illness, cancers, sickle cell anemia, cystic fibrosis, and a variety of genetic and other birth defects (Price et al. 2013).

The AA population in the USA has an increased prevalence of several of these chronic diseases, including stress-related conditions such as blood pressure (BP). Environmental factors, such as low SES and behavioral AND lifestyle factors; as well as genetic variations that affect gene expression and thereby alter physiological functions, may interact with each other and increase disease incidence and mortality rates in this population. One study investigated the role of gene-environment interaction in predicting BP in the AA population; mostly females who were either overweight or obese were part of this study. The study looked at the interaction of low SES and glucocorticoid-receptor genetic variants in waking cortisol levels and BP in a cross sectional observation (Coulon et al. 2016). The results from this study demonstrated that AA individuals with genetic variants that predispose to increased sensitivity to cortisol level had higher waking cortisol in neighborhoods of higher SES and lower cortisol in neighborhood of lower SES, although low SES was associated with higher systolic BP. This finding provides an example of the complex gene-environment interaction underlying disease risks and health disparities. The following sections look at the role of gene-environment interaction and specific disease disparities.

10.6.1 Asthma Disparities

Early-life environmental exposures, including respiratory tract infections, the infant-gut microbiome and airway microbiome, in combination with in utero environmental exposures to smoke or the maternal diet during pregnancy, are associated with increased risk of asthma. Epidemiological observation indicates that exposure to a farming environment remains one of the strongest protective factors against the development of asthma and allergy, suggesting that the exposure to microbial products, such as the ingestion of raw milk and inhalation of microbial molecules in dust, are protective factors (Bonnelykke and Ober 2016). In contrast, living in cities where there is less exposure to microbes may likely contribute to the increased prevalence of asthma in the general population.

In addition to environmental exposures, several genes have been identified that play a role in asthma incidence, and the expression of some of these genes is triggered by environmental exposures. In particular, genes that regulate immunoglobulin E (IgE) expression and allergic inflammation require activation by the environment (Gern et al. 1999). In addition, cockroaches and dust mites, which are more prevalent in low-SES homes, may increase the risk for the development of airway susceptibility to asthma. One potential mechanism for the physical environment and gene interaction in developing pulmonary illness including asthma involves the role of the innate immune system, the first defense against pathogen/allergen attack. The innate immune system uses toll-like receptor (TLR) signals which are sensors for innate immunity. Exposure to environmental allergens sends signals to activate TLR that in turn lead to activating signals of the adaptive immune system by modulating the balance between Th1/Th2 cytokines, where strong Th2 response favors more allergenic response and airway inflammation (Vandenbulcke et al. 2006). Other mediators in the immune signals of asthma include secretion of the cytokines interleukin (IL)-4, and IL-13 induces B cells to produce immunoglobulin E (IgE) antibodies, which, upon binding to allergens, trigger a cascade leading to mucus production and constriction of smooth muscle in the airways. The phenotypic symptoms of asthma include wheezing and chest tightness, as well as shortness of breath. Long-term asthmatic conditions are caused by secretion of IL-5, which in turn activates eosinophils, and consequently increased inflammation and obstruction of the airways, causing the persistent clinical manifestations of asthma.

In one study by Chen et al. (2006), they observed that children with asthma from low-SES families had significantly greater eosinophil counts in comparison with children from high-SES families, even when confounding medical and demographics characteristics are controlled for. In an in vitro experiment to model the body's encounter to allergens, Chen and others demonstrated that, when peripheral blood mononuclear cells (PBMCs) from low-SES children with asthma were stimulated with a mitogen cocktail to mimic the immune cells encounter with allergens in the human body, there was an increased expression of the cytokines implicated in asthma, namely, IL-5, IL-13, and eosinophil counts in comparison with the cytokine-expression pattern observed when PBMCs from high SES were similarly stimulated (Chen et al. 2003, 2006). These observations suggest that a low-SES environment might trigger the immune cells of children with asthma to respond more aggressively to some allergic stimuli.

Other studies to elucidate the molecular mechanisms of asthma have focused on the biological function of transcription factors. These are proteins that can relay external stimuli from the environment outside the cell to cause cellular changes in gene expression inside the cell nucleus. Transcription factors in the nucleus can bind to specific segments of DNA called promoters and switch gene expression on or off. Thus, transcription factors regulate the expression of proteins like cytokines that play an important role in inflammatory responses to asthma attack (Busse and Lemanske 2001). To elucidate the transcription factors that play a major role in asthma, Chen et al. (2009) carried out a genome-wide transcriptional analysis of blood T-lymphocytes (which are involved in allergic diseases including asthma) samples derived from children with asthma who are from low-SES families in comparison with high-SES families. Results from this study demonstrated differences in the transcriptional profile between low-SES children with asthma in comparison with high-SES children with asthma. Overall, the low-SES asthma patients showed increased expression of the nuclear factor kappa B (NF-kB) transcription factor activity and decreased expression of cAMP response element binding (CREB) protein activity in comparison with high-SES patients. NF-kB and CREB are transcription factors that have multiple regulatory functions, including the activation of pro-inflammatory cytokines in inflammatory and immune-signaling pathways. These findings are consistent with other studies that have linked several types of social adversity to gene expression profiles (Cole et al. 2007; Lutgendorf et al. 2009). It is speculated that chronic family stresses in low-SES environments may mediate the increased expression of cytokines in association with asthma risk (Chen et al. 2006), whereas poor family relationships in low-SES environments may increase the expression of pro-inflammatory cytokines, which are associated with the adverse clinical outcomes of asthma (Chen et al. 2007).

The accumulating data from Chen, Miller, and others have established a chain of events that links environmental exposures, SES, and biological signals in the pathophysiology of asthma. This includes expression profiles of asthma-relevant inflammatory markers, increased eosinophil counts, increased expression of IL-5 and other cytokines, and activation of relevant transcription control pathways (e.g., NF-kB and CREB). Importantly, all of these relationships are in a direction that is consistent with the clinical phenomenon of children from lower-SES backgrounds who experience greater asthma impairment.

Despite the important contribution of environmental risk factors in asthma incidence, there are heritable factors, including a high frequency of genetic variants that are associated with asthma risk (discussed in Chap. 2), with differential frequencies in various populations, which is reflected in the differences in susceptibility to asthma risk. The genetic variants associated with asthma incidence explain why some individuals are more susceptible, whereas other individuals have a low risk of developing asthma. Genetic variants on the 5q31 locus and differential environmental exposure (Kauffmann and Demenais 2012) in various racial and ethnic groups can contribute to the disparity associated with asthma incidence.

Genetic variants cannot fully explain the heritable factors associated with asthma risk. On the other hand, differential epigenetic alterations may also account for some of the differences in the susceptibility to asthma risk observed in one population in comparison with another population. A potential role of aberrant epigenetic changes has been proposed for both childhood and adulthood onset of asthma disease in response to environmental exposures. There are reports to indicate that exposures to tobacco smoke and both indoor and outdoor air pollutants, as well as occupational exposure to microbial and viral pathogens, nutrients, and life styles, can induce epigenetic changes including DNA methylation and asthma risk. Recent reports in support of environmentally mediated epigenetic changes and asthma risk is demonstrated for the drug aspirin-exacerbated respiratory disease (AERD) in individuals susceptible to this environmental drug effect. Genome-wide DNA-methylation analysis, using nasal polyps of subjects with AERD and control aspirin-tolerant asthma (ATA) individuals, demonstrated differential methylation profiles for candidate genes involved in the immune-signaling pathways associated with asthma risk. Notably, significant hypermethylation of prostaglandin E synthase and hypomethylation of prostaglandin D synthase, arachidonate 5-lipoxygenase, activating protein leukotriene B4 receptor, have been observed in AERD individuals in comparison with ATA individuals (Lee et al. 2015).

Other studies have reported epigenome-mediated increased risk of asthma in response to environmental and nutritional exposures. One study in mice demonstrated that runt-related transcription factor 3 (RUNX3), a gene known to be a negative regulator in allergic airway disease, was hypermethylated and had reduced expression level in FI progeny when exposed to a diet rich in folic acid (high methyl diet donor), suggesting that dietary factors can modify the heritable risk of allergic airway diseases (Hollingsworth et al. 2008). Thus, in response to some environmental risk factors, differential epigenetic changes and varying frequencies of genetic variants in various racial and ethnic populations may be critical mediators in alterations of gene expression at the transcriptional and protein levels in cells, causing disequilibrium in TH1/TH2 cytokines and consequently increasing risk of asthma and asthma disparities.

10.6.2 Diabetes Disparities

Diabetes is a group of metabolic disorders whereby the body is unable to produce any or sufficient amounts of insulin to regulate blood-glucose levels. There are several types of diabetes, including gestational diabetes whereby a diabetic mother's high blood sugar may disrupt the metabolism of a fetus, and/or other postnatal environmental exposures may predispose individuals to diabetes. This phenomenon has been observed in the Pima Indian population. The Pima Indians of Arizona, originally from Mexico, have a very high incidence of type 2 diabetes (T2D). However, diabetes was uncommon among the Pima Indians until the second half of the twentieth century when their stable diet changed from complex carbohydrates and a diet low in saturated animal fat to one rich in animal fat (Pratley 1998), clearly demonstrating a strong environmental component to the risk of diabetes.

Another type of diabetes is the so-called type 1 diabetes that affects individuals with little or no insulin production and these individuals must receive exogenous insulin to augment for this defect. Type 1 diabetes (T1D) is commonly diagnosed in children and school-age youths. Whereas T2D, a disorder of how the body processes glucose, is typically diagnosed in youths and adults, in particular obese adults (Schulze and Hu 2005). As a result, individuals with T2D may be able to control this condition through healthy diet and exercise, as well as the administration of exogenous insulin. There is also a prediabetic condition whereby an individual has an elevated blood-glucose level, which can lead to full-blown diabetes (Price et al. 2013).

The incidence and mortality rate of diabetes has a strong gene-environment interaction as depicted in Fig. 10.1. Risk factors that are associated with diabetes incidence and mortality rates include genetic, epigenetic changes, race, culture, lifestyle, behavior, and environment, as well as the health-care system. The genetic and epigenetic factors that are associated with diabetes are discussed in Chaps. 2 and 3, respectively, and these factors have been demonstrated to interact with environmental exposures to contribute to diabetes. For instance, the Dutch famine studies discussed previously showed that individuals born to malnourished pregnant mothers during the Dutch famine period were predisposed to obesity and diabetes. A potential mechanism for the environmental nutritional defects that influenced gene alteration (gene expression) is demonstrated for epigenetic DNA methylation of insulin-like growth factor 2 [IGF2] and leptin [LEP] genes, which are involved in pathogenesis of diabetes and obesity. Malnutrition induced significant changes in DNA methylation, including hypomethylation of IGF2 gene. Briefly, hypomethylation of IGF2, a protein that plays a role in growth, suggests that children exposed to famine during gestation may compensate against food scarcity, whereas hypermethylation of LEP and subsequent reduction in expression may compensate towards hyperactive eating. Thus, the epigenetic pattern is programmed to

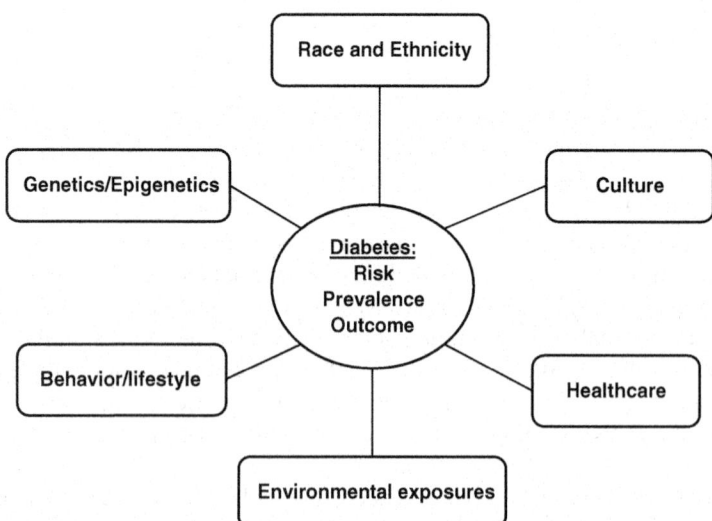

Fig. 10.1 The role of gene-environment interaction in diabetes. Diagram demonstrates several factors that are associated with the risk, prevalence, and outcome of diabetes

10.6 The Role of Gene-Environment Interactions in Disease Disparities

compensate for food scarcity, whereas, under conditions of food abundance, this could lead to obesity (Jackson et al. 2013). Other risk factors, such as lifestyle choices including excessive alcohol consumption and tobacco smoke as well as behavior or dietary habits such as high fat and high energy dense foods as well as a sedentary lifestyle, all contribute to increased risk of diabetes. The environment may also affect diabetes risk either directly or through behavior and life-style modifications. Environmental factors, such as low-SES communities with scarcity of fresh fruits and vegetable supermarkets, absence of safe areas for recreational sports, or lack of access to health care and high rates of neighborhood stresses, are all associated with increased risk of diabetes. Other environmental evidence comes from the observation that low-SES communities that have high numbers of fast-food and convenient stores in comparison with fresh fruits and vegetable supermarkets are also linked with high prevalence of both diabetes and obesity, even after controlling for race/ethnicity, income, age, gender, and physical activity. Several of these environmental, behavioral, and life-style choices are over-represented in poorly educated, low-income populations, such as AA and other minority populations, hence the high prevalence of diabetes in these populations.

10.6.3 Tobacco Smoking and Alcohol Consumption Disparities

Tobacco smoke and excessive alcohol consumption are significantly associated with increased risk of many diseases. It is estimated that the combination of smoking and excessive alcohol consumption accounts for 3.5% of all cases of cancer incidence and mortality rates in USA (Nelson et al. 2013). Tobacco smoking alone, or excessive alcohol consumption or both tobacco smoking and alcohol abuse, are significantly associated with increased risk and mortality of not only cancer but other diseases, such as CVDs, obesity, and diabetes as discussed subsequently.

Tobacco smoking is a major environmental risk factor which is associated with many diseases including cancer, CVD, and obesity. There are over 4000 chemicals including approximately 60 well-known carcinogenic compounds, such as nitrosamines, polycyclic amines, aldehydes, and benzene in tobacco smoke (Taioli 2008). The damaging effects of tobacco smoke occur by inducing cellular and molecular changes via both genetic and epigenetic alterations. Smoking behavior is significantly associated with a genetic component, although the mechanisms are largely unknown.

Through GWAS, nine genetic variants or SNPs in the gene-promoter region of IL15 are associated with the quantity and intensity of tobacco smoking, plus overall dependence (Liu et al. 2009). Several of these genetic variants are located on the transcription factor binding sites of the IL15 promoter and can modulate the transcription, hence the expression of IL15. The IL15 encodes for a key pro-inflammatory cytokine of the immune system and has long been recognized to influence drug-addiction behavior, thus tobacco-smoke addiction also involves the immune modulation via the IL15 signal. Other genetic polymorphism in the cytochrome P450 superfamily of enzymes, which plays an important role in detoxification of carcinogens, has been associated with tobacco smoke and disease (e.g., cancer risk). One study identified SNPs in P450 family of enzymes, CYP29, CYP1B1, CYP2D6, and CYP2E1 and also the glutathione S-transferase (GSTPI) detoxification enzymes, to be associated with increased risk of prostate cancer in AA populations in comparison with EA populations (Ragin et al. 2010), suggesting that the genetic variants in the cytochrome P450 family of enzymes may contribute to prostate cancer disparities in the AA and EA populations. Other GWAS and candidate gene studies and a history of familial dependence and nicotine addiction have identified genetic variance in CHRNA5, CYP2A6, and GABRB1 genes and nicotine dependence. The association was strongest with childhood adversity (loss of parent, experienced violent crime or been sexually abused) linked to increased risk of dependence.

Other studies have investigated epigenetic changes in response to tobacco smoke. One of the best examples of how environmental exposure can alter epigenetic patterns is demonstrated for the tumor suppressor gene p16 which plays a biological function in the regulation of cell cycle and death associated protein (DAP) kinase. In a study by Belinsky et al. (2002) that investigated the DNA methylation of several genes in bronchial-epithelium cells collected in sputum (which contains exfoliated cells from the lower respiratory tract), they observed significant hypermethylation of p16 and DAP kinase in samples collected from current and former smokers with lung cancer and cancer-free smokers in comparison with non-smokers sputum. The hypermethylation of p16 persisted even after tobacco smoke cessation. Gene silencing of p16 expression by hypermethylation in association with tobacco smoke may be an important step in the acquisition of additional genetic and epigenetic aberrations that may contribute to the carcinogenesis of not only lung cancer, but also cancers of the pancreatic and other organs. Though there is no current report of differential methylation of p16 status in various racial and ethnic groups with cancer, such an association would support a role for aberrant p16 epigenetic changes and cancer disparities.

With regards to differential epigenetic changes and tobacco smoke in various racial and ethnic groups, one study has indicated that DNA methylation changes of two smoking-related genes, namely, F2RL3 (factor II receptor-like 3) and GPR15 (G-protein-coupled receptor 15), are significantly associated with tobacco-smoking risk in both AA and EA populations (Sun et al. 2013), suggesting a molecular mechanism involving DNA-methylation changes in response to tobacco smoke exposure. Other reports indicate that smoking could alter the expression of interleukins, such as the observation of decreased IL15 expression mentioned previously and diminished activation of downstream signaling molecules which may culminate in dysfunctional immune response to tobacco smoke (Mian et al. 2009).

Excessive consumption of alcohol is associated with increased risk to many diseases. Alcohol use has both environmental components such as the ease and access in certain low-SES neighborhoods and behavior or life-style choice, as well as genetic component. However, despite alcohol toxicity (e.g., carcinogenic) to the human body, the molecular mechanism whereby alcohol exerts its toxic effect is not fully known. Studies that have investigated alcohol metabolism have focused on the first and most toxic alcohol metabolite, acetaldehyde, which is regarded as carcinogen in both animal and human studies (Woutersen et al. 1986). Acetaldehyde exerts its carcinogenic effects by interfering with DNA synthesis and repair, as well as increasing genomic instability inside the human cell (Seitz and Stickel 2007). Acetaldehyde is metabolized from alcohol by alcohol dehydrogenase (ADH2), which in turn is metabolized to carbon dioxide and water by another enzyme known as acetaldehyde dehydrogenase (ALDH2). Genetic variants in ADH2 and ALDH2 can influence the metabolism of acetaldehyde and can determine alcohol dependence in certain populations (Taqi et al. 2011). Genetic variants of ADH2 and ALDH2 are rare among EA but common in Asian populations. Some genetic variants are linked to blood-acetaldehyde concentration of six-to-19-times higher in comparison with people who have the wild-type gene and consume the same amount of alcohol, suggesting that such variants can increase acetaldehyde toxicity and increase risk to diseases such as esophageal and pancreatic cancers (Zhao et al. 2015). Alcohol consumption can also exert its carcinogenic effects by inducing the activity of cytochrome P450 2E1 (CYP2E1), that generate reactive oxygen species, increase inflammation, and consequently modulate cellular-immune responses (Thapar et al. 2012). In addition, alcohol can disrupt folate uptake and cause nutritional folate deficiencies, although folate deficiencies are primarily due to low dietary intake. Ultimately, destruction of folate uptake by alcohol leads to an imbalance in both S-adenosylmethionine and nucleotide pools, causing aberrant epigenetic changes (discussed subsequently) and other genetic damages that are capable of inducing carcinogenesis (Kim 2007).

While there are numerous reports on the role of genetic alterations and alcohol dependence, the role of epigenetic alterations and alcohol dependence lags behind that of genetic studies. However, there is great interest in elucidating the potential role of epigenetics in organism behavior, physiology, and life-style choices because at least some epigenetic marks are responsive to environmental factors, including drugs of abuse (Feil and Fraga 2011). Animal studies has provided robust evidence for epigenetically mediated changes in gene expression for several candidate transcription factors such as ΔFosB, cAMP-response element-binding protein (CREB), and neuropeptide Y following drug exposure (Starkman et al. 2012). These transcription factors play various biological functions, including neurological signals to suggest that drug exposure (such as alcohol) can induce changes that will ultimately result in functional alterations of critical brain circuitry implicated in addiction (Nestler 2013) or alter gene expression that would culminate in carcinogenesis. Both global hypomethylation and gene-specific promoter hypermethylation are associated with cancer (Ehrlich 2002; Momparler 2003).

One study reported promoter hypermethylation of the HERP gene (homocysteine-induced endoplasmic reticulum protein) in response to alcohol treatment. The HERP encodes for protein that is involved in the intracellular defense system. Hypermethylation of HERP was associated with concomitant and significant down regulation in gene expression in patients with alcohol dependence compared to healthy controls (Bleich et al. 2006), suggesting that excessive alcohol consumption might weaken cellular defense system.

Another study analyzed the methylation status of 82 candidate genes that are involved in several brain neurotransmission system in association with chronic alcohol consumption using peripheral blood genomic DNAs derived from 285 AAs (141 alcohol-dependent (AD) cases and 144 controls) and 249 EAs (144 alcohol-dependent cases and 105 controls) (Zhang et al. 2013). Results demonstrated differential methylation in alcohol-dependent cases in both AAs and EAs cases in comparison with controls. Overall, promoter methylation of HTR3A, whose protein product encodes for a serotonin receptor, was significantly highly methylated in AAs when compared to EAs cases suggesting a role for epigenetic DNA-methylation changes and alcohol dependence in an ethnic/racial-specific manner. There are multiple scenarios that have been described for how alcohol consumption as an environmental exposure could alter DNA-methylation changes. First, alcohol consumption could directly induce DNA-methylation changes (Harlaar and Hutchison 2013). In support of this scenario, one report has demonstrated prenatal alcohol exposure and changes in methylation in the developing hippocampus (Chen et al. 2013). Another scenario posits that DNA methylation is an intermediate step in the disease pathway of alcohol dependence and the epigenetic mechanisms used is altering gene expression in the process (Harlaar and Hutchison 2013). Consistent with this "mediating mechanism" hypothesis, studies on rodents have shown that the anxiolytic effects of alcohol exposure may be due to histone modifications that lead to chromatin remodeling in the amygdala (Pandey et al. 2008). It is hypothesized that excessive alcohol use and its metabolites can disrupt the one carbon metabolic pathway, which as discussed previously is a major source of methyl substrate required for DNA methylation. This disruption can give rise to global hypomethylation (Fowler et al. 2012) that can give rise to potential activation of proto-oncogenes, which are associated with carcinogenesis.

Alcohol-related carcinogens may interact with other factors such as tobacco smoke (common co-occurring disorders) to induce abnormal DNA-methylation changes that are particularly important in carcinogenesis. For instance, the combined alcohol-tobacco smoke event affects enzymes that are involved in drug-metabolizing pathways, and potentially contribute to carcinogenesis. One such enzyme, the π-class glutathione S-transferase (GSTP1), which plays important biological roles in detoxifying electrophilic and oxidative carcinogens, has been observed to be hypermethylated in cancer. The hypermethylation of the GSTP1 gene-promoter region is a common somatic genome alteration reported in more than 90% of prostate cancers (PCa). The GSTP1 hypermethylation appears very early in the disease pathway and is more frequent than other genetic defects (e.g., mutation, gene amplification, or gene fusion) associated with PCa carcinogenesis

(Nelson et al. 2003). This observation suggests that hypermethylation may be particularly important in prostate carcinogenesis (Gonzalgo et al. 1997; Zingg and Jones 1997). DNA methylation is one type of epigenetic change that we and others have observed to increase with age in non-cancer tissues (Issa 2000; Kwabi-Addo et al. 2007). It is very likely that cancer-risk factors including excess alcohol consumption, cigarette smoke, diet, and demographic (age, gender, race) and other environmental exposures (benzene, persistent organic pollutants, lead, arsenic and air pollution) induce aberrant DNA-methylation changes and hence increase cancer risk and cancer disparities (discussed in Sect. 10.6.7).

10.6.4 Hypertension Disparities

Although hypertension is commonly diagnosed in adults, it can be present at any age, including infancy. It is estimated that 5% of children have higher than normal blood pressure (pre-hypertension) with less than 1% of this population reported to have hypertension. There are gender and racial differences in blood-pressure measurement among US children. It has been reported that, among boys of average weight, AAs are significantly more likely to have high blood pressure when compared to other racial and ethnic groups, including Hispanics and EAs (Luma and Spiotta 2006). However, for boys who are overweight or obese, Hispanic boys ranked at the top, followed by AA boys as having higher blood pressure in comparison with EA boys. Among girls of normal weight, AA and Hispanic girls are reported to have higher incidence of prehypertension when compared to EA girls, and although AA girls have higher blood pressure than EA girls, the difference becomes insignificant when variables such as body mass are taken into account (Rosner et al. 2009). A recent report indicates that AA children with high blood pressure are more associated with increased risk to hypertension and high prevalence of obesity than EA children (Brady et al. 2010). There is a general trend for youths with hypertension to have their disease tracked into adulthood. Several risk factors have been identified as associated with increased risk of hypertension, including premature birth, very-low-birth weight, congenital heart disease, obesity, kidney disease, tobacco smoking, and illicit-drug use (steroids, cocaine, etc.) as well as a family history of hypertension (Chobanian et al. 2003).

There is on-going debate between nature and nurture and their roles in disease prevalence that affects AAs and more recent members of the African diaspora in the USA. Are genetic factors more prominent in explaining higher disease risk in AA population or is it rather environmental factors such socio-economic behavioral or life-style risks that explain health disparities in the AA population? One argument in support for both gene-environmental interaction and the difference in rates of hypertension and diabetes in recent members of the African diaspora in the USA and AA populations who are descendants of slaves (more than 400-years ago) is that the novel environments encountered in the African diaspora triggered expression of certain genetic variations quiescent in Africa (Daniel and Rotimi 2003). If genetic factors do explain the increased prevalence of hypertension, HIV/AIDs, diabetes, obesity, and cancer among AAs in the USA, then individuals of African descent living outside the USA should also have increased prevalence of these diseases. However, the prevalence of these conditions is much lower for those of African descent living outside the USA (Cooper et al. 1997b; Woodcock et al. 2001). Thus, for certain diseases, such as hypertension, HIV/AIDs, diabetes, and obesity, and certain types of cancer (non-communicable), there might be a strong environmental component, such as diet, chronic societal stress, segregation of low-SES AAs in poor neighborhoods, and environmental exposures that are not common to Africans on the African continent, whereas such environmental factors would give risk to higher incidence and mortality from hypertension in the US population (Forrester et al. 1998; Kaufman et al. 1999).

Despite the high prevalence of hypertension among individuals of African descent living in the USA, hypertension was not considered a major health risk among individuals in sub-Saharan African until recently (Unwin et al. 2001). The prevalence of complex diseases including hypertension is on the rise on the African continent, which has coincided with the adaptation of urbanization and a sedentary life style, as well as Western dietary life styles, supporting strong environmental risk factors for the increased incidence of hypertension, diabetes, and cancer. One study that investigated hypertension incidence in rural and urban places in Nigeria and Cameroon reported that the incidence of hypertension was 15–20%, and an even higher incidence rate, as high as 20–33%, in Tanzania (Cooper et al. 1997a). In all analyses, the prevalence of hypertension is much higher in urban areas when compared with rural areas, with African women having the highest prevalence of hypertension. These findings confirm the increased prevalence of hypertension in sub-Saharan Africa, especially in urban areas. There are also reports that indicate genetic variations are associated with differential susceptibility to hypertension in various African populations by geographic location, as well as between Africans living on the nascent African continent and AAs in the USA. One study noted that the degree of heritability ranges 45–68% in those of African descent living in sub-Saharan Africa (Gu et al. 1998; Rotimi et al. 1999).

Genetic variation in renin-angiotensin system has been implicated in hypertension. The renin-angiotensin system is a hormonal mechanism whose normal physiological role is to regulate plasma sodium concentration and arterial blood pressure. A major enzyme in the renin-angiotensin pathway is the angiotensin converting enzyme (ACE) responsible for activating angiotensin I and II (AGTI and AGTII) from angiotensinogen (discussed in Chap. 2). Observations reports 67 and 77% heritability of ACE and AGTII variants respectively in the Nigeria population in comparison with 18% heritability of both genetic variants in the AA population (Cooper et al. 2000). The observation of a high prevalence of hypertension in AAs, who have a low frequency of genetic heritability when compared to those of African descent who live in their native African country, with high heritability in genetic variants but low incidence of hypertension further highlights the importance of environmental component in the observed variability across populations and among individuals with regards to the prevalence to hypertension. Thus it is possible to differentiate genetic from environmental risk factors for these diseases.

10.6.5 Cardiovascular Disease Disparities

Cardiovascular diseases (CVDs) have strong genetic and environmental components in the disease etiology. There is abundant published evidence of the fetal origins of CVDs that has been discussed throughout this book. For instance, Barker's hypothesis of the fetal origins to CVDs has been mentioned in Chaps. 2 and 3, and this hypothesis suggests that the in utero environment, such as malnutrition and prenatal exposures to stress, is significantly associated with increased risk of CVDs and other diseases in adulthood (Kuzawa and Adair 2003; Prentice and Moore 2005). This observation suggests that early-life environmental exposures to under-nutrition or stress have long-term impact on adverse health including CVDs. In addition to diet and stress, other behavioral factors that are associated with CVD risk include a sedentary life style and tobacco smoking. Genetic predisposition and/or common environmental exposures in families with a history of CVDs have been suggested for increased risk of CVDs.

Several reports suggest that genetic factors are important contributors in the association of birth weight and CVD risk. Studies in monozygotic- and dizygotic-twin pairs give an opportunity to assess the role of environmental versus genetic contributions to disease incidence. For instance, because monozygotic twins have the same genotype, any differences between them would suggest environmental factors, whereas differences in dizygotic twins would suggest both genetic and non-genetic factors. One study carried out by Ijzerman et al. (2003) found that low birth weight in dizygotic twins, but not in monozygotic twins, was significantly associated with increased blood pressure (a major predictor of CVDs) suggesting a genetic contribution to the increased risk of CVDs.

In terms of genetic contribution and CVDs risk, one study observed genetic variance in fatty acid desaturase (FADs) genes to be associated with increased risk to CVDs (Chilton et al. 2014). In addition, higher frequencies of genetic variants in the arachidonic acid (ARA) gene are associated with increased risk to CVDs. The ARA encodes for a protein with biological function in immunity and inflammation. Certain dietary pattern such as high-fat diets can induce inflammation, and this is associated with multiple conditions including CVDs, diabetes, cancer, and asthma, suggesting a role for environmental (dietary) exposures and ARA expression (gene-environment interaction) in CVDs. Thus, the increase expression of ARA could contribute to CVDs disparities in AA populations, particularly in the presence of dietary fat. Other studies have suggested that dietary metabolism could use epigenetic modification (discussed in Sect. 10.3) to limit CVDs risk in later life, even in individuals exposed to in utero or early-life exposures to environmental diet, stress, behavioral, or other adverse life styles.

10.6.6 HIV Disparities

HIV infection disproportionately affects the most vulnerable in our society, such as the low-SES and poorly educated minority population, which has limited access to prevention and treatment services. Environmental exposures and behavioral, as well as life-style, choices such as cigarette smoking, alcohol abuse, and high-risk sexual behavior including multiple partners are risk factors for HIV infection. For instance, there are disparities in reported high-risk sexual behaviors, with AA male populations reporting higher risk behavior than EA or Hispanic men, which may contribute to the differential prevalence of HIV infection in various US racial and ethnic populations. The HIV infection impacts the immune response, and several cytokines have been identified to play a role in cellular responses to HIV infection, including human leukocyte antigen (HLA), regulatory T cells (Tregs), and the chemokine receptor (CCR). GWAS of the HIV-infected population has identified genetic variation and polymorphisms in HLA-class 1 region and CCR genes to be associated with 25% of the variability in viral load (McLaren et al. 2015). However, these studies were carried out using an only European patient sample, therefore additional GWAS are needed in the non-European-descent population to assess the link of genetic variants and viral load in other populations and whether genetic variants are associated with HIV disparities.

A role for aberrant epigenetic changes during microbial infection such as HIV infection has been suggested by several scientific findings, and this is described in Sect. 3.8. For instance, HIV-1 infection increases DNMTs expression, inducing hypermethylation and silencing of several proteins including interferon-gamma, thereby blocking host immune response (Ay et al. 2013). However a role for environment interaction and epigenetics changes in HIV disparities is not well established.

10.6.7 Alzheimer's Disease Disparities

Alzheimer's disease (AD) is estimated to be diagnosed in every one in nine American over the age of 65 year. Late-onset Alzheimer's disease (LOAD) is the most common cause of dementia and African-Americans and Hispanics are more than twice as likely to develop LOAD in comparison with their EA counterparts (Tang et al. 2001). Environmental factors in both prenatal and postnatal conditions, such as malnutrition, exposure to environment pollutants and toxins, SES, societal stress, and education, have been associated with LOAD.

One study that investigated the role of gene-environment interaction and siblings' differences to Alzheimer's risk noticed that the level of educational attainment correlated with APOE E4 variant and this was associated with cognitive decline, dementia, and LOAD (Cook and Fletcher 2015). In this study, Cook and Fletcher observed that individuals with college degrees and homozygous for the APOE variant E4 did not have declines in cognitive ability. On the other hand,

10.6 The Role of Gene-Environment Interactions in Disease Disparities

among high-school graduates, the APOE homozygous E4 variant lead to cognitive decline, even when other factors such as wealth, marital status, occupation, and health insurance are accounted for. A potential role for APOE in LOAD is the accumulation of amyloid plaques in the brain, a condition that is strongly associated with AD. Individuals with homozygous alleles of the APOE E4 variant are more prone to develop AD than individuals with other variants. Years of education correlates with the increased volume and metabolism of grey matter as well as strengthening neurological connections, thus higher education and years spent schooling may be protective against cognitive decline through altered brain processes and building cognitive reserves, rather than alleviating cognitive decline in old age through other processes such as higher SES and resources over the course of life. Since low-SES AA and other minority populations have significantly lower education attainment in comparison with their EA counterparts, education may be one mediating factor for higher prevalence of AD in these populations, particularly in individuals with APOE E4 variants.

Alzheimer's disease may also have fetal origins of disease risk. Even though Barker's hypothesis of the adverse fetal conditions applied specifically to CVDs, this hypothesis can also be applied to other diseases, including AD. Human studies investigating the effects of in utero adverse exposures and neurodegenerative diseases are limited. However, there are studies in rat models to demonstrate that exposure to a plethora of environmental factors, both in utero and postnatal early years, can adversely affect neurological diseases including AD. Animal studies have shown that in utero exposures to placental insufficiency, maternal malnutrition and hormonal exposure, and toxic exposure to heavy metals, including lead and mercury, pesticides such as organophosphates, and carbonates, as well as life-style choices, such as excess alcohol consumption, tobacco smoking, and drug abuse, are all associated with AD with early-life exposures having more damaging effects than later-life exposures (Modgil et al. 2014).

A potential epigenetic mechanism including DNA-methylation changes and histone modification, as well as non-coding RNAs, has been proposed to mediate the adverse environmental exposures and neurodegenerative diseases. For example, the DNA-methylation pattern in the human brain is responsive to environmental exposures, such as maternal folate deficiency or maternal hormones induce oxidative stress and inflammation (Weaver et al. 2004, 2005), and this could lead to increased risk of neurodegenerative diseases. Alterations in histone modification, including the accumulation of histone acetylation, is associated with age-dependent cognitive decline. In addition, the dysregulation of the histone modification enzymes, specifically HATs, lead to complex changes in the chromatin landscape and consequently alter gene expression profiles associated with cognition. Such negative changes exacerbate an individual's vulnerability to age-related cognitive decline. There is little information on the role of differential epigenetic changes and the prevalence of AD risk in various US populations. However, AA and other minority populations experience more of the adverse environmental factors described here, and this could potentially influence their increase susceptibility to AD.

10.6.8 Cancer Disparities

The accumulating and abundant data on the risk factors associated with cancer demonstrate that most cancers have underlying multifactorial risk factors, including genetic and epigenetics and their interaction with environmental risk factors. Risk factors that are commonly associated with cancer includes race (Shavers and Brown 2002), smoking status (Pfeifer et al. 2002), age (Issa 2000), family history of cancer (Johns and Houlston 2001), poverty (Ward-Smith 2007), alcohol consumption (Hashibe et al. 2007), and a high-fat diet (Popkin 2007). Studies that are intended to investigate the role of gene-environment interaction and cancer risks have focused on the role of genetic variations and environmental factors in population studies. However, most GWAS to elucidate the genetic variants associated with cancer risk have so far focus on the European population, and very few studies have looked at genetic variants in non-European populations including AAs.

One gene-expression analysis in AA and EA populations carried out by Zhang et al. (2008) investigated population differences in gene expression and associations with genetic variations using lymphoblastoid cell lines derived from individuals from African ancestry in comparison with individuals of European ancestry as carried out by GWAS on the same samples. The results from this study identified differential gene expression for several genes enriched in the immune system, such as inflammatory cytokines, receptor signals, vascular endothelial growth factor, and the signaling pathway in these population cohorts. This observation demonstrates that variation in cancer susceptibility genes in various populations may contribute to differential gene expression and, consequently, disparities in cancer incidence and perhaps mortality in various ethnic and racial groups.

As discussed in Chap. 2, there are several published reports of genetic variations in genes that encode for the cytochrome P450 family of enzymes with important biological roles in chemical carcinogens and drug metabolism. Differential frequencies in the genetic variations of the cytochrome P450 genes which affects enzymatic activity may contribute to differences in the metabolism of carcinogens found in tobacco smoke and alcohol, and, consequently, this may be associated with differences in tobacco- and alcohol-associated cancers, such as lung, pancreatic, and liver cancer in various racial and ethnic groups.

Components of one-carbon metabolism, including folate, vitamin B12, choline, betaine, methionine, and cysteine, are directly influenced by dietary intake, and large prospective studies have shown that elevated plasma concentrations of choline and vitamin B2 may be associated with increased risk of prostate cancer (Johansson et al. 2009), colon cancer (Schernhammer et al. 2011), and breast cancer (Deroo et al. 2013). Genetic polymorphisms in genes with biological roles in one-carbon metabolism pathways, including dietary factors such as folic acids, vitamin B, and S-adenosylmethionine have been demonstrated to contribute to cancer risk via dietary intake. For instance, genetic variants in MTR, MTRR, SHMT1, TYMS and SLC19A1 genes were associated with differential breast cancer risk in AAs in comparison with EA women, and the association appeared to be modified by dietary folate intake, suggesting that genetic variants of one carbon-metabolizing genes in the presence of certain diets could contribute to differences in breast cancer risks in AA versus EA women (Gong et al. 2015b).

Other studies have investigated genetic polymorphisms in genes that are responsible for the metabolism of environmental and endogenous carcinogens, such as tobacco smoke and prostate-cancer risk. One candidate gene family is the glutathione S transferases (GSTs) family of phase II detoxification enzymes. The so-called phase II enzymes play a role in transforming carcinogenic compounds and thereby assist in their removal from the cell. One member of the GSTs enzymes, namely, GSTM1, plays a role in DNA-adduct formation that can be caused by benzo (a) pyrene, the main by-product of tobacco smoke, whereas another member of the GSTs, known as GSTT1, conjugates with smaller molecules, such as epoxide during inflammation. Both GSTM1 and GSTT1 are expressed in prostatic epithelial cells, and thus the complete deletion of these enzymes could lead to accumulation of toxic compounds and subsequent DNA genomic instability, which is associated with prostate carcinogenesis. One study showed that deletion of both GSTM1 and GSTT1 was associated with higher risk of prostate cancer in AA men who smoked, suggesting that the gene-environment interaction between smoking and GSTM1 and GSTT1 deletion may play a role in prostate-cancer risk among men of African ancestry (Taioli et al. 2013). Thus genetic variation in GSTM1 and GSTT1, in combination with hypermethylation of GSTP1 under certain environmental exposure, may give rise to increased prostate-cancer risk in the AA population in comparison with the EA population.

Other studies have investigated the role of vitamin D metabolism and diseases, including colorectal cancer incidence and mortality rates because the prevalence of colorectal cancer is higher in the AA population in comparison with other racial and ethnic groups in the USA. The AA population has been reported to have lower serum vitamin D level in comparison with the EA population. GWAS has identified several genetic variants in vitamin D signal pathways in the EA population, but few such studies have been carried out in the AA population. Batai et al. (2014) identified two SNPs as associated with associated with the 20–28% difference in serum vitamin D levels in AAs and EAs, respectively. Other reports have investigated vitamin D receptor (VDR) polymorphisms and colorectal-cancer risk, and one report has suggested an association between one VDR SNP allele and vitamin D intake, indicating a VDR gene-environment interaction in AAs. However, there is no report of significant association between VDR polymorphisms and colorectal cancers in AA or EA populations.

Much of the differential genetic variation observed in various ancestral population are most likely the result of differences in long-term programming of gene functions, suggesting a potential role for epigenetic variations in addition to genetic variation for producing the phenotypic variation associated with health and disease states (Meaney and Szyf 2005). As discussed extensively in Chap. 3, aberrant epigenetic changes are responsible for a plethora of diseases, including prenatal predispositions and diseases evident at birth or infancy, as well as other diseases later on in life.

Epigenetic programming has been associated with life-time health outcomes, as exemplified by aberrant epigenetic changes in prenatal exposures to in utero adverse environmental factors, such as malnutrition and increased risk to CVDs and other diseases. One report by Needham et al. (2015) examined the role of epigenetic-environmental interaction by studying the association of several candidate stress and inflammatory markers that have previously been reported in rodents, primates, and humans to undergo alterations in DNA-methylation levels in response to psychosocial exposures. The study by Needham et al. was a large population-based study of US adults from various ethnic and racial groups including AA, EA, and Hispanic populations with information on their life-course SES. Overall, they found that low SES in childhood was significantly associated with increased DNA-methylation levels of several stress and inflammatory response markers. Because DNA methylation influence gene expression, differential methylation could alter gene expression and consequently physiological response, thus influencing the disease milieu and increasing disease susceptibility in low-SES environment populations and contribute to disparities in disease incidence, as well as mortality rates.

10.7 Summary

It is hard to imagine that pregnant women would knowingly expose their fetuses to environmental pollutants, yet many are unaware of the toxic effects of their environment and otherwise related to their SES that are responsible for harming potentially healthy offspring. Doctors commonly discuss risks associated with smoking, diet, and alcohol consumption with pregnant women, yet exposures to pesticides, BPA, and other environmental pollutants are overlooked. Doctors need to discuss the harms of these environmental pollutants in order to reduce fetal exposure. Yet, other in utero exposures such as estrogens levels are also linked to increased risk of later-life diseases, such as prostate cancer. Epigenetic programming is an important intermediate whereby these environmental exposures to both in utero and postnatally can induce aberrant alterations in gene expression and increase risk of adverse health conditions. Variations in environmental exposures, such as nutritional deprivation and chemical toxins in various ethnic and racial groups during critical developmental and growth periods, could result in epigenetic modification and consequently increased disease risk throughout the life span of an individual and even transmission to progeny and subsequent generations (Fig. 10.2). Additional studies are needed to fully elucidate the role of epigenetic-environmental interactions with regard to social, behavioral, and environmental exposures, as well as cross-generational studies of the interaction between epigenetics and social/behavioral/biological/environmental factors in families of alcoholic dependence throughout life and across generations, and how they influence each other.

10.7 Summary

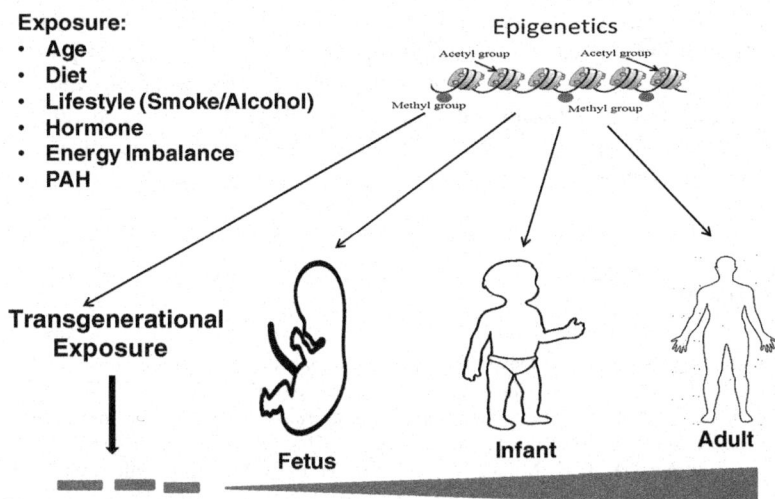

Fig. 10.2 The role of environmental-epigenetic alteration and health. Diagram demonstrates the differential toxic environmental exposures that can induce aberrant epigenetic changes to alter gene expression and physiological responses that can contribute to adverse health effects throughout the life span of an individual and perhaps transgenerationallz. Aberrant epigenetic changes increases as a function of age (indicated in *red*) (Color figure online)

While we cannot do much about individual genotypes, we can in theory reverse somatic epigenetic changes. Epigenetic processes, although stable, are not static and are potentially reversible and therefore amenable to therapeutic intervention (Szyf 2001). Therefore, studies directed towards epigenetic-environmental interactions could lead to reversal of diseases in which epigenetic changes are important, such as drug addiction. Drugs targeting histone deacetylation epigenetic machinery have been developed (Weidle and Grossmann 2000) and used for treatment of psychiatric disorders (Simonini et al. 2006). Knowledge gleaned from the fetal origins of disease may benefit adults who can potentially be at risk of diseases such as CVDs, diabetes, and cancer because of low birth weight or even the awareness of exposures to some in utero adverse condition that can contribute to early detection and/or tailored courses for intervention. This knowledge makes a pregnant mother's womb a critical target for prevention and should be a priority for public-health concern, if obesity and CVDs can be prevented before birth.

In addition to the important role of epigenetic programing and environmental interaction for adverse health outcomes, GWAS is uncovering the role of genetic variation and disease susceptibility or resistance, as well as drug metabolism. However, there is critical need to carry out more studies in non-European populations to fully understand the potential role of genetic polymorphisms and disease disparities. Advances in genomic research would lead to identifying patterns of behavioral addictions, life-style choices, and environmental exposures and their interaction with differences in genetic variation racial and ethnic populations. Such knowledge is fundamental to improving the understanding and explanation and observation of the prevention and management of illness, as well as promotion of optimal health and well-being. Future studies that integrate genetic variation, epigenetic changes, and environmental exposures will provide more insights into the role of gene-environmental interaction in the disproportionate disease burden among AAs and other racial and ethnic groups.

References

Adair, L., & Dahly, D. (2005). Developmental determinants of blood pressure in adults. *Annual Review of Nutrition, 25*, 407–434. Available from: PM:16011473.

Adair, L. S., & Cole, T. J. (2003). Rapid child growth raises blood pressure in adolescent boys who were thin at birth. *Hypertension, 41*(3), 451–456. Available from: PM:12623942.

Aguilera, O., Fernandez, A. F., Munoz, A., & Fraga, M. F. (2010). Epigenetics and environment: A complex relationship. *Journal of Applied Physiology (1985), 109*(1), 243–251. Available from: PM:20378707.

Agyemang, C., Beune, E., Meeks, K., Owusu-Dabo, E., Agyei-Baffour, P., Aikins, A., et al. (2014). Rationale and cross-sectional study design of the Research on Obesity and type 2 Diabetes among African Migrants: The RODAM study. *BMJ Open, 4*(3), e004877. Available from: PM:24657884.

Arenz, S., Ruckerl, R., Koletzko, B., & Von, K. R. (2004). Breast-feeding and childhood obesity–a systematic review. *International Journal of Obesity and Related Metabolic Disorders, 28*(10), 1247–1256. Available from: PM:15314625.

Ay, E., Banati, F., Mezei, M., Bakos, A., Niller, H. H., Buzas, K., et al. (2013). Epigenetics of HIV infection: Promising research areas and implications for therapy. *AIDS Review, 15*(3), 181–188. Available from: PM:24002202.

Batai, K., Murphy, A. B., Shah, E., Ruden, M., Newsome, J., Agate, S., et al. (2014). Common vitamin D pathway gene variants reveal contrasting effects on serum vitamin D levels in African Americans and European Americans. *Human Genetics, 133*(11), 1395–1405. Available from: PM:25085266.

Belinsky, S. A., Palmisano, W. A., Gilliland, F. D., Crooks, L. A., Divine, K. K., Winters, S. A., et al. (2002). Aberrant promoter methylation in bronchial epithelium and sputum from current and former smokers. *Cancer Research, 62*(8), 2370–2377. Available from: PM:11956099.

Bleich, S., Lenz, B., Ziegenbein, M., Beutler, S., Frieling, H., Kornhuber, J., et al. (2006). Epigenetic DNA hypermethylation of the HERP gene promoter induces down-regulation of its mRNA expression in patients with alcohol dependence. *Alcoholism: Clinical and Experimental Research, 30*(4), 587–591. Available from: PM:16573575.

Bonnelykke, K., & Ober, C. (2016). Leveraging gene-environment interactions and endotypes for asthma gene discovery. *Journal of Allergy and Clinical Immunology, 137*(3), 667–679. Available from: PM:26947980.

Brady, T. M., Fivush, B., Parekh, R. S., & Flynn, J. T. (2010). Racial differences among children with primary hypertension. *Pediatrics, 126*(5), 931–937. Available from: PM:20956429.

Brawley, O. W., Knopf, K., & Thompson, I. (1998). The epidemiology of prostate cancer part II: The risk factors. *Seminars in Urologic Oncology, 16*(4), 193–201. Available from: PM:9858325.

Breton, C. V., Byun, H. M., Wenten, M., Pan, F., Yang, A., & Gilliland, F. D. (2009). Prenatal tobacco smoke exposure affects global and gene-specific DNA methylation. *American Journal of Respiratory and Critical Care Medicine, 180*(5), 462–467. Available from: PM:19498054.

Brinkman, H. J., de Pee S., Sanogo, I., Subran, L., & Bloem, M. W. (2010). High food prices and the global financial crisis have reduced access to nutritious food and worsened nutritional status and health. *Journal of Nutrition*, *140*(1), 153S–161S. Available from: PM:19939996.

Bruin, J. E., Gerstein, H. C., & Holloway, A. C. (2010). Long-term consequences of fetal and neonatal nicotine exposure: a critical review. *Toxicological Sciences*, *116*(2), 364–374. Available from: PM:20363831.

Bruniquel, D., & Schwartz, R. H. (2003). Selective, stable demethylation of the interleukin-2 gene enhances transcription by an active process. *Nature Immunology*, *4*(3), 235–240. Available from: PM:12548284.

Burdge, G. C., Slater-Jefferies, J., Torrens, C., Phillips, E. S., Hanson, M. A., & Lillycrop, K. A. (2007). Dietary protein restriction of pregnant rats in the F0 generation induces altered methylation of hepatic gene promoters in the adult male offspring in the F1 and F2 generations. *British Journal of Nutrition*, *97*(3), 435–439. Available from: PM:17313703.

Buss, C., Davis, E. P., Muftuler, L. T., Head, K., & Sandman, C. A. (2010). High pregnancy anxiety during mid-gestation is associated with decreased gray matter density in 6–9-year-old children. *Psychoneuroendocrinology*, *35*(1) 141–153. Available from: PM:19674845.

Busse, W. W., & Lemanske, R. F., Jr. (2001). Asthma. *New England Journal of Medicine*, *344*(5), 350–362. Available from: PM:11172168.

Chen, E., Chim, L. S., Strunk, R. C., & Miller, G. E. (2007). The role of the social environment in children and adolescents with asthma. *American Journal of Respiratory and Critical Care Medicine*, *176*(7), 644–649. Available from: PM:17556714.

Chen, E., Fisher, E. B., Bacharier, L. B., & Strunk, R. C. (2003). Socioeconomic status, stress, and immune markers in adolescents with asthma. *Psychosomatic Medicine*, *65*(6), 984–992. Available from: PM:14645776.

Chen, E., Hanson, M. D., Paterson, L. Q., Griffin, M. J., Walker, H. A., & Miller, G. E. (2006). Socioeconomic status and inflammatory processes in childhood asthma: the role of psychological stress. *Journal of Allergy and Clinical Immunology*, *117*(5), 1014–1020. Available from: PM:16675327.

Chen, E., Miller, G. E., Walker, H. A., Arevalo, J. M., Sung, C. Y., & Cole, S. W. (2009). Genome-wide transcriptional profiling linked to social class in asthma. *Thorax*, *64*(1), 38–43. Available from: PM:19001005.

Chen, Y., Ozturk, N. C., & Zhou, F. C. (2013). DNA methylation program in developing hippocampus and its alteration by alcohol. *PLoS ONE*, *8*(3), e60503. Available from: PM:23544149.

Chilton, F. H., Murphy, R. C., Wilson, B. A., Sergeant, S., Ainsworth, H., Seeds, M. C., et al. (2014). Diet-gene interactions and PUFA metabolism: a potential contributor to health disparities and human diseases. *Nutrients*, *6*(5), 1993–2022. Available from: PM:24853887.

Chobanian, A. V., Bakris, G. L., Black, H. R., Cushman, W. C., Green, L. A., Izzo, J. L., Jr., et al. (2003). Seventh report of the joint national committee on prevention, detection, evaluation, and treatment of high blood pressure. *Hypertension*, *42*(6), 1206–1252. Available from: PM:14656957.

Choi, S. W., & Friso, S. (2010). Epigenetics: A new bridge between nutrition and health. *Advances in Nutrition: An International Review Journal*, *1*(1), 8–16. Available from: PM:22043447.

Coffey, D. S. (2001). Similarities of prostate and breast cancer: Evolution, diet, and estrogens. *Urology*, *57*(4 Suppl 1), 31–38. Available from: PM:11295592.

Cole, S. W., Hawkley, L. C., Arevalo, J. M., Sung, C. Y., Rose, R. M., & Cacioppo, J. T. (2007). Social regulation of gene expression in human leukocytes. *Genome Biology*, *8*(9), R189. Available from: PM:17854483.

Cook, C. J., & Fletcher, J. M. (2015). Can education rescue genetic liability for cognitive decline? *Social Science & Medicine*, *127*, 159–170. Available from: PM:25074513.

Cooper, R., Rotimi, C., Ataman, S., McGee, D., Osotimehin, B., Kadiri, S., et al. (1997a). The prevalence of hypertension in seven populations of West African origin. *American Journal of Public Health*, *87*(2), 160–168. Available from: PM:9103091.

Cooper, R. S., Guo, X., Rotimi, C. N., Luke, A., Ward, R., Adeyemo, A., et al. (2000). Heritability of angiotensin-converting enzyme and angiotensinogen: A comparison of US blacks and Nigerians. *Hypertension, 35*(5), 1141–1147. Available from: PM:10818078.

Cooper, R. S., Rotimi, C. N., Kaufman, J. S., Owoaje, E. E., Fraser, H., Forrester, T., et al. (1997b). Prevalence of NIDDM among populations of the African diaspora. *Diabetes Care, 20* (3), 343–348. Available from: PM:9051385.

Coulon, S. M., Wilson, D. K., Van Horn, M. L., Hand, G. A., & Kresovich, S. (2016). The Association of Neighborhood Gene-Environment Susceptibility with Cortisol and Blood Pressure in African-American Adults. *Annals of Behavioral Medicine, 50*(1), 98–107. Available from: PM:26685668.

Daniel, H. I., & Rotimi, C. N. (2003). Genetic epidemiology of hypertension: An update on the African diaspora. *Ethnicity and Disease, 13*(2 Suppl 2), S53–S66. Available from: PM:13677415.

Davis, E. P., Glynn, L. M., Waffarn, F., & Sandman, C. A. (2011). Prenatal maternal stress programs infant stress regulation. *Journal of Child Psychology and Psychiatry, 52*(2), 119–129. Available from: PM:20854366.

Deroo, L. A., Bolick, S. C., Xu, Z., Umbach, D. M., Shore, D., Weinberg, C. R., et al. (2013). Global DNA methylation and one-carbon metabolism gene polymorphisms and the risk of breast cancer in the Sister Study. *Carcinogenesis.* Available from: PM:24130171.

Duthie, S. J. (2011). Epigenetic modifications and human pathologies: Cancer and CVD. *Proceedings of the Nutrition Society, 70*(1), 47–56. Available from: PM:21067630.

Ehrlich, M. (2002). DNA hypomethylation, cancer, the immunodeficiency, centromeric region instability, facial anomalies syndrome and chromosomal rearrangements. *Journal of Nutrition, 132*(8 Suppl), 2424S–2429S. Available from: PM:12163705.

Falek, P. R., Ben-Sasson, S. Z., & Ariel, M. (2000). Correlation between DNA methylation and murine IFN-gamma and IL-4 expression. *Cytokine, 12*(3), 198–206. Available from: PM:10704246.

Fan, Z., Lipsitz, S., Egan, B., & Lackland, D. (2000). The impact of birth weight on the racial disparity of end-stage renal disease. *Annals of Epidemiology, 10*(7), 459. Available from: PM:11018370.

Feil, R., & Fraga, M. F. (2011). Epigenetics and the environment: Emerging patterns and implications. *Nature Reviews Genetics, 13*(2), 97–109. Available from: PM:22215131.

Fisher, P. A., Lester, B. M., DeGarmo, D. S., Lagasse, L. L., Lin, H., Shankaran, S., et al. (2011). The combined effects of prenatal drug exposure and early adversity on neurobehavioral disinhibition in childhood and adolescence. *Development and Psychopathology, 23*(3), 777–788. Available from: PM:21756431.

Fitzpatrick, D. R., Shirley, K. M., & Kelso, A. (1999). Cutting edge: Stable epigenetic inheritance of regional IFN-gamma promoter demethylation in CD44highCD8+ T lymphocytes. *The Journal of Immunology, 162*(9), 5053–5057. Available from: PM:10227972.

Forrester, T., Cooper, R. S., & Weatherall, D. (1998). Emergence of Western diseases in the tropical world: The experience with chronic cardiovascular diseases. *British Medical Bulletin, 54*(2), 463–473. Available from: PM:9830210.

Fowler, A. K., Hewetson, A., Agrawal, R. G., Dagda, M., Dagda, R., Moaddel, R., et al. (2012). Alcohol-induced one-carbon metabolism impairment promotes dysfunction of DNA base excision repair in adult brain. *Journal of Biological Chemistry, 287*(52), 43533–43542. Available from: PM:23118224.

Francis, D., Diorio, J., Liu, D., & Meaney, M. J. (1999). Nongenomic transmission across generations of maternal behavior and stress responses in the rat. *Science, 286*(5442), 1155–1158. Available from: PM:10550053.

Fuller, K. E. (2000). Low birth-weight infants: The continuing ethnic disparity and the interaction of biology and environment. *Ethnicity & Disease, 10*(3), 432–445. Available from: PM:11110360.

Gern, J. E., Lemanske, R. F., Jr., & Busse, W. W. (1999). Early life origins of asthma. *Journal of Clinical Investigation, 104*(7), 837–843. Available from: PM:10510321.

References

Godfrey, K. M., & Barker, D. J. (2000). Fetal nutrition and adult disease. *American Journal of Clinical Nutrition*, *71*(5 Suppl), 1344S–1352S. Available from: PM:10799412.

Godfrey, K. M., Sheppard, A., Gluckman, P. D., Lillycrop, K. A., Burdge, G. C., McLean, C., et al. (2011). Epigenetic gene promoter methylation at birth is associated with child's later adiposity. *Diabetes*, *60*(5), 1528–1534. Available from: PM:21471513.

Gong, Z., Yao, S., Zirpoli, G., David Cheng, T. Y., Roberts, M., Khoury, T., et al. (2015a). Genetic variants in one-carbon metabolism genes and breast cancer risk in European American and African American women. *International Journal of Cancer*, *137*(3), 666–677. Available from: PM:25598430.

Gong, Z., Yao, S., Zirpoli, G., David Cheng, T. Y., Roberts, M., Khoury, T., et al. (2015b). Genetic variants in one-carbon metabolism genes and breast cancer risk in European American and African American women. *International Journal of Cancer*. Available from: PM:25598430.

Gonzalgo, M. L., Liang, G., Spruck, C. H., III, Zingg, J. M., Rideout, W. M., III, & Jones, P. A. (1997). Identification and characterization of differentially methylated regions of genomic DNA by methylation-sensitive arbitrarily primed PCR. *Cancer Research*, *57*(4), 594–599. Available from: PM:9044832.

Gu, C., Borecki, I., Gagnon, J., Bouchard, C., Leon, A. S., Skinner, J. S., et al. (1998). Familial resemblance for resting blood pressure with particular reference to racial differences: Preliminary analyses from the HERITAGE Family Study. *Human Biology*, *70*(1), 77–90. Available from: PM:9489236.

Gunnar, M. R., Tout, K., de Haan, M., Pierce, S., & Stansbury, K. (1997). Temperament, social competence, and adrenocortical activity in preschoolers. *Developmental Psychobiology*, *31*(1), 65–85. Available from: PM:9222117.

Harlaar, N., & Hutchison, K. E. (2013). Alcohol and the methylome: Design and analysis considerations for research using human samples. *Drug and Alcohol Dependence*. Available from: PM:23968814.

Harrison, M., & Langley-Evans, S. C. (2009). Intergenerational programming of impaired nephrogenesis and hypertension in rats following maternal protein restriction during pregnancy. *British Journal of Nutrition*, *101*(7), 1020–1030. Available from: PM:18778527.

Hashibe, M., Brennan, P., Benhamou, S., Castellsague, X., Chen, C., Curado, M. P., et al. (2007). Alcohol drinking in never users of tobacco, cigarette smoking in never drinkers, and the risk of head and neck cancer: Pooled analysis in the International Head and Neck Cancer Epidemiology Consortium. *Journal of the National Cancer Institute*, *99*(10), 777–789. Available from: PM:17505073.

Heijmans, B. T., Tobi, E. W., Stein, A. D., Putter, H., Blauw, G. J., Susser, E. S., et al. (2008). Persistent epigenetic differences associated with prenatal exposure to famine in humans. *Proceedings of the National Academy of Sciences of the United States of America*, *105*(44), 17046–17049. Available from: PM:18955703.

Henderson, B. E., Bernstein, L., Ross, R. K., Depue, R. H., & Judd, H. L. (1988). The early in utero oestrogen and testosterone environment of blacks and whites: Potential effects on male offspring. *British Journal of Cancer*, *57*(2), 216–218. Available from: PM:3358915.

Ho, S. M., Tang, W. Y., de Belmonte, F. J., & Prins, G. S. (2006). Developmental exposure to estradiol and bisphenol A increases susceptibility to prostate carcinogenesis and epigenetically regulates phosphodiesterase type 4 variant 4. *Cancer Research*, *66*(11), 5624–5632. Available from: PM:16740699.

Hollingsworth, J. W., Maruoka, S., Boon, K., Garantziotis, S., Li, Z., Tomfohr, J., et al. (2008). In utero supplementation with methyl donors enhances allergic airway disease in mice. *Journal of Clinical Investigation*, *118*(10), 3462–3469. Available from: PM:18802477.

Huxley, R., Owen, C. G., Whincup, P. H., Cook, D. G., Rich-Edwards, J., Smith, G. D., et al. (2007). Is birth weight a risk factor for ischemic heart disease in later life? *American Journal of Clinical Nutrition*, *85*(5), 1244–1250. Available from: PM:17490959.

Hyman, S. E. (2009). How adversity gets under the skin. *Nature Neuroscience*, *12*(3), 241–243. Available from: PM:19238182.

Ijzerman, R. G., Stehouwer, C. D., de Geus, E. J., van Weissenbruch, M. M., Delemarre-van de Waal, H. A., & Boomsma, D. I. (2003). Low birth weight is associated with increased sympathetic activity: Dependence on genetic factors. *Circulation, 108*(5), 566–571. Available from: PM:12860905.

Issa, J. P. (2000). CpG-island methylation in aging and cancer. *Current Topics in Microbiology and Immunology, 249*, 101–118. Available from: PM:10802941.

Jackson, F. L., Niculescu, M. D., & Jackson, R. T. (2013). Conceptual shifts needed to understand the dynamic interactions of genes, environment, epigenetics, social processes, and behavioral choices. *American Journal of Public Health, 103*(Suppl 1), S33–S42. Available from: PM:23927503.

Jensen, C. B., Storgaard, H., Madsbad, S., Richter, E. A., & Vaag, A. A. (2007). Altered skeletal muscle fiber composition and size precede whole-body insulin resistance in young men with low birth weight. *The Journal of Clinical Endocrinology & Metabolism, 92*(4), 1530–1534. Available from: PM:17284623.

Johansson, M., van Guelpen, B., Vollset, S. E., Hultdin, J., Bergh, A., Key, T., et al. (2009). One-carbon metabolism and prostate cancer risk: Prospective investigation of seven circulating B vitamins and metabolites. *Cancer Epidemiology and Prevention Biomarkers, 18*(5), 1538–1543. Available from: PM:19423531.

Johns, L. E., & Houlston, R. S. (2001). A systematic review and meta-analysis of familial colorectal cancer risk. *The American Journal of Gastroenterology, 96*(10), 2992–3003. Available from: PM:11693338.

Kaelin, W. G., Jr., & McKnight, S. L. (2013). Influence of metabolism on epigenetics and disease. *Cell, 153*(1), 56–69. Available from: PM:23540690.

Kauffmann, F., & Demenais, F. (2012). Gene-environment interactions in asthma and allergic diseases: Challenges and perspectives. *Journal of Allergy and Clinical Immunology, 130*(6), 1229–1240. Available from: PM:23195523.

Kaufman, J. S., Owoaje, E. E., Rotimi, C. N., & Cooper, R. S. (1999). Blood pressure change in Africa: Case study from Nigeria. *Human Biology, 71*(4), 641–657. Available from: PM:10453105.

Kim, Y. I. (2007). Folate and colorectal cancer: an evidence-based critical review. *Molecular Nutrition & Food Research, 51*(3), 267–292. Available from: PM:17295418.

Koleganova, N., Piecha, G., & Ritz, E. (2009). Prenatal causes of kidney disease. *Blood Purification, 27*(1), 48–52. Available from: PM:19169017.

Konijnenberg, C. (2015). Methodological issues in assessing the impact of prenatal drug exposure. *Substance Abuse: Research and Treatment, 9*(Suppl 2), 39–44. Available from: PM:26604776.

Kuzawa, C. W., & Adair, L. S. (2003). Lipid profiles in adolescent Filipinos: Relation to birth weight and maternal energy status during pregnancy. *American Journal of Clinical Nutrition, 77*(4), 960–966. Available from: PM:12663298.

Kwabi-Addo, B., Chung, W., Shen, L., Ittmann, M., Wheeler, T., Jelinek, J., et al. (2007). Age-related DNA methylation changes in normal human prostate tissues. *Clinical Cancer Research, 13*(13), 3796–3802. Available from: PM:17606710.

Lee, J. U., Kim, J. D., & Park, C. S. (2015). Gene-environment interactions in asthma: Genetic and epigenetic effects. *Yonsei Medical Journal, 56*(4), 877–886. Available from: PM:26069107.

Li, C. C., Maloney, C. A., Cropley, J. E., & Suter, C. M. (2010). Epigenetic programming by maternal nutrition: Shaping future generations. *Epigenomics, 2*(4), 539–549. Available from: PM:22121973.

Liu, Y. Z., Pei, Y. F., Guo, Y. F., Wang, L., Liu, X. G., Yan, H., Xiong, D. H., et al. (2009). Genome-wide association analyses suggested a novel mechanism for smoking behavior regulated by IL15. *Molecular Psychiatry, 14*(7), 668–680. Available from: PM:19188921.

Luma, G. B., & Spiotta, R. T. (2006). Hypertension in children and adolescents. *American Family Physician, 73*(9), 1558–1568. Available from: PM:16719248.

Lutgendorf, S. K., Degeest, K., Sung, C. Y., Arevalo, J. M., Penedo, F., Lucci, J., III, Goodheart, M., et al. (2009). Depression, social support, and beta-adrenergic transcription control in human ovarian cancer. *Brain, Behavior, and Immunity*, 23(2), 176–183. Available from: PM:18550328.

Luyckx, V. A., & Brenner, B. M. (2005). Low birth weight, nephron number, and kidney disease. *Kidney International Supplement* (97), S68–S77. Available from: PM:16014104.

Marchand, L. L. (1999). Combined influence of genetic and dietary factors on colorectal cancer incidence in Japanese Americans. *Journal of the National Cancer Institute. Monographs*, 26, 1–5. Ref Type: Journal (Full).

McGowan, P. O., Sasaki, A., D'Alessio, A. C., Dymov, S., Labonte, B., Szyf, M., et al. (2009). Epigenetic regulation of the glucocorticoid receptor in human brain associates with childhood abuse. *Nature Neuroscience*, 12(3), 342–348. Available from: PM:19234457.

McKay, J. A., & Mathers, J. C. (2016). Maternal folate deficiency and metabolic dysfunction in offspring. *Proceedings of the Nutrition Society*, 75(1), 90–95. Available from: PM:26621202.

McLaren, P. J., Coulonges, C., Bartha, I., Lenz, T. L., Deutsch, A. J., Bashirova, A., et al. (2015). Polymorphisms of large effect explain the majority of the host genetic contribution to variation of HIV-1 virus load. *Proceedings of the National Academy of Sciences of the United States of America*, 112(47), 14658–14663. Available from: PM:26553974.

Meaney, M. J. (2001). Maternal care, gene expression, and the transmission of individual differences in stress reactivity across generations. *Annual Review of Neuroscience*, 24, 1161–1192. Available from: PM:11520931.

Meaney, M. J., & Szyf, M. (2005). Maternal care as a model for experience-dependent chromatin plasticity? *Trends in Neuroscience*, 28(9), 456–463. Available from: PM:16054244.

Mian, M. F., Pek, E. A., Mossman, K. L., Stampfli, M. R., & Ashkar, A. A. (2009). Exposure to cigarette smoke suppresses IL-15 generation and its regulatory NK cell functions in poly I:C-augmented human PBMCs. *Molecular Immunology*, 46(15), 3108–3116. Available from: PM:19592095.

Modgil, S., Lahiri, D. K., Sharma, V. L., & Anand, A. (2014). Role of early life exposure and environment on neurodegeneration: implications on brain disorders. *Translational Neurodegeneration*, 3, 9. Available from: PM:24847438.

Momparler, R. L. (2003). Cancer epigenetics. *Oncogene*, 22(42), 6479–6483. Available from: PM:14528271.

Needham, B. L., Smith, J. A., Zhao, W., Wang, X., Mukherjee, B., Kardia, S. L., et al. (2015). Life course socioeconomic status and DNA methylation in genes related to stress reactivity and inflammation: The multi-ethnic study of atherosclerosis. *Epigenetics*, 10(10), 958–969. Available from: PM:26295359.

Nelson, D. E., Jarman, D. W., Rehm, J., Greenfield, T. K., Rey, G., Kerr, W. C., et al. (2013). Alcohol-attributable cancer deaths and years of potential life lost in the United States. *American Journal of Public Health*, 103(4), 641–648. Available from: PM:23409916.

Nelson, W. G., De Marzo, A. M., & Isaacs, W. B. (2003). Prostate cancer. *New England Journal of Medicine*, 349(4), 366–381. Available from: PM:12878745.

Nestler, E. J. (2013). Epigenetic mechanisms of drug addiction. *Neuropharmacology*. Available from: PM:23643695.

Newbold, R. R., Padilla-Banks, E., & Jefferson, W. N. (2006). Adverse effects of the model environmental estrogen diethylstilbestrol are transmitted to subsequent generations. *Endocrinology*, 147(6 Suppl), S11–S17. Available from: PM:16690809.

Northrop, J. K., Thomas, R. M., Wells, A. D., & Shen, H. (2006). Epigenetic remodeling of the IL-2 and IFN-gamma loci in memory CD8 T cells is influenced by CD4 T cells. *Journal of Immunology*, 177(2), 1062–1069. Available from: PM:16818762.

Oberg, S., Ge, D., Cnattingius, S., Svensson, A., Treiber, F. A., Snieder, H., et al. (2007). Ethnic differences in the association of birth weight and blood pressure: The Georgia cardiovascular twin study. *American Journal of Hypertensions*, 20(12), 1235–1241. Available from: PM:18047911.

Painter, R. C., Osmond, C., Gluckman, P., Hanson, M., Phillips, D. I., & Roseboom, T. J. (2008). Transgenerational effects of prenatal exposure to the Dutch famine on neonatal adiposity and health in later life. *BJOG: An International Journal of Obstetrics & Gynaecology, 115*(10), 1243–1249. Available from: PM:18715409.

Painter, R. C., Roseboom, T. J., & Bleker, O. P. (2005). Prenatal exposure to the Dutch famine and disease in later life: An overview. *Reproductive Toxicology, 20*(3), 345–352. Available from: PM:15893910.

Pandey, S. C., Ugale, R., Zhang, H., Tang, L., & Prakash, A. (2008). Brain chromatin remodeling: A novel mechanism of alcoholism. *Journal of Neuroscience, 28*(14), 3729–3737. Available from: PM:18385331.

Paneth, N., Ahmed, F., & Stein, A. D. (1996). Early nutritional origins of hypertension: A hypothesis still lacking support. *Journal of Hypertensions. Supplement: Official Journal of the International Society of Hypertension, 14*(5), S121–S129. Available from: PM:9120669.

Pawlby, S., Hay, D. F., Sharp, D., Waters, C. S., & O'Keane, V. (2009). Antenatal depression predicts depression in adolescent offspring: Prospective longitudinal community-based study. *Journal of Affective Disorders, 113*(3), 236–243. Available from: PM:18602698.

Pembrey, M. E. (2010). Male-line transgenerational responses in humans. *Human Fertility (Cambridge), 13*(4), 268–271. Available from: PM:21117937.

Pfeifer, G. P., Denissenko, M. F., Olivier, M., Tretyakova, N., Hecht, S. S., & Hainaut, P. (2002). Tobacco smoke carcinogens, DNA damage and p 53 mutations in smoking-associated cancers. *Oncogene, 21*(48), 7435–7451. Available from: PM:12379884.

Pollard, I. (2007). Neuropharmacology of drugs and alcohol in mother and fetus. *Seminars in Fetal and Neonatal Medicine, 12*(2), 106–113. Available from: PM:17240208.

Popkin, B. M. (2007). Understanding global nutrition dynamics as a step towards controlling cancer incidence. *Nature Reviews Cancer, 7*(1), 61–67. Available from: PM:17186019.

Pratley, R. E. (1998). Gene-environment interactions in the pathogenesis of type 2 diabetes mellitus: Lessons learned from the Pima Indians. *Proceedings of the Nutrition Society, 57*(2), 175–181. Available from: PM:9656318.

Prentice, A. M., & Moore, S. E. (2005). Early programming of adult diseases in resource poor countries. *Archives of Disease in Childhood, 90*(4), 429–432. Available from: PM:15781942.

Price, J. H., Khubchandani, J., McKinney, M., & Braun, R. (2013). Racial/ethnic disparities in chronic diseases of youths and access to health care in the United States. *Biomedical Research International, 2013*, 787616. Available from: PM:24175301.

Radtke, K. M., Ruf, M., Gunter, H. M., Dohrmann, K., Schauer, M., Meyer, A., et al. (2011). Transgenerational impact of intimate partner violence on methylation in the promoter of the glucocorticoid receptor. *Translational Psychiatry, 1*, e21. Available from: PM:22832523.

Ragin, C. C., Langevin, S., Rubin, S., & Taioli, E. (2010). Review of studies on metabolic genes and cancer in populations of African descent. *Genetics in Medicine, 12*(1), 12–18. Available from: PM:20027111.

Rosner, B., Cook, N., Portman, R., Daniels, S., & Falkner, B. (2009). Blood pressure differences by ethnic group among United States children and adolescents. *Hypertension, 54*(3), 502–508. Available from: PM:19652080.

Rotimi, C. N., Cooper, R. S., Cao, G., Ogunbiyi, O., Ladipo, M., Owoaje, E., et al. (1999). Maximum-likelihood generalized heritability estimate for blood pressure in Nigerian families. *Hypertension, 33*(3), 874–878. Available from: PM:10082502.

Sandovici, I., Smith, N. H., Nitert, M. D., Ackers-Johnson, M., Uribe-Lewis, S., Ito, Y., et al. (2011). Maternal diet and aging alter the epigenetic control of a promoter-enhancer interaction at the Hnf4a gene in rat pancreatic islets. *Proceedings of the National Academy of Sciences of the United States of America, 108*(13), 5449–5454. Available from: PM:21385945.

Sankar, P., Cho, M. K., Condit, C. M., Hunt, L. M., Koenig, B., Marshall, P., et al. (2004). Genetic research and health disparities. *JAMA, 291*(24), 2985–2989. Available from: PM:15213210.

Schernhammer, E. S., Giovannucci, E., Baba, Y., Fuchs, C. S., & Ogino, S. (2011). B vitamins, methionine and alcohol intake and risk of colon cancer in relation to BRAF mutation and CpG island methylator phenotype (CIMP). *PLoS ONE, 6*(6), e21102. Available from: PM:21738611.

References

Schulze, M. B., & Hu, F. B. (2005). Primary prevention of diabetes: What can be done and how much can be prevented? *Annual Reviews of Public Health*, *26*, 445–467. Available from: PM:15760297.

Seitz, H. K., & Stickel, F. (2007). Molecular mechanisms of alcohol-mediated carcinogenesis. *Nature Reviews Cancer*, *7*(8), 599–612. Available from: PM:17646865.

Shavers, V. L., & Brown, M. L. (2002). Racial and ethnic disparities in the receipt of cancer treatment. *Journal of the National Cancer Institute*, *94*(5), 334–357. Available from: PM:11880473.

Shore, R. (1999). Rethinking the Brain: New insights into early development. Families and Work Institute. Ref Type: Journal (Full).

Simonini, M. V., Camargo, L. M., Dong, E., Maloku, E., Veldic, M., Costa, E., et al. (2006). The benzamide MS-275 is a potent, long-lasting brain region-selective inhibitor of histone deacetylases. *Proceedings of the National Academy of Sciences of the United States of America*, *103*(5), 1587–1592. Available from: PM:16432198.

Singal, R., Das, P. M., Manoharan, M., Reis, I. M., & Schlesselman, J. J. (2005). Polymorphisms in the DNA methyltransferase 3b gene and prostate cancer risk. *Oncology Reports*, *14*(2), 569–573. Available from: PM:16012746.

Starkman, B. G., Sakharkar, A. J., & Pandey, S. C. (2012). Epigenetics-beyond the genome in alcoholism. *Alcohol Research: Current Reviews*, *34*(3), 293–305. Available from: PM:23134045.

Sun, Y. V., Smith, A. K., Conneely, K. N., Chang, Q., Li, W., Lazarus, A., et al. (2013). Epigenomic association analysis identifies smoking-related DNA methylation sites in African Americans. *Human Genetics*, *132*(9), 1027–1037. Available from: PM:23657504.

Susser, E., Hoek, H. W., & Brown, A. (1998). Neurodevelopmental disorders after prenatal famine: The story of the Dutch Famine Study. *American Journal of Epidemiology*, *147*(3), 213–216. Available from: PM:9482494.

Szyf, M. (2001). Towards a pharmacology of DNA methylation. *Trends in Pharmacological Sciences*, *22*(7), 350–354. Available from: PM:11431029.

Szyf, M., Weaver, I., & Meaney, M. (2007). Maternal care, the epigenome and phenotypic differences in behavior. *Reproductive Toxicology*, *24*(1), 9–19. Available from: PM:17561370.

Taioli, E. (2008). Gene-environment interaction in tobacco-related cancers. *Carcinogenesis*, *29*(8), 1467–1474. Available from: PM:18550573.

Taioli, E., Sears, V., Watson, A., Flores-Obando, R. E., Jackson, M. D., Ukoli, F. A., et al. (2013). Polymorphisms in CYP17 and CYP3A4 and prostate cancer in men of African descent. *Prostate*, *73*(6), 668–676. Available from: PM:23129512.

Tang, M. X., Cross, P., Andrews, H., Jacobs, D. M., Small, S., Bell, K., et al. (2001). Incidence of AD in African-Americans, Caribbean Hispanics, and Caucasians in northern Manhattan. *Neurology*, *56*(1), 49–56. Available from: PM:11148235.

Taqi, M. M., Bazov, I., Watanabe, H., Sheedy, D., Harper, C., Alkass, K., et al. (2011). Prodynorphin CpG-SNPs associated with alcohol dependence: Elevated methylation in the brain of human alcoholics. *Addiction Biology*, *16*(3), 499–509. Available from: PM:21521424.

Thapar, M., Covault, J., Hesselbrock, V., & Bonkovsky, H. L. (2012). DNA methylation patterns in alcoholics and family controls. *World Journal Gastrointestinal Oncology*, *4*(6), 138–144. Available from: PM:22737275.

Torrens, C., Poston, L., & Hanson, M. A. (2008). Transmission of raised blood pressure and endothelial dysfunction to the F2 generation induced by maternal protein restriction in the F0, in the absence of dietary challenge in the F1 generation. *British Journal of Nutrition*, *100*(4), 760–766. Available from: PM:18304387.

Unwin, N., Setel, P., Rashid, S., Mugusi, F., Mbanya, J. C., Kitange, H., et al. (2001). Noncommunicable diseases in sub-Saharan Africa: Where do they feature in the health research agenda? *Bulletin of the World Health Organization*, *79*(10), 947–953. Available from: PM:11693977.

Van Guelpen, B. R., Wiren, S. M., Bergh, A. R., Hallmans, G., Stattin, P. E., & Hultdin, J. (2006). Polymorphisms of methylenetetrahydrofolate reductase and the risk of prostate cancer: a nested

case-control study. *European Journal of Cancer Prevention, 15*(1), 46–50. Available from: PM:16374229.
Vandenbulcke, L., Bachert, C., Van, C.P., & Claeys, S. (2006). The innate immune system and its role in allergic disorders. *International Archives of Allergy and Immunology, 139*(2), 159–165. Available from: PM:16388196.
Ward-Smith, P. (2007). The effects of poverty on urologic health. *Urologic Nursing, 27*(5), 445–446. Available from: PM:17990624.
Watters, J. L., Satia, J. A., Kupper, L. L., Swenberg, J. A., Schroeder, J. C., & Switzer, B. R. (2007). Associations of antioxidant nutrients and oxidative DNA damage in healthy African-American and White adults. *Cancer Epidemiology and Prevention Biomarkers, 16* (7), 1428–1436. Available from: PM:17627008.
Weaver, I. C., Cervoni, N., Champagne, F. A., D'Alessio, A. C., Sharma, S., Seckl, J. R., et al. (2004). Epigenetic programming by maternal behavior. *Nature Neuroscience, 7*(8), 847–854. Available from: PM:15220929.
Weaver, I. C., Champagne, F. A., Brown, S. E., Dymov, S., Sharma, S., Meaney, M. J., et al. (2005). Reversal of maternal programming of stress responses in adult offspring through methyl supplementation: Altering epigenetic marking later in life. *Journal of Neuroscience, 25* (47), 11045–11054. Available from: PM:16306417.
Weaver, I. C., Meaney, M. J., & Szyf, M. (2006). Maternal care effects on the hippocampal transcriptome and anxiety-mediated behaviors in the offspring that are reversible in adulthood. *Proceedings of the National Academy of Sciences of the United States of America, 103*(9), 3480–3485. Available from: PM:16484373.
Weidle, U. H., & Grossmann, A. (2000). Inhibition of histone deacetylases: A new strategy to target epigenetic modifications for anticancer treatment. *Anticancer Research, 20*(3A), 1471–1485. Available from: PM:10928059.
Weidman, J. R., Dolinoy, D. C., Murphy, S. K., & Jirtle, R. L. (2007). Cancer susceptibility: Epigenetic manifestation of environmental exposures. *The Cancer Journal, 13*(1), 9–16. Available from: PM:17464241.
Werner, E. A., Myers, M. M., Fifer, W. P., Cheng, B., Fang, Y., Allen, R., et al. (2007). Prenatal predictors of infant temperament. *Developmental Psychobiology, 49*(5), 474–484. Available from: PM:17577231.
Woodcock, A., Addo-Yobo, E. O., Taggart, S. C., Craven, M., & Custovic, A. (2001). Pet allergen levels in homes in Ghana and the United Kingdom. *Journal of Allergy and Clinical Immunology, 108*(3), 463–465. Available from: PM:11544469.
Woutersen, R. A., Appelman, L. M., Van Garderen-Hoetmer, A., & Feron, V. J. (1986). Inhalation toxicity of acetaldehyde in rats. III. Carcinogenicity study. *Toxicology, 41*(2), 213–231. Available from: PM:3764943.
Xu, M. Q., Sun, W. S., Liu, B. X., Feng, G. Y., Yu, L., Yang, L., et al. (2009). Prenatal malnutrition and adult schizophrenia: Further evidence from the 1959–1961 Chinese famine. *Schizophrenia Bulletin, 35*(3), 568–576. Available from: PM:19155344.
Xu, X., Sharma, R. K., Talbott, E. O., Zborowski, J. V., Rager, J., Arena, V. C., et al. (2011). PM10 air pollution exposure during pregnancy and term low birth weight in Allegheny County, PA, 1994–2000. *International Archives of Occupational and Environmental Health, 84*(3), 251–257. Available from: PM:20496078.
Yajnik, C. S. (2004). Early life origins of insulin resistance and type 2 diabetes in India and other Asian countries. *Journal of Nutrition, 134*(1), 205–210. Available from: PM:14704320.
Zhang, H., Herman, A. I., Kranzler, H. R., Anton, R. F., Zhao, H., Zheng, W., et al. (2013). Array-based profiling of DNA methylation changes associated with alcohol dependence. *Alcoholism: Clinical and Experimental Research, 37*(Suppl 1), E108–E115. Available from: PM:22924764.
Zhang, T., Guan, H., Arany, E., Hill, D. J., & Yang, K. (2007). Maternal protein restriction permanently programs adipocyte growth and development in adult male rat offspring. *Journal of Cellular Biochemistry, 101*(2), 381–388. Available from: PM:17230459.

Zhang, W., Duan, S., Kistner, E. O., Bleibel, W. K., Huang, R. S., Clark, T. A., et al. (2008). Evaluation of genetic variation contributing to differences in gene expression between populations. *American Journal of Human Genetics*, *82*(3), 631–640. Available from: PM:18313023.

Zhao, T., Wang, C., Shen, L., Gu, D., Xu, Z., Zhang, X., et al. (2015). Clinical significance of ALDH2 rs671 polymorphism in esophageal cancer: evidence from 31 case-control studies. *OncoTargets and Therapy*, *8*, 649–659.

Zingg, J. M., & Jones, P. A. (1997). Genetic and epigenetic aspects of DNA methylation on genome expression, evolution, mutation and carcinogenesis. *Carcinogenesis*, *18*(5), 869–882. Available from: PM:9163670.

Chapter 11
Race: a Biological or Social Concept

Abstract Race was once thought to be a real biological concept when anthropologists used study of the human skull as a way to justify racial differences and social inequality. Scientists no longer believe there is a biological basis to distinguish racial groups, rather, race is a social, cultural, and/or political construct wherein racial segregation has real consequences on health and health disparities. The biological basis of differential prevalence of disease susceptibility or resistance is due to genetic variations that exist in various racial and ethnic groups. Thus, race as a social concept can be used to categorize populations or groups based on disease susceptibility or resistance, and this offers promise for personalized/precision medicine as it applies to human health.

11.1 Introduction

A lot has been written about the historical basis of race, whether there is biological evidence in support of race or whether this is a social concept. The word race came into existence following the arrival of the first Africans to the European colonies in the Americas in the early 1600s. It is believed that the first Africans who arrived in the territories now constituting the USA had Spanish and Portuguese names, and these individuals were already familiar with European culture. The culture of Englishmen at this time was synonymous with a free society based on free labor, and historians believe that true slavery did not exist following the arrival of the first Africans to the Americas.

The Europeans were prejudiced towards these Africans however, because of their physical features, specifically their dark skin, and there was some forms of servitude, although these individuals were in general not considered as slaves because they enjoyed similar rights and privileges as other ethnic populations in the New World. However, there was no clear distinction between slaves and servants at this time, as the terms were often used interchangeably (Fredrickson 2002;

Morgan 1998; Allen 1997). Over a period of time, several laws were enacted that separated Europeans from Africans. The tendencies of the governing bodies in America was to categorize different populations based on physical features, such as notably skin color, which became markers of racial (social) status. As Virginia's governor William Gooch asserted, the assembly sought to "fix a perpetual brand upon Free Negroes and Mulattos" (Allen 1997). Under newly enacted laws, European settlers in America for the first time were now grouped together as "whites," regardless of ethnicity, socioeconomic status, or religious beliefs, rather than as Christians as it formerly was noted in public records. Africans and their descendants increasingly experienced restrictions on their rights and mobility and eventually a condition of permanent slavery was imposed on them.

Towards the end of the Seventeenth century and during the early eighteenth century, several amendments were made to the existing laws in the British colonies, including a law passed in 1691 that prohibited the marriage of Europeans and Negroes, Indians, and Mulattoes (Smedley 2007). Many of the decisions made by the sovereign powers who ruled the colonies, i.e., Europeans, was to manage and to subjugate the Africans as subordinate to the Europeans, including even the free Negroes, and laws were passed that prohibited Africans from voting. These changes to the status quo formed the basis of racism and the subsequent racial slavery that forced several millions of Africans from their native African continent to the Americas to work on plantations or as artisans, beginning the racialization that has persisted to this day. From the early eighteenth century on, race classification negatively categorized Africans as inferior to Europeans, and this provided a rationale for enslavement, creating unequal groups and imposing pejorative social identities on Africans. In the USA, slavery was eventually abolished in the 1860s, but "race" as a social concept and a basis for discrimination and prejudice, embodied in a social hierarchical system that treats Africans as inferior and relegated to the bottom rung and Caucasians as superior and placed at the top, has remained until today (Smedley 2007).

The past three centuries have witnessed the use of various scientific approaches, including the measurement of various aspects of the human body (e.g., the skull) and IQ tests as a means to measure human differences in intelligence, all in search of scientific evidence to support a biological basis for differences between Africans and Caucasians, as well as to justify maintaining the established status quo of racial categories that are, in reality, based on phenotypical features.

11.2 Anthropological Rationale for the Scientific Basis of Human Classification

The nineteenth and early twentieth centuries witnessed studies in physical anthropology, such as the attempt to equate measurement of the size of human skull with the range of human intelligence. The hypothesis was that Caucasians had larger skull (brains) and were therefore smarter, whereas Africans had smaller skull (brains) and therefore less intelligent. This resulted in the creation of a hierarchical rankings of the human race, with the Caucasian predecessor known as the Caucasoids referred to as the biological standard of normalcy at the top and the African (Negroids) at the bottom. Additional bases for these racial categorizations included traits such as skin color and facial features, as well as the shape and size of the head, body and underlying skeleton. In all, a total of five categories were created, with Caucasoids at the top, Negroids at the bottom and Asians and Native Americans, known as Mongoloids, as intermediates (Blakey 1996, 2001). Each racial category was believed to possess distinct heritable, physical, intellectual, and behavioral traits, however, as we now know, such distinctions based on biological evidence do not exist. Categorizing races based on the size of the skull and supposedly their corresponding intelligence meant that one race is endowed with superior traits that the others do not match, creating the stereotype that Caucasians are intellectually superior, whereas African-American are intellectually inferior. Physical anthropology has a deplorable history of racism because it created the ideology that justifies racial segregation, colonialism, eugenics, and class, as well as gender, inequality.

Several other studies have been reported that contradicted and challenged the dominant racial trend in early physical anthropological analysis. Studies carried out by T. Wingate Todd on macerated cadavers at the Western Research University in the 1930s measured and examined the growth and maturation of a number of children on the basis of which he suggested that environmental factors make an important contribution to the differences in the skull sizes between Africans and Caucasians and that there was no real comparative differences between their skull sizes. Moreover, he came to the conclusion that both racial groups have an equal potential for achievement (Blakey 2001) regardless of the size of skull. Other supporting data for Todd's observations came from the studies carried out by Todd's protégé, WM Cobb (Blakey 2001). Dr. William Montague Cobb, the then distinguished professor at Howard University, carried out anthropological studies on skeletal collections and living populations. He performed comparative analysis of various bones used in running and jumping from Caucasians and Africans, and he did not observe any significant differences between the two groups. He argued that the incredible athletic ability of African Americans (AAs), such as Jesse Owens, a four-time Olympic gold medalist, was the result of athleticism and not due to their cognitive intelligence or some form of endowed athletic genes, but perhaps selection through slavery. Furthermore, other socioeconomic and demographic factors would indicate that, rather than AAs being considered as an inferior race, their high adaptability to harsh conditions, such as social and economic barriers and racial segregation in the USA, would suggest that intellectual achievements of AAs are rather extraordinary (Blakey 2001). Unfortunately, many of these studies had little impact on the field of anthropology at that time.

Other studies reported greater skeletal size in the AA population in comparison to Caucasians, and these few reports appeared only in the African diasporic bioarcheological publications until the 1970s (Blakey 2001). The measurement of skulls meant to justify racial hierarchical ranking and the evolutionary basis of social inequalities with the focus on physical anthropology of Negroes would continue until World War II, except in forensic science, where the measure of skull is still in use for the identification of crime victims and missing persons. However, forensic anthropologists cannot determine race from bones, and their findings tends to be based on estimates and probabilities that rely on pre-existing information, such as self-reporting censuses (Konigsberg et al. 2009). Thus, analyses of continuous variations in skin tones, bones, and skull size do not confirm traditional race classification, and neither can the observed genetic diversity offer proof of, or support for, race classification.

In 1912, Franz Boas, known as the father of anthropology, collected and carried out cranial measurements on over 13,000 subjects from US-born children of immigrants and their European-born parents. His findings of differences in the sizes of skulls, comparing pre-adult children and their parents, led him to hypothesize that the human skeleton is largely plastic, practically shaped by the environment, which is, in turn, determined by social forces. He advocated that the sizes of human skulls could not be used reliably to distinguish race, let alone intellect. However, recent findings by two physical anthropologists, namely, Corey Sparks and Richard Jantz, who re-analyzed Boas data, have challenged his conclusion. In a 2002 PNAS article, Sparks and Jantz (2002) asserted that Boaz had measured the ratio of head width to head length for a cranial index, and, in many cases, the had compared pre-adult children with their parents, without taking into consideration cranial changes as an individual develops into maturity. The reanalysis carried out by Sparks and Jantz suggests an overall stability of the cranial index even under changing environments and circumstances and argue that the differences in the observed skull sizes between same-age related individuals born in Europe and American are negligible when compared to the differences observed between various ethnic and racial groups, suggesting that differences could be genetic.

A recent article published by Bejan and Jones (2010) has gone as far as to suggest that even athleticism is, in part, based on genetic traits, noting that some of the world's fastest athletes are of African origin. They suggests that athleticism could be reflected in the differences in body composition, whereby AAs supposedly have longer limbs with smaller circumferences, which means that their centers of gravity are higher compared to Caucasian of the same height. Others have suggested that there may be genes that encode for fast muscle switches in athletes of African descent, e.g., the likes of Usain Bolt, a Jamaican runner who currently holds the world record in the 100-m event. Yet, there are reports of the world's fastest long-distance runners originating from Finland; these are Caucasians in a different racial category compared to long-distance runners from East Africa, refuting the argument of preferential genetic traits among Africans that predisposes them to athleticism. Others suggest that Asians and Caucasian tend to have longer torsos, so their centers of gravity are lower and that having a higher center of gravity means an individual will hit the ground faster than someone with a lower center of gravity. On the other hand, Caucasian tends to have the advantage in swimming, where a longer torso enables faster speeds. Some view this new concept about bone density, more muscle in legs and athleticism as pseudoscience, whether there is any scientific basis to this observation remains to be proven.

11.3 Skin Color as Basis for Racial Classification

The nineteenth century definition of race was not based on skin color, but rather a social-hierarchy classification. Variation in skin color is historically an adaptive trait that has been used to define a "racial trait" in humans. Skin color is an adaptive trait to environmental factors and interaction with human polymorphisms. Charles Darwin, the world-renowned evolutionist, observed that the variation that existed in human-skin color is an adaptive phenomenon to the environment, and he opposed the notion that this, or any other difference in physical features, could be the basis for distinguishing between human races (Darwin 1871). Darwin argued that differences between the races, such as color of skin, eyes, or hair, are the result of sexual selection with natural selection producing the gradient of skin-tones groups observed in the human race. As humans recently expanded within and out of Africa, they encountered novel physical and cultural environments to which they likely had to adapt by local natural selection. Interestingly, recent studies by Relethford (2002) suggests that the genetic variations that exist between various racial and ethnic groups shows patterns opposite to skin-color diversity. Relethford noted that the majority of genetic variation (craniometric measurements of 57 traits) exist within racial populations (approximately 85%), whereas only about 5% of genetic variation existed between different racial and ethnic groups. On the other hand, the variation in skin pigmentation was approximately 88% among various racial and ethnic groups, whereas only about 9% of diversity in skin pigmentation existed within any racial or ethnic group. Therefore, the discordance between genetic variation and the diversity in skin pigmentation cannot be used to support a biological basis for race classification based on skin-color traits.

Skin, hair, and eye color is the visible phenotype of human variability, whereas the genetic basis for skin, hair, and eye coloration are pigmentations produced by melanin, a biopolymer produced by cells called melanocytes. Skin color is the result of two contrasting forms of melanin: the darker eumelanin which is associated with brown/black skin phenotype and the lighter phaeomelanin which is associated with yellow/red skin phenotype. The phaeomelanin pigmentation is the result of a switching mechanism from eumelanin, a process catalyzed by the alpha-melanocyte-stimulating hormone receptor (MC1R). Melanin plays an important role in the protection of the human body from damage by UV radiation. Skin color highly correlates with latitude and UVR, and variation in skin-melanin production arose as various populations adopted diverse biological processes to handle exposure to solar radiation. Thus, the exposure to UV intensity is a predictor of skin color since people living at various latitudes adapted to their environmental UV intensity. People living near the equator have darker skin to absorb UV radiation, whereas people at higher altitude have lighter skin. While several hypotheses have been postulated to explain variations in skin color, dark-skin pigmentation is an adaptive trait in high UV environments in order to protect against the UV radiation damage to the skin DNA, if not protected by melanin. Light skin pigmentation is adaptation in low UV environments in order to make sufficient vitamin D, which requires UV radiation (Jablonski and Chaplin 2010). Vitamin D is an essential nutrient in the body's metabolism of calcium. Vitamin D is not common in nature, and the body, with the help of UV, is able to synthesize vitamin D in the skin. The importance of vitamin D is recognized in that too much can be toxic to the body and is implicated in diseases including cancer, whereas too little of vitamin D can cause debilitating diseases such as rickets.

DNA sequencing and GWAS has identified a plethora of genetic variants in several genes that are associated with skin pigmentation. The selection to maintain darker skin in high UVR environment is expected to constrain pigmentation phenotype and variation in pigmentation loci. Of interest is the MC1R gene which shows less sequence variation in the AA population, suggesting a strong negative selection against any alleles that alters dark skin. There is evidence of differential variation in the MC1R gene in various populations, as shown for high variation of the MCIR gene in non-African populations living in low-UVR regions, whereas there is low variation of MCIR gene in African populations living in high-UVR regions (Norton et al. 2015), suggesting a strong selective pressure on the wild-type MC1R gene in high-UVR regions.

Interestingly, the Melanesian population from the islands of Melanesia (including the Solomon Islands archipelago), a region where UVR is high, are of dark complexion. The Melanesians appears closely related to Africans who also live in high-UVR regions than with populations with whom they share a common recent ancestry (East Asians). The East Asian populations live on the opposite sides of the world and are more likely to have high variations in their genetic makeup, even though they have skin color similar to the Melanesians. Despite experiencing high levels of UVR, the Melanesian population displays a wide variation in skin and hair pigmentation. What is even more unusual is the observation that some Melanesians have "blond hair" as evidenced in the Melanesian population from the Solomon Islands. It is unlikely that genetic variation could suggest very-fine-scale adaptation in UVR differences in the Melanesian population, rather the differences suggests that even in a high-UVR environment, pigmentation phenotype may vary, so long as it is maintained above a protective melanin threshold. Even though genetic variation in MC1R appears to have a strong influence on pigmentation in several non-African populations, this does not seem to be the case for the Melanesian population from the Northern Island of Melanesia. There may be other as yet unidentified pigmentation-candidate genes that may be responsible for phenotypic skin-pigmentation diversity in this population.

As people migrate away from the equator to higher latitudes where there is less UV radiation, the selective pressure on MCIR becomes less, as evidenced by the plethora of variation in the MCIR gene in non-African populations. At higher latitudes, UVB becomes important for the synthesis of vitamin D. Variation in melanin is important for the biological synthesis of vitamin D, as studies have shown that indigenous people in high altitude with diet rich in vitamin D have darker pigmentation. What different skin color teaches us about is adaptation; thus red/yellow skin people are more susceptible to skin cancer in low-latitude regions, and, on the other hand, dark/brown skinned people are more susceptible to vitamin D deficiencies in high-latitude regions, and they therefore need to supplement their diet with vitamin D. Skin color is not associated with human intelligence, but, rather, a product of evolution that is linked to vitamin D synthesis. The genetic variation that gives rise to differences in skin color is clearly not a reliable indicator of overall genetic diversity in various racial and ethnic populations, thus, there is no biological basis for the use of skin color as a defining physical trait for race.

11.4 The Human Genome Sequence and Race Classification

The completion of the human genome sequencing in 2003 has been revolutionary in understanding the sequence variation that exists among various racial and ethnic populations. It is now known that all human beings, regardless of race or ethnicity, share at least 99.5% similarity in their DNA sequences. Any two people from the African continent are more genetically diverse than any differences that exist with other racial and ethnic group such as Caucasians. The high diversity among Africans is because they are the oldest human population, whereas all other racial and ethnic groups migrated out of Africa. The genetic diversity in humans is extremely low, such that for any two randomly chosen individuals, they differ in about one in 1000 nucleotide pairs. Most of these variations are neutral, without any biological impact, but a fraction has biological function that can influence gene expression, physiology, and consequently phenotypic differences that exist between various racial and ethnic populations, including susceptibility and resistance to diseases. Overall, the vast majority of this diversity reflects individual uniqueness and not race (Templeton 2013).

As already pointed out, the vast majority of human genetic variation seen in various ethnic and racial groups does not support a genetic basis for race, rather the phenotypic manifestation of genetic variation reflects local adaptations, and, most of all, individual uniqueness. These genetic variations arise as a result of natural selection as seen for the MC1R genetic variation and skin pigmentation (Sect. 11.3), during DNA recombination, mutation, and adaptation due to distinct environmental pressures and diseases such as lactase persistence, malaria, and kidney disease. The difference in genetic variation in various populations is what gives rise to differences in phenotypic response to the same environmental exposures (Colilla et al. 2000; Morris et al. 2010).

Rosenberg et al. (2002) studied genetic variation in 1056 individuals from 52 populations using 377 autosomal microsatellite loci. They identified 93–95% frequencies of genetic variation within populations as compared to only 35% variation differences among major population groups. Using computer algorithms, they sorted individuals into five groups, namely: (1) sub-Saharan Africans; (2) Europeans, Near, and Middle Easterners, and Central Asians; (3) East Asians; (4) Pacific populations; and (5) Americans. They also proved that the genetic ancestry of most individuals came from just one group. This article was very widely cited and generated an interest in the scientific community because it was believed to give support for the idea of a biological basis for race. But, Rosenberg et al. (2002) did not make such an assertion, noting that, if they increased the number of groups beyond five, they would be able to expand the classification into smaller groups, demonstrating that, with enough genetic markers, it is possible to discriminate most local human populations from one another. Thus, while the genetic differences alone do not mean that any of these groups are races, it indicates that genetic variations can give information about disease phenotype and adverse drug response that varies across populations. Lessons learned from genetic data can be used to distinguish groups and allocate individuals into groups, and this can lead to more accurate prediction of health-related traits, such as disease susceptibility and resistance, as well as response to drugs.

11.5 Racism and Health Disparities

Racism is real even though there is no scientific or biological evidence to suggest that there are differences in intellectual characteristics and abilities between individuals or populations based on different skin or hair color, whereby one race is superior to the other. However, race has arisen as a result of social rather than biological constructs to categorize people into social groups, based on their skin color, common cultural heritage, or common language, or even religious beliefs which enforces an oppressive hierarchical system in which one race is dominant and subjugates other races to justify their racist ideology. Racism is a man-made institution that benefits the dominant group based on selective and arbitrary physical attributes, such as skin color, and discriminates against another race by oppression and restrictions, which adversely affect the lives and health of the oppressed race or ethnic groups.

Five pathways have been identified through which racism can have adverse effect on the health outcomes of minority individuals or populations that faces racism. (1) Barriers to economic and social opportunities. (2) Racial segregation of minorities into poor neighborhoods where there is pollution, toxic substances, and hazardous conditions. (3) Adverse psychological effects such as mental, physical, and verbal threats or making minority individuals who experience racism the victims of violence. (4) Targeted marketing of tobacco and alcohol industries, as well as easy access to junk food and psychoactive substances (licit and illicit drugs). (5) Lack of access to, or inadequate, medical care (Krieger 2000).

Racism affects every aspect of the racial minority population, and many studies have documented that racial and ethnic minorities who report experiencing racism are at a greater risk of experiencing poorer health in comparison with individuals who do not report experiencing racism. There are numerous reports to suggest that the long-term effects of racism may affect AAs' health and that racism in part may contribute to adverse health among US racial and ethnic populations, and hence create health disparities. Data from National Survey of Black Americans showed that perceptions of racism and racial discrimination were associated with poorer mental health (Jackson 1996). One cross-sectional study carried out by Kwate et al. (2003) investigated recent and the long-term effects of racism on health of 71 AA women recruited from an urban cancer-screening program. The study was based upon self-reported health in response to several racist events, including: unfair treatment; discrimination by colleagues, employer, professor, and physician; being called by a racist name; or accused unfairly. Results showed a strong association between racism and self-reported poor health, even when demographic variables, such as income and education, were accounted for. In this study, AA women who smoked and drank alcohol reported increased numbers of cigarette smoked and alcohol consumed, in response to racism. The study demonstrates that recent experience of racism was associated with the common cold, whereas the long-term experiences of racism were significantly associated with a life-time history of adverse health. Because this was a cross-sectional study, there may be biases in the self-reported data. A more accurate measurement would have been measures of allostatic predictors (i.e., endocrine measures, such as cortisol). Also, other factors such as insurance and generational wealth, not accounted for in this study, may have confounded the outcome. Nevertheless, this report demonstrates an association between racism and adverse psychological distress in AA and other minority populations, which supports other studies of the impact of racism and adverse psychological well-being discussed in Chap. 9. Overall, racial and ethnic minorities bear a disproportionate burden of mortality and morbidity as documented throughout this book, and racism is one important cause of the health disparity documented in AA and other minority populations. Other observations suggest that racism and low SES are the major contributors to health disparity in the USA. Thus eliminating health disparity cannot be realistically accomplished without addressing and undoing this institution of racism.

Racism operates not only at the individual level but also at the local, community, and state levels. At the local or community level, the segregation of racial and ethnic minorities into poor residential areas, such as inner city communities, where there is high concentration of poverty, environmental pollution, and violence, as well as high rates of exposure to infectious disease and limited access to healthcare resources, affects health. At the local or state level, policies influence the quality of education in poor communities, such that inner city schools do not provide the same quality education as do the suburban schools where high-SES families tend to live. Furthermore, there are limited job opportunities, and minorities may find themselves more often in low-paying jobs with fewer benefits and more hazardous working environments. Racial segregation also limits access and the quality of health-care resources, which all may contribute to the well-documented health disparities that exist between AA and EA populations (Ofili 2001). Racism may also be manifest as psychosocial factors (stress and low self-worth) that are linked with stigmas of inferiority (Williams 1999).

African-American and other minority communities are also heavily targeted by advertisements by the alcohol and tobacco industries, which are often designed to match the demographic make-up and SES of the community to encourage the alcohol and tobacco consumption or other licit or illicit drugs. In addition, there is easy access to fast foods, instead of fresh fruits and vegetable in such communities. There are also convenient shops where alcohol and tobacco smoke is easily available. The convenience and consequences of the use of alcohol, tobacco products, and illicit drugs as a coping mechanism against racial discrimination can help explain why the health- associated problems of alcohol use and tobacco smoke are so high in AA and other minority communities, with low-SES and less-educated AA individuals more likely to smoke and consume alcohol excessively.

11.6 Race Categorization and Health Disparities

If there is any biological difference between various races, then this would imply that destiny is written in our genes and everything is out of our control (the worse form of racism). Thus, one racial group would be endowed with intelligent genes and great skills, and this group would be the superior racial group, whereas the inferior group would have none of these traits. Clearly, there is no evidence or biological biases in our genes towards preferential endowment of intelligence.

Yet, we use racial categories to define ourselves, and we use racial categories to understand our culture, disease risk, etc. While we cannot seem to get away from using racial categorization, the use of race can better serve as surrogate markers for a group of individuals or populations at a higher risk of a particular disease, based on sharing certain genetic variations from genetic data, and this could lead to identify or characterize disease genes in order to improve disease detection and to develop more efficacious therapeutic drugs. At the same time, the diversity that exists among individuals belonging to one racial group or population, such as the AA population, clearly demonstrates that, to target one treatment to the AA population, underestimates the extent of true genetic diversity present within people of African descent.

Race is included in hospital patient's chart to obtain information about ethnicity, disease risk, and mortality rates by geographic and cultural groups. However, race statistics from hospital charts are based on self-identified race or ethnicity (SIRE), which is primarily sociocultural rather than a biological entity, and their use in genetic research is invalid (Cardon and Palmer 2003). Many AA individuals whose SIRE is African ancestry are often of admixture populations (AAs are estimated to have at least 20% EA ancestry), which can confound biological correlations with race. Nonetheless, there are some biological correlations with SIRE. Nowadays, the ethnicity of any individual can be tested by sequence analysis based on autosomal

11.6 Race Categorization and Health Disparities

ancestry informative markers (AIMs) that analyze for unique polymorphic markers with different frequencies in various racial or ethnic groups. When AIMs is used to check for the ethnicity of the AA population, the results support the genetic make-up of AAs to have admixture with the EA population.

The use of race in health-care can lead to the assumption that poor health has a genetic/biologic basis (although this may be the case for a few number of diseases), rather than social or political factors. A danger of the use of genetics as the major determinants of health disparities is that certain populations such as AA and other minority groups may be stereotyped as predisposed to certain diseases, thereby ignoring environmental factors that underlie increased disease prevalence and necessitating alternative solutions to bridge health disparities. For instance, the increase incidence of obesity and associated diabetes among people of African descent in the UK, Caribbean, and the USA, as well as in Africa, can be explained by changes in environmental exposures, such as poor diet and a sedentary life style, and this has no genetic basis whatsoever. In this case, the increased incidence of adverse health can be explained solely by social determinants that have been discussed throughout this book. Similarly, there is no genetic basis for a high incidence of alcoholism in Native American populations. Thus, trying to use a genetic basis to explain poor health in minority racial groups can stigmatize populations, who are already prone to adverse health outcomes, based on social determinants, behavioral/life-style choices, or other environmental factors. In other cases, adverse health such as increased incidence of hypertension in the AA population is associated with low SES, poor diet, and their interaction with genetic susceptibility loci. Yet, myriad epidemiological analyses continues to use race as the genetic variable in seeking to explain health disparities and, in so doing, takes attention away from what might be seen as racism (segregation, stress, poor food, and adaptation to environment). Despite the abundant evidence and the demonstrated importance of social determinants and environmental factors for adverse health in the AA population, there is still the tendency to use self-identified race as a predictor of disease outcomes in epidemiological studies. Race is still used even when the findings from epidemiological analysis points to social determinants, such as life styles and SES, to be significantly associated with disease incidence and mortality rates (Pappas et al. 1993), and scientist continues to interpret differences in health outcomes as indirect support for genetic position of race (Kistka et al. 2007).

Because race is a not a genetically meaningful concept, some scholars have opted to use the term ethnicity or population to describe various groups by their geographic or cultural identity. Others continue to use the term race when referring to the social phenomenon of historically constructed racial categories, but, for the sake of argument, this book uses both race and ethnicity to mean the same thing, a socially constructed category of different populations based on skin color or other phenotypic characteristics that has no biological implications, rather than a genetically justified criteria for classifying human genetic variation (Cooper 1986).

11.7 Genetic Variation and Race Categorization

Many GWAS have reported differential allelic variations in various racial and ethnic groups, refuting those who reject any genetic basis for the phenotypic differences in various races and ethnic populations. Indeed the studies carried out by Rosenberg et al. (2002) were able to categorize their study population into racial and ethnic groups, based on genetic variation that existed in this study cohort.

Being able to categorize populations into different racial and ethnic groups is important because it helps to identify disease traits in particular groups and how environment, as well as culture or behavior, can influence their health outcomes. For instance, certain disease phenotypes are predominantly found in one population compared to other populations, such as the Tay-Sachs disease, a fatal genetic condition commonly found in the Ashkenazi Jewish population. The Tay-Sachs disease is caused by a deficiency in an enzyme called hexosaminidase and leads to the accumulation of glucocerebroside in nerve cells, causing deafness and progressive blindness. Genetic screening for this condition has been available to the Ashkenazi Jews since the 1970s (Kaback 2001). Several thousands of people have benefited from screening for this genetic trait, including pregnant women, couples intending to start a family, and even orthodox Jewish men and women who are contemplating marriage are often advised to obtain genetic counseling about Tay-Sachs condition before developing a serious relationship. As a result, more than one million people have had Tay-Sachs-carrier testing, and this has decreased the number on Tay-Sachs births. Currently, less than five children are born each year with Tay-Sachs disease, in comparison with the more than 40 annual births prior to genetic screening.

Another genetic condition commonly found in the Ashkenazi Jew population is BRCA1 or BRCA2 germline mutation, which causes defects in DNA repair and is associated with increased susceptibility to breast, ovarian, and prostate cancers. Clustering of some of these cancers occurs in not only the Ashkenazi Jewish population but other European families, such that some women or men who come from high-risk families with mothers and sisters, aunts, and cousins affected with breast and/or ovarian or other cancers carry BRCA1 or BRCA2 mutations. Genetic testing for members of such families has led to prevention of cancers through life-preserving prophylactic oophorectomy and mastectomy.

While the Ashkenazi Jew population may be the avant-garde for population-based genetic screening for breast and ovarian cancer risk, Rubinstein et al. (2009) found that almost half of Ashkenazi Jews that tested positive for BRCA1 or BRCA2 mutations did not have any family histories of cancer. The absence of a family history confounds efforts toward presymptomatic carrier identification for prophylactic treatments (Rubinstein et al. 2009), thus, as yet, unidentified additional environmental factors must be taken into consideration for the identification of at-risk individuals who carry these genetic mutations and are likely to develop cancer. Ashkenazi Jews are now screened for 18 conditions, and this number is increasing.

A common autosomal recessive genetic disease often detected in people of African ancestry is sickle cell anemia (SCA) disease that has risen as a natural selection in response to malaria (discussed in Sect. 2.5.2). Individuals with the full-blown disease have their normal blood cells become "sickled" impeding blood flow and experiencing severe pain in their bones that, in some extreme cases, can cause death. There is genetic screening available for this condition, and, currently, it is common for men and women of African descent with a family history of SCA and who are contemplating marriage to obtain genetic counseling before developing a serious relationship. However, malaria is widespread in other areas outside of Africa, and non-African populations in these regions who have developed resistance to malaria also have the sickle-cell trait. For example, there is high frequency of the sickle-cell trait on the Arabian Peninsula and among the Indian population, despite SCA referred to as "black" disease.

Just as the SCA trait is common not only in the African population, Tay-Sachs disease is also not only common in the Ashkenazi Jew population, but is also found in the Gentile population in the Middle East. Thus, the genetic variants/adaptive traits that are associated with diseases point to geographic distribution of the underlying environmental factor for which it is adaptive. Putting labels and associating certain diseases or traits with one racial or ethnic group means that other groups with the same trait may not benefit from screening or treatment for the condition. For instance, by labeling SCA as a disorder found only in people of African descent means that large groups of AAs, Indians, or Arab who resides in the USA and suffer from SCA are ignored because they are the minority group. We see that the use of genetic variation as a biological basis to define race clearly raises problems, at least from the health perspective and will not warrant the full benefit of the scientific breakthroughs in genetic screening or prophylactic measures to minimize diseases in all susceptible populations. Perhaps a better way to define population categorization is one based on shared genetic or some adaptive traits. This will ensure that individuals with high-risk genetic profiles, not based on race or ethnicity can take full advantage of all known prevention strategies.

In the USA, where you live based on SES and health-care access may be a better determinant of health outcomes than race. This is because of the importance of environmental exposures and their interactions with genetic (variants) which underlies health disparities. Therefore, disparities in highly prevalent disease may help trace differential exposure to environmental risk factors that increase the risk of disease. However, if the relevant susceptibility variant is common to most populations and interactions with different environmental risk factors are ignored, the underlying causes of differential disease burdens may be overlooked, and effective intervention opportunities missed. On the other hand, there may be certain susceptibility variants that are disproportionately prevalent among persons of AA or EA descent, which, independently or in relationship to common environmental exposures, affect disease etiology.

Multiple GWAS for common diseases holds the prospect of uncovering all of the genetic variants that are associated with various diseases with differential prevalence in various races and ethnic groups. Technological advances, such as whole-exome and whole genome sequencing and discoveries of genetic basis for heritable diseases, can only increase public initiatives in genetic testing for various diseases and for the development of a battery of tests for the accurate prenatal and postnatal diagnoses of genetic conditions, consequently paving the way for the development of effective therapies for genetic conditions.

Genomics has the potential for early diagnosis of diseases. For instance, prophylactic therapy involves the prevention of symptoms before they occur. In order for such therapy to be effective, pre-symptomatic diagnosis needs to be performed. This means that a test has to be performed on an individual to determine whether they have a genetic condition before they develop any symptoms. One of the best known forms of prophylactic therapy for a genetic condition is for phenylketonuria (PKU). PKU is an autosomal recessive condition caused by mutations in the gene for phenylalanine hydroxylase, which is the enzyme that converts phenylalanine to tyrosine. Few physical signs of PKU are evident in a newborn baby, but, with the ever-increasing levels of phenyl-alanine accumulating in the body and with the absence of tyrosine, severe mental retardation results. A baby with PKU will, however, develop normally and have a normal life span if fed a diet very early in infancy that is low in phenylalanine and supplemented with tyrosine. Thus, both early diagnosis and therapy of PKU are mandatory if normal development is to occur. All babies in the UK are tested a few days after birth for PKU. A blood spot from a heel-prick is collected on a card (the Guthrie card) during a home visit and sent to a central laboratory where the phenylalanine level in the blood is measured. Babies whose levels are above a threshold are called in for further tests to confirm the finding. If the result is positive, the baby can be put on the correct diet immediately.

Pre-symptomatic diagnosis is now also possible for some inherited forms of cancer, such as breast cancer and colon cancer. For familial breast cancer, it is possible to test individuals with a family history of early-onset breast cancer to determine whether they have inherited one of the predisposing mutations. If they have inherited one of these mutations, then their risk of developing breast cancer is about 80%. In the event of a positive result, some women may opt to undergo a double mastectomy to ensure that they will not develop breast cancer. Likewise, individuals who have tested positive for colon cancer susceptibility mutations, such as p53 or k-ras, have elected to undergo a colectomy at the first sign of symptoms.

Knowledge from GWAS has several benefits in advancing medical care but also has the potential to exacerbate health disparities if the benefits are not realized equally among various racial and ethnic groups, or if the information is used only for research and treatment of rare disease or the information is used to discriminate and stigmatize the already disenfranchised minorities in society. There is also the concern for the misuse of genetic information or stigmatization of individuals with horrible diseases based on genetic testing. However, the success of whole-genome research is in the clinical setting, where findings from genomic research can be used not only in screening, but also for diagnosis and the development of efficacious therapies.

11.8 Race-Based Genetic Testing and Personalized Medicine

There is increasing understanding of the multifactorial and complex gene-environment basis underlying some disease etiology, as well as progression. In addition, GWAS is uncovering genetic variation associated with poor treatment response and/or increased toxicities found in some "high risk" groups. The observed differences in response to disease treatment in various ethnic and racial groups, as determined by variance in metabolic genotypes, suggests that we are ushering in the era of medicinal treatment based on individuals belonging to the same or different ethnic groups (Helgason et al. 2005). Thus pharmacogenetics is likely to contribute to improved, targeted drug treatment for individuals, rather than race-specific treatment. The goal of pharmacogenomics is to optimize the use of drug dosage and treatment that is driving a new era of drug treatment tailored specifically to individuals, instead of the current one-size-fits-all approach of drug therapy. Today, the prospect of personalized medicine with drugs designed to suit individual patient's genetic profile is considered to be just around the corner. Advances in pharmacogenomics would also reduce the number of people who die from adverse drug reaction each year.

For instance, complications associated with blood coagulation are responsible for the death of one million people in the USA annually, and one of the most effective anti-coagulants on the market is warfarin. However, warfarin has a very narrow therapeutic index and there is about 20-fold differences in sensitivity between different individuals and populations (Jonas and McLeod 2009). The differences observed in warfarin sensitivity are due to genetic variations in CYP2C9, a type of cytochrome P450 drug metabolizing enzymes and the VKORC1 (vitamin K-epoxide reductase) gene, which encodes for the enzyme responsible for reducing vitamin K to its potent and active form and which is also the target for warfarin. Genetic variants in CYP2C9 are present in 1–15% of the US population and results in 15–40% reduced activity of the enzyme, whereas genetic variants in VKORC1, which also reduces the enzyme activity, are more frequent in the general population, about 40% in the EA but much less in the AA population, about 12%. Individuals with genetic variants in CYP2C9 and VKORC1 may need lower warfarin doses as higher doses could lead to excessive bleeding that can even prove fatal.

Different frequencies in genetic variations of genes associated with disease risk, or drug metabolism and/or drug toxicity that are observed in individuals belonging to one population or different populations are driving the field of pharmacogenetics and personalized or precision medicine. An example of a drug that was specifically designed and reported to achieve efficacy in the AA population is BiDil. In 2005, the FDA approved a vasodilator heart drug called BiDil, which was specifically designed for the AA population with heart disease. BiDil was designed as a combined drug of two vasodilators: hydralazine hydrochloride and isosorbide dinitrate. Clinical trials for this drug were carried out in 1050 self-identified AA men and women, and the results showed a 43% reduction in mortality and a 39% reduction in risk of hospitalization against a placebo (Krimsky 2012). Three clinical trials showed clear therapeutic value in AA patients, and, as a result, the FDA approved BiDil as a secondary treatment for heart failure in self-identified AAs with heart disease.

While some in the scientific community viewed the approval of BiDil as a race-specific drug as great news and heralded an era of drug treatment driven by genetic knowledge of a particular group, others raised disapproval of a drug designed and targeted towards one particular population based on old racial category because there are no racial genes or clear genomic divide. Some question whether the success of BiDil with self-identified AA was a statistical accident or due to some unknown factor(s). Others questioned why additional clinical trials had not been done in non-AA populations to assess the efficacy of BiDil in other ethnic and racial populations. In addition, there were no genetic markers in the population samples involved in the clinical trials, thus BiDil is not targeted to detect any genetic variation with high prevalence in the AA population.

BiDil cannot be considered a pharmacogenetic drug target because its efficacy was not based differential genetic variants and high disease prevalence in one population as compared to the general population. For personalized medicine, drug efficacy is due to genetics and physiology of the patients, thus, for BiDil, even though it was effective, the premise for approving this drug was based on the misuse of human-race classification and questionable science. The controversy surrounding BiDil can be resolved if, for instance, there are high genetic variations with a high prevalence and increased risk of heart disease in AA populations that specifically respond to BiDil treatment. Although, BiDil remains a treatment option, there is no marketing effort to promote its use.

When it comes to the potential benefits and the economic opportunities of genomic research and race as regards to personalized medicine, there are varied interests in the private sector, pharmaceutical companies, economists, and policy makers. A marketing strategy for a population with unique health issues requires an understanding of factors such as human behaviors, cultural as well as psycho-social association, and how these factors are also impacted by political factors in order to design targeted and efficacious interventions. Clearly, there are biological contributions in health disparities, such that drug companies can manufacture drugs that can specifically target at-risk populations who would respond to the drug treatment based on genetic variations, whereas other industries can seize this opportunity to target the design of specific products for unique features of racial and ethnic groups, such as Nike's design of bigger shoes for Native Americans because they have bigger feet.

Society must decide how best to promote equality in this context. Which group will drug companies' targets to maximize their profits? Clearly, the answer is the groups that are more likely to afford the drug treatment. In that case, what happens to the non-targeted groups for drug design, especially if there are no available alternatives? Would the current therapeutic drive towards personalized medicine create winners and losers? These are some questions that must be addressed in this new era of pharmacogenomics, so that the creation of a pharmaceutical apartheid, in which the price and availability of a needed drug are a function of genetics and race, can be avoided. There are also significant legal, ethical, and social issues that must be resolved with regards to privacy issues with individual genetic information, inequalities in access to genetic tests, use of genetic information in the legal system, and discrimination based on genetic information. Is there danger in overemphasizing genetics as compared to other social determinants, such as environmental influence and behavioral patterns, in addressing health disparities? These are a few of the areas that must be addressed by health officials, lawmakers, scientists, government regulators, and policy makers.

11.9 Summary

According to the Institute of Medicine, disparities are on the rise despite advances in prevention, diagnosis, and disease treatment (www.nationalacademies.org). Individuals of low SES and who are less educated are least likely to benefit from the advances that have been made in medicine. Race and ethnicity matters for health, and this book has examined several factors that contribute to the persistent racial disparity in the prevalence of diseases.

The debates surrounding race and health are often embroiled in controversy with regards to the relative contribution of individual life styles and behavioral factors versus social factors. While individual choice matters with regards to health, these are less consequential for understanding population patterns in disease distribution and racial health disparities. This chapter has looked at racism at multiple levels, such as SES, segregation, and inequities in education and job opportunities that are driving psychobiological behavioral and interactions with genes to cause increased biological vulnerability to a plethora of diseases in minority populations. For example, racism faced by minorities with regards to employment discrimination, residential segregation, excessive police violence, cognitive stigmatization, and daily indignities (microaggressions) is significantly associated with increased incidence of CVDs in AA populations. Cumulative racial stresses on minority populations affect all aspects of their lives: premature births, high-infant-mortality rates, and life times of poor health outcomes for individuals who experience racism.

In the quest to address health issues that uniquely affect the AA population and other minorities, there is a need to move away from the use of race to categorize individual populations based on their skin color, geographic origin, or culture. The US Census Bureau has classified the US population into five predominant groups: whites; AA or Blacks; American Indian or Alaska Natives; Asian; and Native Hawaiian or other Pacific Islander, and people have the option to report more than one race which is indicative of racial mixture. Data from such categories are used in the sociological and political arenas and in epidemiological studies to discover health disparities. However, this is a very crude classification of the US population, as there are significant differences within each racial group. The Asian group, for example, has great diversity in terms of genetic variations, behavior, culture, diet, and so forth. Similarly, there are huge differences in the AA populations. From health perspectives, a better definition of various populations calls for the use of Ancestry Informative Markers (AIMs) to provide new insights into the role of ancestral genetic make-up and environmental interactions in diseases that exhibit differential rates among various populations (Stefflova et al. 2011). This will be potentially important in the field of pharmacogenomics in designing targeted therapies that would specifically benefit populations based on genetic variants that are associated with adverse health risks and health disparities.

References

Allen, T. W. (1997). *The invention of the white race* (Vol. 2). London: Verso.
Bejan, A., & Jones, E. (2010). Scientist theorizr that black athletes run fast. *The International Journal of Design and Nature and Ecodynamics*.
Blakey, M. L. (1996). Skull doctors revisited: Intrinsic social and political bias in the history of American physical anthropology, with special reference to the work of Ales Hrdlicka. In L. Reynolds, & L. Lieberman (Eds.), Race and other misadventures: Essays in Honor of Ashley Montagu in his ninetieth year, 1996 (pp. 64–95). New York: General Hall.
Blakey, M. L. (2001). Bioarchaeology of the African Diaspora in the Americas: Its origins and scope. *Annual Review of Anthropology, 30*, 387–422.
Cardon, L. R. & Palmer, L. J. (2003). Population stratification and spurious allelic association. *Lancet, 361*(9357), 598–604. Available from: PM:12598158.
Colilla, S., Rotimi, C., Cooper, R., Goldberg, J., & Cox, N. (2000). Genetic inheritance of body mass index in African-American and African families. *Genetic Epidemiology, 18*(4), 360–376. Available from: PM:10797595.
Cooper, R. D. R. (1986). The biological concept of race and its application to public health and epidemiology. *Journal of Health Politics, Policy and Law, 11*, 97–116.
Darwin, C. (1871). *The descent of man*. Princeton: Princeton University Press.
Fredrickson, G. M. (2002). *Racism: A short history*. Princeton: Princeton University Press.
Helgason, A., Yngvadottir, B., Hrafnkelsson, B., Gulcher, J., & Stefansson, K. (2005). An Icelandic example of the impact of population structure on association studies. *Nature Genetics, 37*(1), 90–95. Available from: PM:15608637.
Jablonski, N. G. & Chaplin, G. (2010). Colloquium paper: Human skin pigmentation as an adaptation to UV radiation. *Proceedings of the National Academic Sciences of United States America, 107*(Suppl 2), 8962–8968. Available from: PM:20445093.
Jackson, J. S. B. T. W. D. T. M. S. S. B. K. (1996). Racism and the physical and mental health status of African-Americans. *Ethnicity and Disease, 6*, 132–147.
Jonas, D. E., & McLeod, H. L. (2009). Genetic and clinical factors relating to warfarin dosing. *Trends Pharmacological Sciences, 30*(7), 375–386. Available from: PM:19540002.
Kaback, M. M. (2001). Screening and prevention in Tay-Sachs disease: Origins, update, and impact. *Advances Genetics, 44*, 253–265. Available from: PM:11596988.
Kistka, Z. A., Palomar, L., Lee, K. A., Boslaugh, S. E., Wangler, M. F., Cole, F. S., DeBaun, M. R., & Muglia, L. J. (2007). Racial disparity in the frequency of recurrence of preterm birth. *American Journal of Obstetrics Gynecology, 196*(2), 131–136. Available from: PM:17306652.
Konigsberg, L. W., Algee-Hewitt, B. F., Steadman, D. W. (2009). Estimation and evidence in forensic anthropology: sex and race. *American Journal of Physical Anthropology, 139*, 77–90.
Krieger, N. (2000). Discrimination and health. In: L. Berkman, I. Kawachi (Eds.), Social epidemiology. Oxford, England: Oxford University Press Inc., pp. 36–75.

Krimsky, S. (2012). The short life of a race drug. *Lancet, 379,* 114–115.

Kwate, N. O., Valdimarsdottir, H. B., Guevarra, J. S., & Bovbjerg, D. H. (2003). Experiences of racist events are associated with negative health consequences for African American women. *Journal of the National Medical Association, 95*(6), 450–460. Available from: PM:12856911.

Morgan, D. M. (1998). *Slave counterpoint: Black culture in the 18th century chesapeake & low country.* Chapel Hill: University of North Carolina Press.

Morris, M. R., Ricketts, C., Gentle, D., Abdulrahman, M., Clarke, N., Brown, M., et al. (2010). Identification of candidate tumour suppressor genes frequently methylated in renal cell carcinoma. *Oncogene, 29*(14), 2104–2117. Available from: PM:20154727.

Norton, H. L., Werren, E., & Friedlaender, J. (2015). MC1R diversity in Northern Island Melanesia has not been constrained by strong purifying selection and cannot explain pigmentation phenotype variation in the region. *BMC Genetics, 16,* 122. Available from: PM:26482799.

Ofili, E. (2001). Ethnic disparities in cardiovascular health. *Ethnicity & Disease, 11*(4), 838–840. Available from: PM:11763309.

Pappas, G., Queen, S., Hadden, W., & Fisher, G. (1993). The increasing disparity in mortality between socioeconomic groups in the United States, 1960 and 1986. The *New England Journal Medicine, 329*(2), 103–109. Available from: PM:8510686.

Relethford, J. H. (2002). Apportionment of global human genetic diversity based on craniometrics and skin color. *American Journal of Physical Anthropology, 118*(4), 393–398. Available from: PM:12124919.

Rosenberg, N. A., Pritchard, J. K., Weber, J. L., Cann, H. M., Kidd, K. K., Zhivotovsky, L. A., & Feldman, M. W. (2002). Genetic structure of human populations. *Science, 298*(5602), 2381–2385. Available from: PM:12493913.

Rubinstein, W. S., Jiang, H., Dellefave, L., & Rademaker, A. W. (2009). Cost-effectiveness of population-based BRCA1/2 testing and ovarian cancer prevention for Ashkenazi Jews: a call for dialogue. *Genetics Medicine, 11*(9), 629–639. Available from: PM:19606050.

Smedley, A. (2007). Race in North America: Origin and evolution of a worldview. Third Edition. 2007. Boulder, CO: Westview Press.

Sparks, C. S., & Jantz, R. L. (2002). A reassessment of human cranial plasticity: Boas revisited. *Proceedings of the National Academic of Sciences United States of America, 99*(23), 14636–14639. Available from: PM:12374854.

Stefflova, K., Dulik, M. C., Barnholtz-Sloan, J. S., Pai, A. A., Walker, A. H., & Rebbeck, T. R. (2011). Dissecting the within-Africa ancestry of populations of African descent in the Americas. *PLoS One, 6*(1), e14495. Available from: PM:21253579.

Templeton, A. R. (2013). Biological races in humans. *Studies in History and Philosophy of Biological and Biomedical Sciences, 44*(3), 262–271. Available from: PM:23684745.

Williams, D. R. (1999). Race, socioeconomic status, and health. The added effects of racism and discrimination. *The Annals of the New York Academy of Sciences, 896,* 173–188. Available from: PM:10681897.

Chapter 12
Translating Health Disparities

Abstract In order to effectively reduce and/or eliminate health disparities, scientifically based remedies have to be implemented in broad/based behavioral interventions that are focused on changing conditions at the community, state, and governmental levels, in addition to the individual level. Infrastructure, such as social networks involving community-health representatives, peer-outreach workers, community-health aides, and peer educators and their interactions with health-care professionals needs to be established.

12.1 Introduction

The overall health status of all Americans has improved tremendously since the beginning of the 21st century. According to the National Vital Statistics Reports (ftp://ftp.cdc.gov/pub/Health_Statistics/NCHS/Publications/NVSR/61_03/Table21.xls), in 1900, the average life expectancy for EAs in the USA was 47.3 years, and for AAs it was much lower at 33 years. The leading causes of deaths in the 1900s were influenza, pneumonia, diphtheria, tuberculosis, and gastrointestinal infections. However, improvements in sanitation, better nutrition, and immunizations in the first half of the twenty first century have resulted in the drastic decline of infectious diseases. Today, such diseases cause a fraction of the deaths compared to the beginning of the 1900s. Scientific advances in understanding the causes of diseases and therapeutic interventions have significantly improved the health status and longevity of the US people. Consequently, the life expectancy for the average American was 79 years in 2011 (Hoyert and Xu 2012) (see Fig. 12.1).

Americans are living longer and infant mortality has also continued to decline. However, despite the generally positive upward trend in the overall health condition of the US population, there is disparity in the mortality rate in African Americans (AAs) and other minorities in comparison with the European-American (EA) population, a disparity that has persisted since accurate federal record keeping began in 1950. According to the Center for Disease Control (CDC) report on minority health (http://www.cdc.gov/minorityhealth/populations/REMP/black.html), the

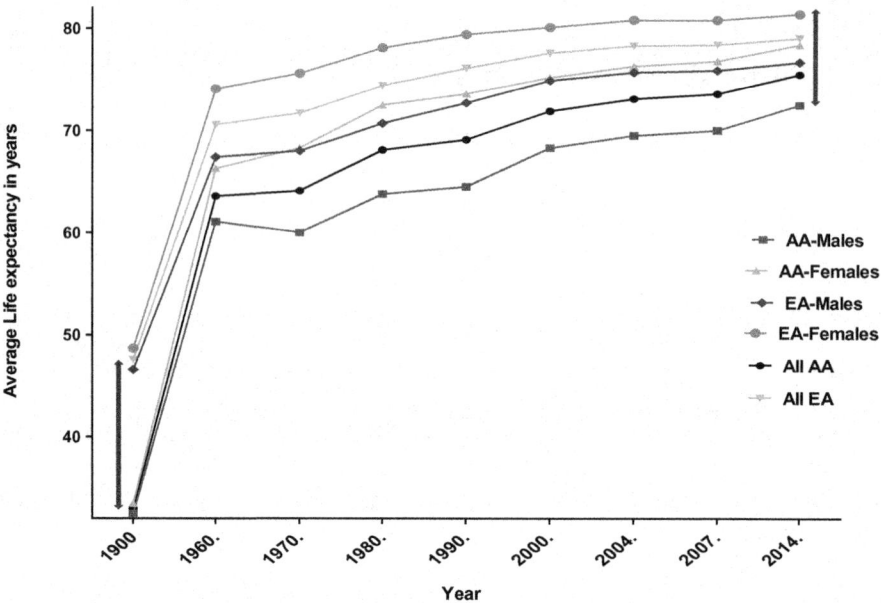

Fig. 12.1 Comparison of average life expectancy in the USA by race and gender 1900–2014. *Arrows* indicate disparities. Data used to generate graph is obtained from the Center for Disease Control/National Center for Health Statistics

average life expectancy for AA men and women combined was 75 years in 2009. This is roughly the same as the average life expectancy for white men and women in 1979, some 30 years earlier. The average life expectancy of black men in 2009 was just 71, compared to 76 for white men (see Fig. 12.1).

In 1985, there was a landmark report published by the Secretary of the Department of Health and Human Services (DHHS), then the honorable Margaret M. Heckler. This report is referred to as the Heckler Report (http://minorityhealth.hhs.gov/assets/pdf/checked/1/ANDERSON.pdf) which consolidated, for the first time, the minority health issues in one report. Six health problems were identified in this report to disproportionally affect minorities, namely: (1) cancer; (2) cardiovascular diseases and stroke; (3) chemical dependency as measured by deaths due to cirrhosis; (4) diabetes; (5) homicide and accidents (unintentional injuries); and (6) infant mortality. As a result of these findings, a taskforce was set up that comprised subcommittees to address each disease area with the mandate to identify the causal factors underlying high prevalence of disease risk in minorities and to come up with intervention approaches. The findings from the task force studies indicated that the factors responsible for the health disparity are complex and defy simplistic solutions and that health status is influenced by the interaction of physiological, cultural, psychological, and societal factors that are poorly understood for the general population and even less so for minorities.

12.1 Introduction

As a result of the taskforce investigations, eight main recommendations were made. The first involved the design of outreach programs to disseminate health information and programs that specifically target minority populations such as AAs, Hispanics and Asian/Pacific Islanders, or Native American. The objective of this recommendation was to make minorities aware of specific disease area that greatly impacted their communities (such as cancer and CVDs) and to provide culturally sensitive health information to promote preventative aspects of disease areas that have the highest mortality and morbidity rates in these populations. Such outreach programs should involve local community leaders, families, and church and other community organizations. The second recommendation was to provide patient education on specific health issues such as diabetes, obesity, and hypertension that is linked to medical care delivery. This recommendation was based on studies that have shown that patient education in health care was cost effective. For instance, education in self-management skills has been demonstrated to reduce complications associated with diabetes. The third was the recommendation that scientific research agenda should emphasize the identification of risk factors associated with increased disparities in minority population and the prevalence of diseases in minority populations. In addition, scientific research should also focus on providing health education and interventions, such as the best way to deliver treatment services in order to identify the socio-cultural factors associated with health outcomes. The fourth recommendation concerned the delivery and financing of health services. The task-force review showed that minorities are disproportionately represented among impoverished Americans and that economic hardship, as well as the lack of health insurance, was a major barrier to seeking health care. The task-force findings also indicated that many minorities tend to rely on Medicaid and charity care for their medical treatment because they have no other sources of care or ways to finance that care. Elderly minority people are less like than elderly EAs to supplement Medicare with additional private insurance. The task force therefore recommended increase flexibility in health-care delivery and the fair apportionment of the costs associated with uncompensated hospital care.

The findings and recommendations from the Heckler Report and subsequent health-care priorities formed the basis for the initiative known as "Healthy People". One of the overarching objectives of the DHHS Healthy People agenda is disease prevention. The disease prevention objective forms a road map and a compass for the country's health with strategic interventions for improving the health of Americans by the end of the century. This initiative formed a framework of public-health priorities and actions. i.e., where we need to go and set priorities and guidelines and actions for the future. Healthy People comprises a set of 10-year objectives for national health that are monitored and reviewed at the end of the 10-year period. Healthy People 2000 (http://www.cdc.gov/nchs/healthy_people/hp2000.htm) was launched by DHHS in 1990. At the end of the 10 year period, there was assessment of the progress made for each objectives, as well as identification of challenges and the setting of future objectives.

This paragraph summarizes some of the Health People objectives that have been set up over the past 30 years beginning in 1990. The overarching goal for Healthy People 1990 was to decrease mortality rates. Reduction in infant mortality rates was to be accomplished through childhood vaccination and immunization and by addressing the numerous factors that would help reduce adult mortality rates. In 2000, the overarching goals were to increase life expectancy, reduce health disparities, and improve access to preventive services for the entire American population. The overarching goals for Healthy People 2010 were to improve the quality and years of life, and the current on-going overarching goals for 2020 are to promote quality of life through the creation of social and physical environments that promote good health, promote disease prevention, and continue to promote quality of life and healthy development, as well as healthy behaviors across all life stages.

How far have we come? The Healthy People agenda over the past 30 years was set out to accomplish several hundred objectives. A subset of objectives addresses the following areas: physical activity, nutrition and obesity, tobacco use, substance abuse, responsible sexual behavior, mental health, injury and violence, environmental quality, immunization, and access to healthcare. These represents major public health concerns. Overall, there has been significant progress in increased life expectancy at birth and in old age and improved better quality of life for children and adolescents. Significant progress has also been made controlling high blood pressure, but this has not reached the targeted goal. There has also been progress through public campaigns, such as the spread of understanding about the harms associated with tobacco smoke in order to reduce tobacco smoking among adults and adolescents.

Unfortunately, one major objective, i.e., to reduce adult obesity, has substantially missed its target. Obesity stands out as the risk factor that has proven most resistant to reduction, even increasing, and has stubbornly persisted as a health disparity. Obesity incidence is on the rise in the USA, and many other parts of the world, due to dietary factors such as high-energy, processed foods in combination with a sedentary life style. It is estimated that 50% of the US population, as a whole, is obese. About two-thirds of the risk factors associated with obesity is genetic, but genetics cannot explain the increase incidence in obesity over the past 15 years, indicating that this risk is expressed only with interaction to environmental factors, such as diet and behavioral/life-style factors that are controllable (McGinnis et al. 2002).

Overall assessment of US minority health since the initial Heckler Report indicates that health disparities are not going away. Disparities are on the rise over the past 50 years despite advances in prevention, diagnosis, and disease treatment (Institute of Medicine 2003), suggesting that other factors that determine health outcomes are beyond the scope of the health-care system. Major contributing factors include social determinants such as socioeconomic status, racial discrimination, residential segregation, and education, as well as behavioral and life-style factors. The following sections discuss some of the intervention approaches for reducing health disparities.

12.2 Life Course Programs

Throughout this book, evidence has been presented for the association of adverse childhood experiences, and indeed adverse prenatal experiences, with adult diseases, including CVDs, obesity, diabetes, and cancer, suggesting that early intervention is critical in order to delay or prevent adult diseases. Family history of health may reflect both shared genetic and behavioral, as well as environmental, risks. Therefore it is important to understand how family history is associated with disease-preventive behaviors in families. Cheng and Solomon (2014) have proposed life-course theory (LCT), a framework designed for the whole person, whole family and community health for the life-time improvement of health for individuals and families over generations. Such LCT can begin with improved access to prenatal care at the time of conception, in which obstetricians, gynecologists, pediatricians, and internal medicine physicians collaborate together to provide the pregnant women with preconception health information on poor nutrition, substance abuse, stress, and poor physical activity, factors that can harm babies. The LCT model should also allow for postpartum visits, family planning for the next pregnancy, and smooth transitions through a life course and across generations. Families with young children should be assisted with on-site, health-related services, including medical and dental care, as well as mental-health evaluations. Also, young parents should be provided with the information and help that is needed to prevent childhood overweight and obesity through healthy diet and physical activity, which will ultimately reduce the risk of adult obesity and associated morbidities. Government-run programs, such as Assistance Developmental evaluations, nutrition and lactation services including the women, infant, and children (WIC), supplemental food, and nutrition programs, as well as screening for family social needs and risk assessments, are some measures that will improve health for low-SES individuals from the time of conception, through childhood, and into adulthood. Low-SES populations such as AAs and other minorities in cities can prioritize the needed services that improve health including health insurance, housing vouchers, adult education, environmental safety, job training and placement, dental care, and counseling, as well as healthy behavior incentives.

12.3 Community-Based Participatory Research (CBPR)

Community-based participatory research CBPR brings together academicians and community members as equal partners in research and education about health care and prevention in the community. In addition, there is a role for lay health advisors (LHA) or peer educators, also known as peer outreach workers or community-health aides, who live in the community and can all play roles in interventions that will help in navigating the health-care system in low-SES communities. The role of LHA can be paid or unpaid and be formulated under the terms health and screening educator, member of a care delivery team, or even as patient-navigator outreach worker. A natural resource that is available in most communities is social networks through which community members can offer and receive social support from each other. Another potential asset are natural helpers who are individuals to whom people in their community turn to for advice and assistance because they have a reputation for good judgment, offering a listening ear and caring shoulder, discreteness, stability in their lives, and contacts with groups outside their community. Furthermore, the church and other religious centers can play pivotal roles in CBPR as discussed in Chap. 8.

12.3.1 CBPR for Hypertension

Based on DHHS recommendations, outreach programs to disseminate health information and programs that specifically target minority populations such as AAs have proven successful, and several studies have evolved as efficacious non-pharmacological, life-style, and behavioral interventions that address health disparities. One such community-based participatory research (CBPR) was designed to address the prevalence of hypertension in the AA community (Zoellner et al. 2014). The incidence of hypertension is very high in the US population, but the AA population is disproportionally affected by this condition. Zoellner et al. enrolled 269 paid participants, mostly AAs (94% of the total and 85% female) from Hattiesburg, a mid-size Mississippi city of approximately 45,000 residents (53% AAs and 42% CAU); the median household income was $27,144, with a 43% incidence of hypertension rates in the population. This was a six-month study designed to measure body waist circumference, BMI, total cholesterol, low and high-density lipoproteins, blood glucose, and dietary intake (fruits and vegetables, fibre, sugar, calcium, and dairy products), both at the start of the study and throughout the study period. Ninety- minute monthly educational sessions were held with a focus on the principle of dietary approaches to stop hypertension (the DASH diet). Participants included in the study were individuals with BP $\leq$ 180/110 and any medication regimen was not taken into account. Participants also had to be free from caffeine and tobacco and were asked to exercise for one hour prior to each assessment. Even though the study lacked a controlled randomized design, at the end of the six-month study, the participants exhibited significant decreases in both the systolic and diastolic BP, and sugar intake was also significantly reduced. This study provided one piece of evidence in support of CBPR as an effective and viable approach for implementing non-pharmacological multicomponent, life-style interventions to help reduce the disparities associated with not only hypertension but also numerous other diseases that disproportionately affect AA populations. These were short-term positive effects, however, and more research is needed to determine long-term effectiveness, as well as more studies among male populations and targeting macro-level interventions.

12.4 Diabetes Outcomes

Diabetes continues to be a major public-health concern. There are 28 million people at risk of this condition, and the cost associated with diabetes was estimated to be $245 billion (US dollars), and it is estimated that one in three individuals in the USA by 2050 will be diagnosed with this condition. There are programs, such as for diabetes prevention and randomized clinical trials with weight watchers, that prove to work in reducing the incidence and morbidities associated with diabetes. The prevalence of diabetes is higher in the AA population in comparison with the EA population. Several diabetic-related intermediate outcomes, such as hemoglobin A1c (HbA1c), systolic blood pressure (SBP), and low-density lipoprotein (LDL) cholesterol are significantly higher in AA in comparison with EA patients and are likely contributing to the increased prevalence of diabetes in the AA population. Diabetes-prevention programs must also teach diabetic patients and, in particular, AA patients to be able to self-manage the condition in order to avoid complications such as blindness, coronary artery disease, stroke, low cases of extremities amputation, and kidney failure. There are several adverse factors that may contribute to the reduced ability to self-manage diabetes. One case-control study was designed to assess which adverse factor were associated with patients' inability to self-manage diabetes. This study enrolled 764 respondents' from both AA and EA populations. Cases were patients with poor control of at least two of three intermediate outcomes (HbA1c $\geq$ 8.0%, SBP $\geq$ 140 mmHg, LDL cholesterol $\geq$ 130 mg/dl), whereas the control patient samples had good control of all three intermediates outcome (HbA1c < 8.0%, SBP < 140 mmHg, LDL $\leq$ 130 mg/dl) (Duru et al. 2009). Multivariant analysis of adverse factors such as depression, low health literacy, incomplete medication adherence, low self-efficacy for reducing cardiovascular risk, and poor patient-physician communication were analyzed in association with the intermediate outcomes. Duru et al. (2009) observed that depression and missing doses of medication were significantly associated with poor diabetes control in AA but not EA population. While this study may lack the sample power to detect associations between other factors, the findings suggests that targeting depression and missing doses of medication, both potentially modifiable intermediates, may contribute to reducing the disparities associated with diabetes in AA and other minority populations.

12.5 Behavioral Intervention Approaches

Since tobacco smoke and its carcinogens are associated with many diseases, it is estimated that one third of all types of cancers can be avoided if people did not smoke cigarettes or otherwise use tobacco. In the USA, the burden of tobacco addiction falls heavily on low SES, low-educated minorities, therefore tobacco deserves our highest commitment for behavior intervention in order to eliminate health disparities. Several effective prevention and cessation programs have been initiated in many states. California and Massachusetts were among the first to integrate the media tools by creating counter advertisement to the tobacco industry. Other initiative includes governmental policies, such as increasing price and taxes on tobacco, introducing smoke-free environment in many government and public areas, providing assistance to help individuals quit, such as counseling, nicotine replacement therapy, provision of free or low cost cessation mechanisms, and other tactics to help communities, schools, and families, as well as individuals quit smoking (Koh et al. 2010). Several behavioral interventions rooted in CBPR include building and revitalizing an anti-violence environment (project BRAVE), for example, an intervention in schools in New Orleans, which is a partnership between school-based organizations, community organizers, and local public-health researchers to reduce violence in schools. This has produced positive trend in school attendance.

Other behavioral-intervention programs should target the reduction of blood pressure and stress level by monitoring physiological stress-response hormones. As discussed in Chap. 9, the levels of several candidate hormone (including cortisol and epinephrine) and other endocrine hormones (dopamine, insulin-like growth factors, and dehydroepiandrosterone sulphate (DHEA-s)) are indicators of physiological stress levels and can be appropriate targets for intervention. In addition, allostatic load markers or metabolic markers, such as systolic and diastolic blood pressure, HDL, and total cholesterol, can be monitored as these are CVDs predictors. Furthermore, inflammatory markers including C-reactive protein, interleukin-6, and tumor necrosis factor can be monitored for immune function, whereas creatinine and homocysteine are potential targets for monitoring kidney functions.

12.6 Cancer

Cancer is ranked as the second highest cause of mortality in the USA, and disparities associated with cancer incidence and mortality rates continues to be a major challenge in the USA and globally. Although there is a decline in cancer incidence and mortality rates for several cancers, racial and ethnic disparities associated with incidence and mortality continue to persist. The disparities for cancer, as with other diseases, may be associated with the stage of detection and management, including screening, diagnosis after screening, access to quality care during cancer treatment, and follow up after completion of therapy. There are several barriers associated with cancer screening, detection, diagnosis, and care of which perhaps the most significant are financial barriers as discussed in Sect. 12.9.

Extensive research coupled with the completion of the human genome sequencing has advanced our understanding of cancer etiology, disease progression, and the challenges associated with developing efficacious therapeutic interventions. It is time to implement actions based on research finding at the translational level to eliminate disparities through developing community-academic networks to address cancer disparities issues, which is the mission of the National Institute on Minority Health and Health Disparities.

In order to translate health disparities into public-health action, there is a need to translate the genetic variants associated with drug addiction into public-health interventions, such as affordable testing to identify individuals who are susceptible to addiction, and then to tailor them to various groups for the necessary interventions. Similar community-academic networks can make data on health information usable at the community level through health-literacy education. Education/advocacy awareness programs should also disseminate efficacious interventions for cancer screening, such as providing mammography services to low-SES communities and increasing access to tobacco cessation programs, among other approaches.

12.7 Importance of Health Literacy

As discussed in Chap. 7, individuals with low health literacy are associated with poor health outcomes. In the US alone, 36% of the adult population is considered to have poor health literacy, and there is a high propensity of poor health illiteracy among AA and other minority populations. To the extent that health literacy involves engaging in written materials, there is the need to enroll adults in educational programs organized by educators-community workers. These need to be designed to fit with the community's social and cultural settings to educate individuals in basic language, literacy, and numeracy programs, such as in adult education settings or colleges. Such education will focus on the ability to read a thermometer and take temperatures, read and interpret food and medicine labels, understand nutritional information, check prescriptions, dosage, and communicate with doctors, among others.

12.8 Financial Cost of Insurance

Lack of insurance continues to be a persistent and a major barrier to eliminating health disparities. As discussed throughout this book, there are several identified barriers that are associated with disease detection, treatment, and mortality rates in various racial and ethnic groups, including lack of knowledge about disease, low health literacy, cultural and language barriers, logistics such as transportation to healthcare centers, and the list goes on. But perhaps one of the most important barriers is financial constraints. Out-of-pocket cost and lack of insurance are huge problems preventing annual physical exams, age-appropriate screening, and obtaining quality health-care diagnoses and disease treatment. One review of systematic studies to identify interventions that best promote breast-cancer screening found that culturally tailored screening that addressed financial barriers, especially amongst low-SES women who had Medicare, Medicaid, or no insurance, was more effective than reminder-based interventions (Masi et al. 2007).

The historic Massachusetts Health Care reform, a bipartisan act, was signed into law in April 2006 and implemented a new universal health-care coverage, making Massachusetts the state with the lowest rate of uninsured residents. Within this law are provisions for increasing health-insurance coverage to reduce health disparities in rates of uninsured groups and improve preventions and treatment services for underserved populations. One recent report on the impact of Massachusetts Health Care reforms investigated the frequency of hospital admissions for ambulatory-care sensitive conditions (ACSC), which are potentially preventable, with quality access to the outpatient health-care system. This report did not find any significant decrease in the number of racial and ethnic minorities being admitted to hospitals for ACSC (McCormick et al. 2015), suggesting that additional efforts are needed for racial and ethnic minorities to obtain quality outpatient care in order to reduce preventable admissions. Positive evidence for the Massachusetts Health Care reform was reported for surgical-resection rates for pancreatic cancer. One study reported the number of racial and ethnic minorities receiving surgical resection (the only cure for cancer) compared to before the Massachusetts Health Care reform, indicating that the increase in insurance coverage can help bridge the disparities associated with pancreatic cancer (Loehrer et al. 2015).

San Francisco has also created government initiatives to reduce disparities by making health-care services accessible and affordable for uninsured residents. Although, this does not provide health insurance, it offers universal access to primary and preventive care for uninsured residents.

The US Universal Care Act also known as Affordable Care Act (ACA) or nicknamed Obama Care was signed into law by the US President Barack Obama on March 23, 2010. The healthcare reform holds the promise of a phenomenal step in the right direction towards eliminating health disparities. Parts of the ACA are designed to provide more Americans with affordable quality health-care insurance, and several reforms, including additional benefits, rights protection, and improved quality and efficiency of health-care, as well, address health disparities and increase quality of life overall. However, ACA has with a backlash, predominantly from the Republican Party which plans to repeal the ACA, now that they are in power. One of their ongoing arguments is that the ACA is too expensive and that tax payers would end up paying for it, but we are already paying for it with crime, unemployment, addiction, physical and mental illness that are all the result of health disparities.

12.9 Precision Medicine

Technological advances in genomic research have revolutionized health-care delivery. Advances in genomic research, such as candidate-gene studies and GWAS, have led to the identification of genetic variations in numerous genes that are associated with differential disease susceptibility in various racial and ethnic populations as discussed extensively in Chap. 2. Several of these genetic variants are beginning to be associated with clinical outcomes. The clinical applications of genetic testing include diagnostic testing, prenatal diagnosis, newborn screening, cancer screening, predictive testing, and pharmacogenomics. They each promise substantial benefits for better disease management and intervention, as well as early detection. For example, clinical laboratories are running genetic tests such as BRCA1 and 2 for predicting breast and ovarian cancers, or K-ras mutation for predicting colon cancers, whereas lipid laboratories are running low-density lipoprotein (LDL) cholesterol and LDL genetic variants to assess risk of CVDs.

Individual genomic information, in combination with other medical information such as socio-demographic and environmental information and family histories, as well as disease treatment and disease response and other molecular and cellular profiling information, altogether make up patient medical record that can be stored electronically, known as electronic health records (HER), which are increasing being used for targeted disease treatment. The HER data is composed of integrated environmental, lifestyle, genome, epigenome, proteomic markers or other molecular profiles that tell us who we are, what is the disease, diagnosis/prognosis, and treatment options. These are driving the area of precision medicine. The current health-are approach is to use individual genomic information, i.e., pharmacogenomics analysis, in combination with HER for the tailored medical treatment to individual characteristics known as precision medicine. Precision medicine has the potential for a physician now to more effectively target the physiological and pharmacological responses to a specific therapeutic treatment for an individual patient based on their genetic and HER data. Based on the tremendous benefits and potential of precision medicine, President Barak Obama in 2015 announced a precision-medicine initiative to develop innovative technologies to improve individual and national health. For instance, it is now well established that BRCA1 and 2 mutations are associated with a predisposition to breast and ovarian cancers. Based on family history and personal history of BRCA1 and 2 mutations, a physician can now order testing for these mutations in order to assist in making decisions on how to reduce risks of breast or ovarian cancers.

Other interventions based on individual genetic variants to medical treatment are the pharmacogenetics dosing algorithms for warfarin as discussed in Sect. 11.6. Further benefits of precision medicine are pharmacogenomics in drug metabolizing enzymes, such as allelic variants in the cytochrome P450 drug metabolizers that can indicate individuals as either poor or elevated drug metabolizers, and this can guide the application of an appropriate drug dosage to be administered to enhance personalized therapies as cost effective and clinically efficacious alternative. The future of health care is to use this genomic information, in addition to transcriptomic (gene expression), proteomics (protein expression), metabolomics (metabolic profiles), the so called "OMICs", in addition to HER and biobank repository data as well as next generation sequencing and GWAS data testing includes sequencing for a single gene, a panel of gene, the whole exome, or the whole genome to determine whether responses to certain drugs can be predicted by HER linked genomic data. This so-called big data has the potential to change the way patients are treated. There are several challenges however: the sheer size, lack of standardization for generating sequencing data, bioinformatics processing data storage, and these issues may compromise the quality of data. It remains to be seen if there will be equitable benefits of personalized medicine made available to all racial and ethnic groups in the USA.

12.10 Summary

We face a mammoth challenge in health disparities, and there is no single element or factor to explain all the incidence and mortality rates associated with disparities. Interventions to reduce or eliminate health disparities must be approached from multiple angles (Fig. 12.2). While some believed that universal care would resolve

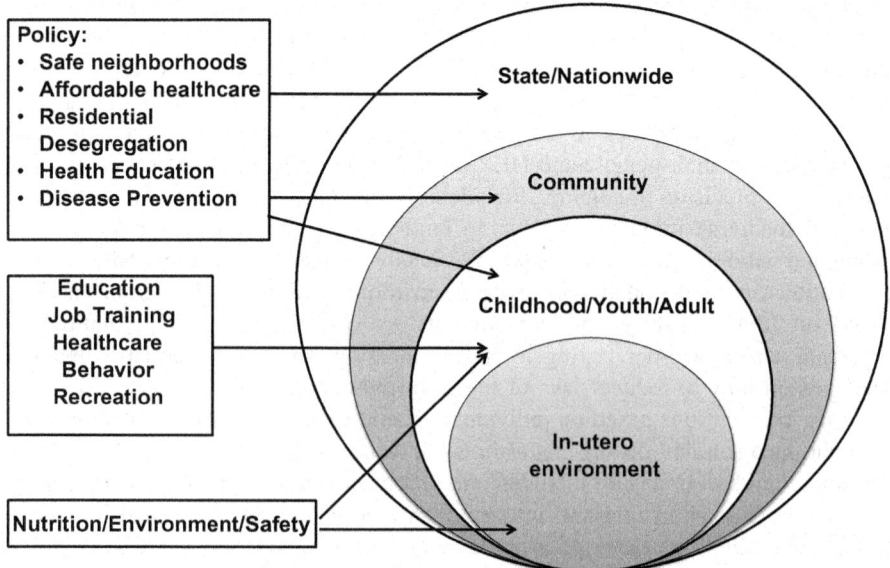

Fig. 12.2 Translating health disparities. *Arrows* indicates some of the factors that can be targeted for intervention throughout the life course of an individual, or family or population

disparities, this model has not worked in some countries, such as the UK, because health care alone does not solve problems, such as residential segregation and employment opportunities which are important determinants for heath. Addressing health disparities requires concerted efforts at the individual, family, community, local, and state levels, as well as government policies with strategic interventions directed towards communities or populations at great risk.

References

Cheng, T. L., & Solomon, B. S. (2014). Translating life course theory to clinical practice to address health disparities. *Maternal and Child Health Journal, 18*(2), 389–395. Available from: PM:23677685.

Duru, O. K., Gerzoff, R. B., Selby, J. V., Brown, A. F., Ackermann, R. T., Karter, A. J., et al. (2009). Identifying risk factors for racial disparities in diabetes outcomes: The translating research into action for diabetes study. *Med Care, 47*(6), 700–706. Available from: PM:19480090.

Hoyert, D. L. & Xu, J. (2012). Deaths: Preliminary data for 2011. *National Vital Statistics Report, 61*(6), 1–51. Available from: PM:24984457.

Institute of Medicine. (2003). Unequal treatment: Confronting racial and ethnic disparities in Healthcare. National Academy Press.

Koh, H. K., Oppenheimer, S. C., Massin-Short, S. B., Emmons, K. M., Geller, A. C., & Viswanath, K. (2010). Translating research evidence into practice to reduce health disparities: A social determinants approach. *American Journal of Public Health, 100*(Suppl 1), S72–S80. Available from: PM:20147686.

Loehrer, A. P., Chang, D. C., Hutter, M. M., Song, Z., Lillemoe, K. D., Warshaw, A. L., & Ferrone, C. R. (2015). Health insurance expansion and treatment of pancreatic cancer: Does increased access lead to improved care? *Journal of American College Surgeons, 221*(6), 1015–1022. Available from: PM:26611798.

Masi, C. M., Blackman, D. J., & Peek, M.E. 2007. Interventions to enhance breast cancer screening, diagnosis, and treatment among racial and ethnic minority women. *Medical Care Research and Review, 64*(5 Suppl), 195S–242S. Available from: PM:17881627.

McCormick, D., Hanchate, A. D., Lasser, K. E., Manze, M. G., Lin, M., Chu, C., & Kressin, N. R. (2015). Effect of Massachusetts healthcare reform on racial and ethnic disparities in admissions to hospital for ambulatory care sensitive conditions: retrospective analysis of hospital episode statistics. *BMJ, 350*, h1480. Available from: PM:25833157.

McGinnis, J. M., Williams-Russo, P., & Knickman, J. R. (2002). The case for more active policy attention to health promotion. *Health Affairs (Millwood), 21*(2), 78–93. Available from: PM:11900188.

Zoellner, J., Connell, C., Madson, M. B., Thomson, J. L., Landry, A. S., et al. (2014). HUB city steps: A 6-month lifestyle intervention improves blood pressure among a primarily African-American community. *Journal of the Academy Nutrition and Dietetics, 114*(4), 603–612. Available from: PM:24534602.

Glossary

Diaspora Migration of people away from their ancestral homeland

Health disparity Markedly distinct differences in health outcomes

Race or ethnicity A social construct that categorizes various populations based on skin color or other phenotypic characteristics

Epigenome Modification of the DNA sequence (genome) with consequences in gene expression

Epigenetics Molecular mechanisms that are mitotically stable and regulate gene expression or cellular phenotypes without altering the DNA sequence

Genome Genetic information in the form of a DNA sequence

GWAS Comprehensive sequence approach that analyzes the entire human genome for the detection of genetic variations

Haplotype A set of genes that are inherited together from a single parent

In-utero The environment in the womb

Linkage disequilibrium Frequency of association of various genes that are inherited together more often than would be expected by chance

DNA methylation A chemical modification whereby a methyl group is added to a cytosine nucleotide (which precedes guanine) in the DNA sequence

Minority population Underrepresented group within various different racial and ethnic populations

Noncoding RNA An RNA molecule that is not translated into a protein

Slavery Subjugation of one racial or ethnic group by another

Social advantage One's relative positive position in a social hierarchy determined by wealth, power, and/or prestige

Index

Note: Page numbers followed by indicate figures

A
Acculturation, 180, 191
Acetaldehyde, 161, 257
Acetaldehyde dehydrogenase (ALDH2), 257
Acquired immunodeficiency syndrome (AIDS). *See* HIV/AIDS
Acute kidney injury (AKI), 91
ADIPOQ gene, 44
Adverse childhood experiences and health disparities, 139
Adverse health outcomes
　in AAs, psychosocial factors and, 215
　allostatic load and SES, 207
　environmental stress, 199, 213–214
　family SES, 145
　financial hardships, 117, 122
　education attainment, 133
　low birth weight, 117
　low paying jobs, 130
　maternal smoking 243
　physical features of housing, 140
　psychological stress in, 10
　small size in infancy, 249
　unemployment, 135
Affordable Care Act (ACA), 12, 144, 308
Africa diaspora, 1–2
　disease-specific disparities of, 2–7
　disparity in health, 7–9
　genetic variation in, 33–34
　health disparities, 9
　　environmental quality, 10
　　genetics, 10–11
　　social effects, 10
African-American diabetes mellitus (AADM), 42

African-Americans (AAs), 4–5, 6, 7, 112
　cardiovascular disease and stroke in, 3
　income level in, 115
　infant death rate among, 120
　leading causes of death among, 3*f*
　psychosocial factors and adverse health outcomes in, 215
　racial segregation of, 112
African migrants, 192
African populations, infectious diseases in, 27
　glucose 6-phosphate dehydrogenase, 30
　HIV/AIDS, 31–32
　malaria, 28–29
　sickle cell disease, 29–30
　tuberculosis, 30–31
Age-related diseases, 5, 84
Aging, epigenetic changes with, 83–84
AGO4 genes, 98
Air pollution, 242
Alcohol consumption
　gene-environment interaction in, 255–259
　and health disparities, 160–161
Alcohol dehydrogenase (ADH), 243–244
Alcohol-related carcinogens, 258
Aldehyde dehydrogenase (ALDH), 243, 257
Allostatic load, 206–207, 219
Alternative medicines and health disparities, cultural behavior in, 189–191
Alzheimer's disease (AD)
　gene-environment interaction in, 262–263
　genetic variants in, 46–48
Ambulatory-care sensitive conditions (ACSC), 308
Amygdala, 258
Ancestry informative markers (AIMs), 288–289, 296
Angiotensin converting enzyme (ACE), 38, 260
Angiotensin II (AGTII), 38, 260

Angiotensinogen, 37
Anthropological rationale, scientific basis of human classification, 280–283
  athleticism, 282, 283
  Boas, father of anthropology, 282
  Caucasoids, 281
  Mongoloids, 281
  Negroids, 281
  skeletal size, 281
  skull size, 280–281
Apolipoprotein E (APOE), 46–47
Apolipoprotein L1 (APOL1) gene, 45
Arachidonic acid (ARA) gene, 261
Aspirin-exacerbated respiratory disease (AERD), 253
Aspirin-tolerant asthma (ATA), 253
Asthma Coalition on Community Environment and Social Stress (ACCESS) project, 208
Asthma disparities, gene-environment interaction in, 250–253
Atherosclerosis Risk in Community (ARIC) study, 88
Atrial fibrillation, 7
Atrial natriuretic peptide (ANP), 87
ATR(-)X syndrome, 82
Attention-deficit/hyperactivity disorder (ADHD), 217, 242–243
Autosomal informatics markers (AIMs), 58
5-Aza-deoxycytidine, 83

B
Behavior and health disparities, 153
  alcohol consumption behavior, 160–161
  dietary behavior, 154–155
  physical activity behavior, 155–157
  tobacco-use behavior, 157–160
Behavior-based counseling, 176
Behavior in post-genome era, 165–166
Behavioral intervention, 162
  affording, 162–163
  health disparities
    government policies and, 164
    individual and community behavioral intervention, 163–164
    translating, 305–306
  obesity and, 164–165
Beta-globin protein, 18
Beta-type natriuretic peptide (BNP), 87
BiDil, 293–294
Big data, 310
Bladder cancer, 59
Blood pressure, 259
  psychological stress and, 221

Boas, Franz, 282
Bonesetters, 190
BRCA2 gene, 57
Breast cancer, 4, 51–53
  disparity, 97–98
Breast feeding and health disparities, 121

C
Caenorhabditis elegans, 86
CAMP-response element-binding protein (CREB), 252, 257
Cancer, 4, 50, 59
  bladder cancer, 59
  breast cancer, 51–53
  colorectal cancer, 53–55
  lung cancer, 55–56
  prostate cancer, 56–59
  translating health disparities in, 306–307
Cancer disparities, epigenetics and, 92–95
  breast cancer disparity, 97–98
  colorectal-cancer disparity, 98
  gene-environment interaction, 264–266
  prostate-cancer disparity, 95–97
Cancer-specific differential DNA methylation regions (cDMRs), 93
CANDLE (Conditions Affecting Neurocognitive Development and Learning in Early Childhood) study, 100
Cardiovascular diseases (CVDs), 212
  in AA population, 3–4
  disparities, 34
    cardiovascular tissue remodeling and, 35–36
    endocrine signaling, 35
    epigenetics and, 87
    gene-environment interaction in, 261
    heart failure, 36
    hypertension, 37–38
Caucasoids, 281
CDH5, methylation of, 98
Chadwick report, 7–8
Chemokine receptor (CCR), 262
Childhood and health disparities
  economic investment in, 120
    breast feeding of infants, 121
    childhood poverty, 121–123
    infant gene-environmental conditions, 249–250
Childhood mortality, 119, 136
Childhood poverty, 121–123
Chronic kidney disease (CKD), 5, 44–45
  disparity, epigenetics and, 90–91
Chronic lower-respiratory disease (COPD), 6
Churches, 187–188

Cigarette smoking, 136, 262
Colonization, 1
Colorectal cancer, 53–55, 265
  disparity, 98
Community-academic networks, 307
Community-based participatory research (CBPR), 303–304
  for hypertension, 304
Community behavioral intervention and health disparities, 163–164
Community-health aides, 303
Community stressors and health, 211–212
Comorbid psychiatric disorders, 217
Comparative genomic hybridization (CGH) arrays, 57
Complementary or alternative medicine (CAM), 189
Corticotrophin releasing factor (CRF), 203
Corticotrophin releasing hormone (CRH), 202, 208, 247
CpG-island methylator phenotype (CIMP), 93
Crohn's disease, 25
Cultural competency, 180
Cultural impact on health disparities, 185
  alternative medicines and, 189–191
  cultural competence, linguistics, and, 191–192
  cultural sensitive medical care and, 193
  diet and, 186
  religion and cultural impact, 187–189
Culture, health literacy and, 179–180
Curanderismo, folk medicine, 190
CYP2C9, genetic variations in, 293
CYP3A4-V, 57–58
Cystic FΔ508, 19
Cystic fibrosis, 11, 19
Cystic fibrosis transmembrane conductance regulator (CFTR) gene, 19
Cytidine deaminase enzymes, 32
Cytochrome P450 2E1 (CYP2E1), 257
Cytosine-phosphate-guanine (CpG), 78, 79–80, 99

D

DASH (dietary approaches to stop hypertension) diet, 176
Death associated protein (DAP) kinase, 256
Dementia, genetic variants in, 46–48
Deoxyribonucleic acid (DNA)
  sequencing, 22–23
  structure, 18
Department of Health and Human Services (DHHS) Healthy People agenda, 301
Depression, 198, 216, 218, 245, 305
Diabetes disparities, gene-environment interaction in, 253–255, 254f
Diabetes mellitus (DM), 4–5, 38, 90, 176
  genetic factors associated
    with type 1 DM, 40–41
    with type 2 DM, 41–42
  obesity and, 156
  translating health disparities in, 305
Diabetes Prevention Program (DPP), 162–163
Diaspora, defined, 1
Diet
  and cultural impact, 186–187
  DASH diet, 176
  role for, 236–240
Dietary behavior and health disparities, 154–155
Diethylstilbestrol (DES), 234
Discrimination
  perceived, 219
  racial, 219, 280, 287–288
Disease-associated genes, 99
Disease-specific disparities of African diaspora, 2–7
DNA methylation, 78–80, 80f, 81, 85, 93, 94, 96, 98, 238, 247–248, 259
DNA methyltransferases (DMNTs), 78, 79, 84
DNA sequencing, 20, 22–23, 284
Double stranded RNA (dsRNA), 78f, 81
Duchenne muscular dystrophy (DMD), 11, 19
Duffy signaling, 28

E

Early-life adversity, 207, 209
Economic factors and health disparities, 111, 113–114
  health and human capital, 114
  health capital and health disparities, 114–116
  infant mortality, 119–120
Economic investment
  in adult and health disparities, 124
  in childhood and health disparities, 120
    breast feeding of infants, 121
    childhood poverty, 121–123
  in children and youths' health and health disparities, 123–124
  in intrauterine environment and health disparities, 117–119
Education, 112, 114, 172
  /advocacy awareness program, 307
  for economic success, 124
  health and, 113
  as social determinant of health, 131–133
Electronic health records (HER), 309, 310

Embryogenesis, 80
Emotions, 198, 199
Employment status, 130
Endocrine hormones, 306
Endothelial nitric oxide synthase (eNOS), 50
End-stage renal disease (ESRD), 44, 45
Environmental stress, 199–200
   body's response to, 202, 203f
   and health disparity, 199–200
Environmental toxins, 236, 244, 247
Epigenetic gate keepers, 93
Epigenetic processes, 11
Epigenetic programming, 266
   in early life, 248–249
   and maternal care and health disparities, 247–248
Epigenetics, 75
   and cancer disparities, 92–95
      breast cancer disparity, 97–98
      colorectal-cancer disparity, 98
      prostate-cancer disparity, 95–97
   and cardiovascular disease disparity, 87
   changes, aging, and disease disparities, 83–86
   and chronic kidney disease disparity, 90–91
   and development, 80–81
   DNA methylation, 78–80
   and genetic association and natural human variation, 99–100
   histone modification, 76–77
   and HIV disease disparity, 91–92
   microRNAs, 77–78
   and obesity disparity, 87–89
   in neuronal development and disease, 82–83
   and type 2 diabetes disparity, 89–90
Epigenome, 234, 235
Epigenome-wide-association-study (EWAS) analysis, 88, 100
Epstein-Barr virus (EBV), 91
Euchromatin, 77f
Eumelanin, 283
European-Americans (EAs), 2, 4–5, 6
   cancer deaths, 4

F

Familial adenomatous polyposis (FAP), 53
Family conflict, SES and, 137–139
Family values, interaction of, 142
Fatty acid desaturase (FADs) genes, 261
Fetal-alcohol-spectrum disorder (FASD), 243
Fetal origin, maternal stress and, 244–246
Folate, 95, 100

"Food deserts" of low-income communities, 130, 141
FTO gene, 43, 44

G

Gates Foundation, 31
Gene-environment interaction, 9
   in Alzheimer's disease, 262–263
   in asthma disparities, 250–253
   in cancer disparities, 264–266
   in CVD disparities, 261
   in diabetes disparities, 253–255, 254f
   and fetal origin of health disparities, role for, 236
      air pollution, 242
      diet, 236–240
      hormonal exposure, 241
      maternal stress, 244–246
      parental substance abuse, 242–244
      and prenatal predisposition to kidney diseases, 246–247
   in HIV disparities, 262
   in hypertension disparity, 259–260
   in tobacco smoking, alcohol consumption, and health disparities, 255–259
Gene expression, 234–236, 238–239, 264
Gene–gene interactions, 9
Genes, defined, 17
Genetic association and natural human variation, 99–100
Genetic basis to health disparity, 17
   cancer, 50, 59
      breast cancer, 51–53
      colorectal cancer, 53–55
      lung cancer, 55–56
      prostate cancer, 56–59
   cardiovascular disease disparities, 34
      cardiovascular tissue remodeling and, 35–36
      heart failure, 36
      hypertension, 37–38
   diabetes, 38
      type 1 diabetes, 40–41
      type 2 diabetes, 41–42
   genetic variants in dementia, 46–48
   genetic variation, 20–21
      in African diaspora, 33–34
      in African population, 25–27
   GWAS in African population, 32–33
   human diseases, 17–20
   infectious diseases in African populations, 27
      glucose 6-phosphate dehydrogenase, 30
      HIV/AIDS, 31–32

Index

malaria, 28–29
sickle cell disease, 29–30
tuberculosis, 30–31
kidney disease, 44–46
non-communicable diseases, 32
obesity, 42–44
pneumonia and influenza, 49–50
septicemia-sepsis, 48–49
tools for studying genetic variants, 21–25
Genetic Epidemiology Network of Arteriopathy (GENOA) study, 91
Genetic research, 10–11
Genetic variants
    in dementia, 46–48
    tools for studying, 21–25
Genetic variation, 20–21
    in African diaspora, 33–34
    in African population, 25–27
    in human population, causes of, 25–27
    and race categorization, 290–292
Genome-wide association studies (GWAS), 23–25, 42, 256, 262, 284, 290, 292, 293
    in African population, 32–33, 60
Genome-wide DNA methylation analysis, 84
Glucagon-like peptide-1 (GLP-1), ethnic differences in, 40
Glucocorticoid receptors (GR), 247
    gene-promoter regions, 238
Glucose 6-phosphate dehydrogenase (G6PD), 30
Glutathione S-transferase
    GSTP1, 93, 95, 256, 265
    GSTPπ, 240
    hypermethylation, 258
Government policies and behavioral intervention, 164
G protein beta 3-subunit (GNB3), 44
Gross domestic product (GDP), 111

H

Haplotype, 20–21
Health and education, 113
Health and human capital, 114
    and health disparities, 114–116
Health and wealth, 112
Health behaviors and health disparities, 142–143
Health-care professionals, 178–179
Health-care system and health-literacy deficit, 177–178
Health disparities, 7–11
    environmental quality, 10

genetics, 10–11
psychosocial factors and psychological implications of, 215
    anxiety and depression, 215–216
    mental health, 216–219
    prejudice and discrimination, 221
    psychological stressors and stigma, 219–220
    racism and health, 219
social effects, 10
Health literacy deficits, 171
    cultural competence and acculturation, 180
    health literacy
        and culture, 179–180
        and professionals, 178–179
    individual self-care and, 174
        individual preventative measures, 175–177
    patient navigation system, 177
    mistrust of health-care system and health-literacy deficit, 177–178
Health-stock accumulation, 112–113
Healthy-immigrant effects, 192
Healthy People 2000, 301
Healthy People 2010, 302
Heart diseases, 118. *See also* Cardiovascular diseases (CVDs)
    in African Americans, 3
Heart failure (HF), 36
Heckler Report, 300
Helicobacter pylori, 91, 122
Hemoglobin C (HbC), 29
Hepatocellular cancer, 59
Hereditary non-polyposis colorectal cancer (HNPCC), 53–54
Hispanics migrants, 192
Histone acetyltransferases (HATs), 76
Histone deacetylases (HDACs), 76, 81
Histone modification, 76–77, 93, 263
Histone modifying enzymes, 89
HIV/AIDS, 6, 31–32, 92
HIV disease disparity
    epigenetics and, 91–92
    gene-environment interaction in, 262
Home environment cognitive stimulation, 210–211
Homelessness, 141
Homicide rates, 5–6
Homo sapiens, 21. *See also* Human classification, anthropological rationale for scientific basis of
Hormonal exposure, role for, 241

Household income, 113
    measurement of, 116–117
Human-capital theory, 114
Human classification, anthropological rationale for scientific basis of, 280–283
    athleticism, 282, 283
    Boas, father of anthropology, 282
    Caucasoids, 281
    Mongoloids, 281
    Negroids, 281
    skeletal size, 281
    skull size, 280–281
Human diseases, genetic basis of, 17
Human DNA sequence analysis, 21
Human genome project, 23
Human genome sequence and race classification, 285–286
Human leukocyte antigen (HLA), 26–27, 262
Hutchinson-Gilford progeria (HGP), 84
Hypertension, 37–38, 246
    community-based participatory research for, 303–304
Hypertension disparity, gene environment in, 259–260
Hypothalamic-pituitary-adrenal (HPA) axis system, 202, 209, 210, 247

I
Immunoglobulin E (IgE)
    antibodies, 251
    expression, 251
Income
    level of, and health outcomes, 113
    as social determinant of health, 133–134
Individual and community behavioral intervention, 163–164
Infant death rate. *See* Infant-mortality rate (IMR)
Infant gene-environmental conditions and health disparities, 249–250
Infant mortality, 6, 119–120
    among AAs, 120
Infant-mortality rate (IMR), 119
Infectious diseases, 6
Influenza, 49–50
Insulin growth factor (*IGF2*) gene, 237, 245
Insurance, financial cost of, 307–308
Interferon gamma (IFNγ) expression, 92
Interferon regulatory factor 1 (IRF1), 31
Intergenerational wealth and health transfer, 115
Interleukin 1 (IL-1) gene, 49
    IL1B, 31
Interleukin-10 (IL-10), 50

International HapMap project, 33
Intervention approaches, 300, 301, 304, 305–307, 309
Intrauterine environment and health disparities, economic investment in, 117–119
In utero environment, 236–237, 241, 245–246, 250, 261
In utero exposures, 241, 243, 244, 246, 263, 266
Investing
    in adult and health disparities, 124
    in children and youths' health and health disparities, 123–124

J
Job-related stress, 134, 201

K
Kidney diseases, 44–46
    chronic kidney disease, 5, 44–45
    disparity, epigenetics and, 90–91
    gene-environment interaction and prenatal predisposition to, 246–247

L
Late-onset Alzheimer's disease (LOAD), 46, 262
Lay health advisors (LHA), 303–304
Lead poisoning, 10
Life-course theory (LCT), 303
Lifestyle choices, 130, 143
Lifestyle-intervention strategies, 164
Linguistics, cultural competence and and health disparities, 191–192
Linkage disequilibrium (LD), 24
Low birth weight, 117–118
    socioeconomic status and, 136
Low-density lipoprotein (LDL) cholesterol, 309
Lung cancer, 55–56
Lynch syndrome, 53–54

M
Malaria, 27, 28–29
MalariaGEN initiative, 31
Massachusetts Health Care reform, 308
Maternal care, epigenetic programming and, 247–248
Maternal malnutrition, 117, 245
Maternal stress
    and fetal origin, 244–246
    during pregnancy, 207
MC1R gene, 284–285
Mediating mechanism hypothesis, 258

Medical care, cultural sensitive, 193
Melanesian population, 284
Melanin, 283
Melanocyte-stimulating hormone receptor (MC1R), 283
Melanoma, malignant, 6–7
Mendelian laws of heredity, 17
Mental health, psychosocial factors and, 216–219
Metabolic syndrome, 5, 132, 200, 201
Metabolomics, 310
Metastasis-associated protein 1 (MTA1), 96
Methylated CpG-island amplification (MCA), 93
Methyl-CpG-binding protein 2 (MeCP2), 82
Methylenetetrahydrofolate reductase (MTHFR), 240
MicroRNAs (miRNAs), 77–78
Middle Passage, journey, 2
Midwifes, 190
Mir-99, 96–97
MiR-375, 90
Mongoloids, 281
Moods and physical health, 198–199
Myosin heavy chain type II isoform A (MYH9), 45

N
National Adult Literacy Survey (NALS), 171
National Association for Advancement of Colored People (NAACP), 115
National Health and Nutrition Examination Survey (NHANES III), 206
National Health Interview Survey (NHIS), 190
National Institute on Alcohol Abuse and Alcoholism (NIAAA), 160
Natural human variation, genes associated with, 99–100
Natural selection, 20, 21, 26, 27, 283
Negative emotions, 222
Negroids, 281
Neighborhood norms, 142
Neighborhood segregation and lower-income families, 124
Neighborhood violence, 141
and health disparities, 141–142
Neonatal abstinence syndrome (NAS), 243
Nerve growth factor-inducible protein A (NGFI-A), 248
Nicotinamide adenine dinucleotide phosphate (NADPH), 30
Nicotine addiction, 176
Non-communicable diseases, 32
Non-genetic factors affecting health, 129–131

North American Association of Central Cancer Registries (NAACCR) organization, 51
NR3C1 gene, 246
Nuclear factor kappa B (NF-kB) transcription factor activity, 252

O
Obesity, 39–40, 42, 302
and behavioral intervention and health disparities, 164–165
and diabetes, 156
genetic factors associated with, 43–44
Obesity disparity
epigenetics and, 87–89
epigenome-wide-association-study (EWAS) analysis, 88
Occupation as a social determinant of health, 134–135
OMICs, 310

P
Parental substance abuse, role for, 242–244
Parenting, SES and, 136–137
Patient navigation system, 177
Peer educators, 303
Peer outreach workers, 303
Peripheral blood mononuclear cells (PBMCs), 251
Peroxisome proliferator activated-receptor gamma (PPAR-gamma), 35, 238
coactivator 1 (PPARGC1), 42
Persistence, 214
Personalized medicine, race-based genetic testing and, 293–295
Phaeomelanin, 283
Phenylketonuria (PKU), 292
Physical activity behavior and health disparities, 155–157
Pituitary adenylate cyclase activating polypeptide (PACAP), 42
Placenta, 245
Plasminogen activator inhibitor (PAI), 49
type 1 (PAI1), 36
Plasmodium falciparum, 28, 30
Plasmodium vivax, 28
Pneumococcal infection, 6
Pneumonia, 49–50
Positive psychosocial behavior, 210
Positive stress, 205
Post-translational modification (PTMs), 77f
Poverty level, childhood, 121
Precision medicine, 309–310
Prejudice and discrimination, 221
Premature death, risk factors and, 166, 166f

Prenatal predisposition, and kidney diseases, 246–247
Prenatal stress and health disparity, 207–209
Professionals, health literacy and, 178–179
Prolonged stresses, 205–206
Prostate cancer, 4, 56–59, 258
  disparity, 95–97
Protein kinase C (PKC) epsilon type, 244
Proteomics, 310
Psychological characteristics and SES and health disparities, 145–146
Psychological factors and health disparities, 197
  adverse health outcomes in AAs, 215
  categories of stress, 205
    positive stress, 205
    prolonged stresses, 205–206
    tolerable stress, 205
  community stressors and health, 211–212
  environmental stresses, 199–200
  home environment cognitive stimulation, 210–211
  measurement of stress indicator, 206–207
  parental care, 209–210
  prejudice and discrimination, 221
  prenatal stress, 207–209
  psychological stress, 10
    biological mechanism of, 202–205
    and blood pressure, 221
    and socioeconomic status, 200–202
    and stroke, 222
  psychological stressors and stigma, 219–220
  psychosocial factors
    anxiety and depression, 215–216
    and mental health, 216–219
  psychosocial relationships in community and health, 212–213
  racism and health, psychological effects of, 219
  resilience and psychological impact on health, 213–214
Psychosocial factors
  anxiety and depression, 215–216
  and mental health, 216–219
  and SES and health disparities, 145

R
Race, 279
  anthropological rationale for human classification, 280–283
  categorization/classification (*see* Race categorization and health disparities)
  race-based genetic testing and personalized medicine, 293–295
  racism and health disparities, 286–288
Race categorization and health disparities, 288–289
  genetic variation, 290–292
  and health disparities, 288–289
  human genome sequence and, 285–286
  racism, 286–288
  skin color as basis for, 283–285
Racial segregation, 112, 281, 287
Racial trait, 281, 283
Racism and health
  and health disparities, 286–288
  psychological effects of, 219
RE1-silencing transcription factor (REST), 82
Red blood cells (RBCs), 28
Regulatory T cells (Tregs), 262
Religion and cultural impact, 187–189
Renin-angiotensin-aldosterone system (RAAS), 35
Renin-angiotensin system, 260
Resilience and psychological impact on health, 213–214
Retinoid X receptor alpha (RXRA) gene, 239
Rett syndrome, 82
Runt-related transcription factor 3 (RUNX3), 253

S
S-adenosylmethionine (SAM), 237
Sanger, Frederick, 22
Schizophrenia, 83, 117, 245
Segregation, racial, 281, 287
Self-care, individual, 174
  individual preventative measures and health-literacy deficit, 175–177
  patient navigation system, 177
Self-identified race or ethnicity (SIRE), 288
Sepsis, 48
Septicemia, 6
Septicemia-sepsis, 48–49
Serotonin transporter protein (SLC6A4) locus, 204
Serpin peptidase inhibitor, 36
Sexual behavior, 161, 165
Shift-and-persist approach, 213
Shift strategies, 214
Sickle cell anemia (SCA), 18, 291
Sickle cell disease, 29–30
Single nucleotide polymorphisms (SNPs), 20–21, 57
Sirtuin 1, 89

Sirtuin protein family of deacetylase, 85
Skin color for racial classification, 283–285
Slavery, 2, 112, 280
SLC11A1, 31
Small gestational age (SGA), 237
SNF2, 82
Sobadores, 190
Social determinants and health disparities, 129
  adverse childhood experiences, 139
  education, 131–133
  income, 133–134
  non-genetic factors affecting health, 129–131
  occupation, 134–135
  SES
    psychological characteristics, 145–146
    psychosocial factors and, 145
Social psychology, 212
Social relationships and support, importance of, 212
Socioeconomic status (SES), 129, 131, 136, 154, 199, 200–202
  association on cognitive ability in children, 210
  and family conflict, 137–139
  health disparities
    access to health care and, 143–145
    adverse childhood experiences and, 139
    health behaviors and, 142–143
    interaction of family values, neighborhood norms, and, 142
    neighborhood housing and, 140–141
    neighborhood violence and, 141–142
    transportation and, 143
  and parenting, 136–137
Spirituality, 187
Stigmatization, 219–220
Stress, 199
  categories of, 205
    positive stress, 205
    prolonged stresses, 205–206
    tolerable stress, 205
  prenatal stress, 207–209
  and psychological distress, 219
  psychological stress
    biological mechanism of, 202–205
    and blood pressure, 221
    and socioeconomic status, 200–202
    and stroke, 222
Stress indicator, measurement of, 206–207
Stress-response hormones, 306
Stroke, 3, 4, 222

T
Taskforce investigations, 300–301
Tay-Sachs disease, 290, 291
Thrifty phenotype, 118
Tissue plasminogen activator (PLAT), 36
Tobacco smoke, 55, 305
  gene-environment interaction, 255–259
Tobacco-use behavior and health disparities, 157–160
Tolerable stress, 205
Toll-like receptor (TLR) signals, 251
Transcriptomic, 310
Translating health disparities, 299–302, 310*f*
  in behavioral intervention approaches, 305–306
  in cancer, 306–307
  community-based participatory research, 303–304
    for hypertension, 304
  in diabetes outcomes, 305
  financial cost of insurance, 307–308
  importance of health literacy, 307
  by life-course programs, 303
  precision medicine, 309–310
Transportation and health disparities, 143
Transposons, 80
Trichostatin A, 83
Triglycerides (TGs), ethnic differences in, 40
Tuberculosis (TB), 30–31
Tumor necrosis factor-alpha (TNF-alpha), 50
Type 1 diabetes mellitus (T1DM), 39, 254
  genetic factors associated with, 40–41
Type 2 diabetes mellitus (T2DM), 39, 253
  disparity, epigenetics and, 89–90
  genetics factors associated with, 41–42

U
Ultraviolet B (UVB) radiation, 241, 284
Uncoupling protein 3 (UCP3) gene, 43
Unemployment, 115, 124, 135
US Universal Care Act, 308

V
Vaccination, 119–120
Vitamin B, 284–285
Vitamin D, 54–55
Vitamin D receptor (VDR), 31
  polymorphisms, 265
Vitamin E, 239
VKORC1 (vitamin K-epoxide reductase) gene, 293

W
Wealth, health and, 112
Wellcome Trust Case Control Consortium, 25
Werner syndrome (WS), 84
Willowbrook study, 178
Wnt signaling pathway, 91

World War II (WWII), 1
 after effect, 193, 282

Y
Youth Risk Behavior Surveillance System (YRBSS), 217

CPSIA information can be obtained
at www.ICGtesting.com
Printed in the USA
LVOW06*2108151017
552529LV00001B/61/P